Immunological Aspects of Rheumatology

Immunological Aspects of Rheumatology

W. CARSON DICK
University Department of Rheumatology
The Royal Victoria Infirmary
Newcastle upon Tyne

Elsevier/North-Holland

Published in the USA and Canada by
Elsevier/North-Holland
52 Vanderbilt Avenue
New York NY 10017

Published in the UK and Europe by
MTP Press Limited
Falcon House
Lancaster, England

Copyright © 1981 MTP Press Limited
Softcover reprint of the hardcover 1st edition 1981

ISBN-13: 978-94-011-6626-3   e-ISBN-13: 978-94-011-6624-9
DOI:10.1007/978-94-011-6624-9

LCCN: 81-69112

Contents

Contents

List of Contributors

P. A. Bacon
ARC Research Group,
Royal National Hospital for Rheumatic
    Diseases, Bath,
and Pharmacology Group,
University of Bath

A. G. Bird
Regional Department of Immunology,
East Birmingham Hospital,
Birmingham

W. G. Chin
Department of Pathology,
University of Toronto,
Ontario M5S 1A8. Canada

P. Davis
Rheumatic Disease Unit,
University of Alberta,
Edmonton, Alberta, Canada

A. M. Denman
Connective Tissue Diseases Research Group,
Clinical Research Centre,
Watford Road,
Harrow, Middlesex

M. E. Devey
Immunology Unit,
Department of Medical Microbiology,
London School of Hygiene and Tropical
    Medicine,
London

A. El-Ghobarey
University Department of Medicine,
Azhar University,
Cairo, Egypt

J. N. Fordham
Bone and Joint Research Unit,
The London Hospital Medical College,
London

I. D. Griffiths
Department of Rheumatology,
Royal Victoria Infirmary,
Newcastle upon Tyne

N. D. Hall
ARC Research Group,
Royal National Hospital for Rheumatic
    Diseases, Bath,
and Pharmacology Group,
University of Bath

J. B. Hay
Department of Pathology,
University of Toronto,
Ontario M5S 1A8. Canada

G. B. Howe
Department of Medicine,
The Westmead Hospital,
Westmead, NSW 2145, Australia

N. Hurst
Rheumatic Diseases Unit,
University of Edinburgh,
Northern General Hospital,
Edinburgh, Scotland

T. B. Issekutz
Department of Pathology,
University of Toronto,
Ontario M5S 1A8, Canada

G. Nuki
Rheumatic Diseases Unit,
University of Edinburgh,
Northern General Hospital,
Edinburgh, Scotland

D. F. Roberts
Department of Human Genetics,
University of Newcastle upon Tyne

LIST OF CONTRIBUTORS

M. W. Steward
Immunology Unit,
Department of Medical Microbiology,
London School of Hygiene and Tropical
  Medicine,
London

J. Wentzel
Department of Human Genetics,
University of Newcastle upon Tyne

K. Whaley
Department of Immunology,
Western Infirmary,
Glasgow, Scotland

Preface

This is an exciting era in medicine and in science. Successive waves of advance in knowledge gather, break and recede uncovering fresh challenges and new opportunities. Each plays its part in eroding the tidemark of yesterday's ignorance. Many involved in the day-to-day management of patients, ill-prepared and ill-equipped by the training which they received as under-graduate students, find it difficult to retain contact with the advances in medical science and feel uncomfortable on the shifting sands of uncertainty upon which we now stand. Which of the new ideas is sound? Upon which data may we rely? How may we distinguish the real from the unreal, the true from the false, recent advances from recent retreats? These are the anxieties, often either unstated or alternatively expressed in terms of an attitude of total opposition to 'all of this research rubbish' which are widespread in medical circles today. It is for these individuals who are not themselves directly involved in the immunology of rheumatic diseases but who, nevertheless, recognize the importance of this subject to their patients and, in particular, to tomorrow's patients, that this book has been written.

There are two points that I believe to be of central concern. Firstly, I think it important to recognize that the intellectual basis of most of the research work being generated today is actually extremely simple. If an audience is left feeling that it is all too complex for them, then it is likely that the fault lies with the communicator.

Secondly, I believe that it is of extreme importance that all clinicians, whether in general practice or in hospital, be aware of the opportunity made available to them by the flowering of technology in medicine. It is a matter of vital importance that those observing and caring for patients should be closely involved in the work of recognizing, defining and exploring areas of advance in medicine. Knowledge is anything which reduced the arbitrariness of man's understanding. Knowledge may be gained by inductive or deductive thinking but very often advances in medicine owe their origin to lateral thinking or to serendipity. For such serendipity to be fruitful it is essential that those in a position to observe are also in a position to recognize the significance of their own observations. The proper sequence of advance in medicine ought to stem

PREFACE

from clinical observation made at the bedside. This should then stimulate the clinician to communicate either directly or through applied science to the basic scientist most involved in that area. This presupposes that the clinician be aware of both the applied and the basic science relevant to his area since it is unrealistic to expect a basic scientist to be aware of the far-flung implications of the very restricted field in which he is working. Thus I believe it is a duty of the clinician to be conversant with both the applied and basic science of his subject. Only in this way can there be a secure base for the recognition of disease and the management of patients in the future. Should this atmosphere prevail, then the opportunities for further advance in the future are limitless. Should we fail in this endeavour, future patients are condemned to be categorized and managed on the basis of yesterday's ignorance.

This book represents a collection of essays on areas of importance to the immunopathogenesis of rheumatic diseases. In each chapter the author has given sufficient of the groundwork and of the source reference of his field for the interested observer to learn the background to the subject. He has then continued by delineating the present state of knowledge and closed by providing pointers to potential areas of importance in the future. There is no attempt to be comprehensive and it is certain that much of the content of this book will be overtaken by future knowledge. The most obvious area in which this is certain to occur is that of monoclonal antibodies which will almost certainly revolutionize both the practice and theory of immunology in the future. This book was conceived and it was written just before the introduction of monocloncal antibodies and is a summary of the state of the art up to that time.

CARSON DICK, MD, FRCP
Reader in Rheumatology

1
Lymphocyte Subpopulations and their Role in the Rheumatic Diseases

N. D. HALL and P. A. BACON

LYMPHOCYTE SUBPOPULATIONS IN HEALTHY INDIVIDUALS

Introduction

The study of lymphocyte subpopulations in man has in general followed a path worn smooth by the passage of many workers in a wide range of subjects from molecular biology to motor mechanics. This comprises an initial dissection of the major and minor components of the system, followed by attempts to make these components work in isolation. The separated parts may be identified by their appearance and by their function, although there may be little apparent connection between the two. The final phase is a slow, complicated reassembly of the individual components into something resembling the original. The analysis of lymphocyte function has progressed rapidly from the initial separation of the immune system into two major pathways— thymus-derived (mediated by T lymphocytes) and bursa or bone marrow-derived (mediated by B lymphocytes). More recently, a third, non-T, non-B, lymphocyte population—'null' cells—has been identified. It is not feasible to provide an extensive survey of T-, B- and null-cell properties here but these are well covered both in immunological textbooks[1,2] and in review articles[3,4]. An outline summary of the surface markers and functions of the major lymphocyte classes and monocytes is given in Table 1.1.

Lymphocyte subpopulations in mice have been extensively characterized in terms of functional activity associated with the expression of specific surface markers, in particular Ly antigens[5]. In man, understanding the specific functions of defined groups of lymphocytes has been hampered by the lack of

1

suitable markers of particular cell subpopulations. This problem is now being resolved and this review is written at a time of rapid progress, with functional subsets of human lymphocytes being analysed for specific surface markers. The advance has been most marked for T cells, but analysis of the null cell population is also being pursued.

Table 1.1 Characteristics of major lymphocyte classes

T cells	form spontaneous rosettes with sheep red blood cells (E rosettes)
	mediate delayed hypersensitivity and graft-versus-host reactions
	regulate B cell activity by both helper and suppressor mechanisms
	proliferate in response to soluble antigens and in the mixed lymphocyte culture (MLC)
	secrete lymphokines
	may become cytotoxic
B cells	express surface immunoglobulin (sIg) and receptors for C3 (EAC rosettes) and Epstein–Barr virus (EBV)
	may express Fc receptors (binding of heat-aggregated IgG)
	synthesize and secrete immunoglobulin
Null cells	express Fc receptors (EA rosettes)
	are cytotoxic (antibody-dependent cellular cytotoxicity, ADCC, K cells)
	may contain immature B cells and monocytes
	may have suppressor activity and helper activity
Monocytes*	express Fc receptors and C3 receptors
	are adherent and phagocytic
	may be cytotoxic
	show helper function (antigen presentation)
	may show suppressor activity

* Included for comparative purposes.

T lymphocytes

Two distinct systems for fractionating T cells in terms of surface characteristics have been identified. First, this population has been found to contain cells with Fc receptors for IgM[6] or IgG[7, 8]. Of particular importance was the discovery that these subpopulations—T_μ and T_γ—possess distinct functions. T_μ cells provide help for, and T_γ cells suppress the polyclonal activation of, B cells by pokeweed mitogen (PWM)[9]. The T_γ cell has also been shown to be active in a K cell assay[10]. The Fc receptor on the T_γ cell is lost following interaction with immune complexes[11, 12], a process which also leads to the loss of K cell activity[11]. The apparently clear distinction between T_μ and T_γ cells has been blurred by the findings that T_γ cells may express receptors for IgM (i.e. become T_μ after losing their Fc_γ receptor[13] and that T_μ cells generate suppressor activity under certain conditions[14].

Lymphocyte subpopulations have also been analysed utilizing antibodies raised against cell surface antigens. This approach has been followed particularly by Schlossman's group in Boston who have amassed considerable data from the use of heteroantisera, naturally occurring autoantibodies and, more recently, monoclonal antibodies, in conjunction with a fluorescence-activated cell sorter. This approach has allowed them to examine the relationships of surface markers and functional activities of lymphoid cell populations and has led to an immunochemical marker system for cells with discrete helper, suppressor and cytotoxic functions. Initial evidence for functional T cell subsets has come from antisera raised against human lymphocytes in rabbits and rendered specific for T cells by absorption. One antiserum detects a marker (TH_1)[15] present on 50–60% peripheral blood T cells which proliferate in a mixed-lymphocyte culture (MLC) and generate lymphokine, but do not respond to soluble antigens. Another antiserum (anti-TH_2) reacts with cells which are relatively inactive in the MLC, but which are active as suppressor cells and as effector cells in a cytotoxicity assay[16–19]. A different subpopulation of regulatory T cells express surface antigen (JRA) identified by autoantibodies present in the sera of patients with active juvenile rheumatoid arthritis[17, 20]. Further analysis of human lymphocyte subsets has been made possible by the production of hybridomas secreting monoclonal antibodies against various cellular antigens. The series of T-cell-specific monoclonal antibodies includes OKT1[21] and OKT3[22, 23] reactive against all peripheral blood T cells, OKT4[24–26] marking helper cells and OKT5[19] identifying a subpopulation of suppressor/cytotoxic T cells equivalent to that previously defined by TH_2. Other monoclonal antibodies have been shown to recognize monocytes and granulocytes (OKM1)[27] and the Ia antigen complex found on human B cells and activated T cells (OKI1)[23].

A comparison of the human T cell subsets identified by monoclonal antibodies or by Fc receptors shows little correlation between these two assay systems[28]. T_μ cells contain both helper and suppressor cells as defined by OKT4 and OKT5 respectively with no enrichment of either over the total T cell preparation. In contrast, only 15% T_γ cells react with the T-cell-specific antibody OKT3. The authors[28] suggest that many of the T_γ cells may be natural killer (NK) cells, a function not demonstrated by OKT5$^+$ cells. Human NK cells have been shown to express T cell markers[29, 30]. The finding of so few T cells (as defined by OKT3) in the T_γ cell population may be a technical problem resulting from the use of neuraminidase-treated sheep erythrocytes during the T cell preparation. The enzyme treatment increases the stability of E rosettes but may cause a loss of specificity for T cells.

The application of hybridoma technology to the study of human lymphocyte subsets is heralding a major step forward in our understanding of the many interactions involved in the regulation of the immune response in healthy individuals. A number of reports have already illustrated the usefulness of this approach in the study of immunological disorders[31–33]. The extension of this work to include patients with rheumatoid arthritis and other connective tissue diseases should provide a valuable means of analysing the aberrant immune systems in these patients.

Null lymphocytes

The null lymphocyte population in man may be defined as containing non-phagocytic cells lacking surface immunoglobulin and failing to form E rosettes with sheep erythrocytes. Most of these cells have receptors for the Fc portion of IgG (FcR) detected either by binding of aggregated IgG[34] or by EA rosette formation with IgG-coated human erythrocytes[35]. The ease of detecting FcR on null cells distinguishes them from mature B cells[36, 37]. Null cells with FcR have been termed non-T, non-B, third-population cells[3], UL cells[38] and L cells[39]. In comparison to T and B cells, null lymphocytes appear to show a far less exquisite immunological specificity. The major function attributed to these cells is antibody-dependent cell-mediated (K cell) cytotoxicity[40–42]. Other activities have however been characterized, and it is clear that the non-T, non-B lymphocyte pool is heterogeneous both for surface markers and functions[43]. Some null cells may suppress immune responses[44] whereas, under different conditions, they act as accessory cells in lymphocyte blastogenesis[45, 46]. A number of authors have questioned the true non-T, non-B nature of null cells. Thus, many null cells are considered to be of B cell lineage[47, 48] or to express T lymphocyte differentiation antigens[49]. Such observations illustrate the methodological problems which play a major role in clouding the definition of human lymphocyte subsets.

Although monocytes are not the subject of this chapter, it is necessary to consider briefly some properties of these cells which overlap with the lymphocyte subpopulations discussed above. It is well known that monocytes express receptors for the Fc region of IgG and for the third component of complement[50]. The FcR on monocytes may be detected using the human EA (Ripley) rosette assay usually employed to study FcR on null cells[51]. Monocytes adhere firmly to a variety of surfaces but this property is shared by B lymphocytes[3] and by some T cells[17]. Functionally, monocytes are phagocytic, cytotoxic[52], act as accessory cells (antigen presentation) in lymphocyte proliferation[53] and may also suppress lymphocyte activity in certain circumstances[54]. These observations suggest that monocytes share many surface markers and functions associated with lymphocyte subpopulations. This may result in monocyte contamination of lymphocyte preparations and vice versa, as illustrated by the recent demonstration of monocyte-specific markers and lack of T cell markers (as defined by monoclonal antibody) on the majority of purified T_γ lymphocytes[28]. Thus, a comparison of cell markers and functions indicates that phagocytosis is the only property which clearly separates monocytes from other mononuclear cells.

SYSTEMIC LUPUS ERYTHEMATOSUS (SLE)

Introduction

SLE is a condition characterized by an excessive production of immunoglobulin, a significant proportion of which is directed against self components including DNA, extractable nuclear antigens and lymphocytes. These auto-antibodies may be responsible for many of the clinical features of SLE either directly or by participating in immune complexes. The synthesis of autoantibodies in SLE has been considered to result from a generalized abnormality of immune regulation in these patients. Such a general defect is, however, unlikely, since other self-reactive antibodies, notably organ-specific autoantibodies, are not prevalent in SLE, nor is the response to exogenous antigen necessarily abnormal[55]. It is clear nevertheless that some perturbation of immune regulation does occur in SLE patients and a number of papers have appeared recently demonstrating altered suppressor cell function in this disease. These abnormalities may reflect changes within the cells themselves, or interactions with various humoral factors or, most probably, both. The disturbances of immune regulation in SLE are not immutable but are clearly linked to disease activity.

T lymphocytes

Suppressor cell activity

A possible lack of suppressor cell activity in SLE is suggested by the observations of several groups that B lymphocytes from SLE patients spontaneously synthesize larger amounts of immunoglobulin in culture than the corresponding cells from healthy controls[56–60]. These results have been obtained using assays of both non-specific[58] and specific (anti-TNP)[57] antibody synthesis and by the enumeration of both non-specific[56, 60] and specific (anti-TNP)[59] antibody-secreting cells. The number of lymphocytes secreting IgG, IgM and IgA are all increased in SLE with the greatest increase being seen with IgG-secreting cells[60]. Increased immunoglobulin production is most marked in cells from patients with clinically active disease[56, 59, 60]. A lack of functional suppressor cells has been implicated in this by the finding[59] that normal T cells can suppress the activity of anti-TNP antibody-secreting cells whereas SLE T cells cannot. The inhibitory effect of healthy T cells in this assay is increased following activation of the lymphocytes by concanavalin A (Con A) but this treatment is unable to generate suppressor cells from SLE T cells[59].

Activation of suppressor cells by Con A[61] has been used extensively to study the function of these cells in SLE. All the reports show a deficiency of Con A-inducible suppressor cells in active disease[59, 62–66]. This deficiency is clearly in the induction of the suppressor lymphocytes, since SLE B cells are readily inhibited by suppressor cells from healthy donors[59, 62, 64]. SLE T cells do not generate soluble immune-response suppressor (SIRS) on incubation with Con A[63]. The failure of Con A to induce suppressor activity in SLE lymphocytes is associated temporally with assessments of disease activity. Thus this effect is more marked in patients with active rather than inactive disease[65] and in serial studies the ability of individual patients to develop suppressor cell functions in response to Con A correlated with disease activity as determined on clinical grounds and by anti-DNA antibody titres[66]. During the inactive phases of the disease, Con A-induced suppressor cells were similar to those of normal controls.

Several studies of surface markers on T lymphocyte subpopulations have shown a reduction in the proportion of T_γ cells in the circulation of SLE patients[64, 67, 68]. In contrast, T cells with receptors for IgM (T_μ cells) are essentially normal in this disease[64, 68]. Levels of T_γ cells have been shown to fluctuate with disease activity, being most depressed in patients with active disease[67, 68]. One paper has failed to find consistently low levels of T_γ cells in SLE compared with healthy controls[69]. However no information concerning the activity of the disease in these patients was included in the report.

The mechanism involved in the loss of Con A-inducible suppressor cells in active SLE is still uncertain, but may be related to the presence of anti-lymphocyte antibodies in this disease[70–74]. Much of this antibody is IgM[73] and is active in complement-dependent lympholysis. Optimal activity is achieved at 15 °C but some reactivity remains at 37 °C[71, 73]. Treatment of normal lymphocytes with the antilymphocyte antibodies from active SLE serum inhibits the generation of suppressor cells following Con A activation[70, 72] and blastogenesis induced by Con A[71]. Other T cell functions, namely activation by phytohaemagglutinin (PHA)[71], PWM[71] or allogeneic cells[71, 72] are less sensitive to treatment with antibody plus complement than the Con A-dependent assays. The SLE sera do not block cell function if added to the culture after Con A, suggesting that the prime target of the antibody is the precursor cell responsive to Con A activation[65, 70]. The majority (64%) of active SLE sera preferentially killed T_γ cells[73], although some sera (14%) showed the opposite specificity indicating the heterogeneity of anti-T cell antibodies in SLE[73, 74].

In addition to antilymphocyte antibodies, immune complexes may also be important in the modulation of lymphocyte subpopulations in SLE, since they can cause a loss of Fc receptors from T_γ cells[11, 12]. This is associated with a failure to generate suppressor activity following incubation with Con A[75]. However, this immune complex mechanism cannot fully explain the lack of Con A-inducible suppressor activity in SLE, since the cells activated by Con A are clearly heterogeneous[75, 76] with distinct cell types showing activity in PWM- and mixed lymphocyte culture (MLC)-activated systems. It has been shown that only T_γ lymphocytes are precursors for cells which can suppress the MLC[65] but both T_γ and $T_{non-\gamma}$ may be activated to suppress the PWM response[65, 75]. These results are in agreement with other data discussed in the section on T lymphocytes[14].

An alternative means of assessing immunoregulatory mechanisms *in vitro* is the autologous mixed-lymphocyte culture (auto-MLC) in which the patients' T cells respond to their own non-T cells[77]. This has been applied to the study of immune regulation and T cell function in SLE. Although SLE lymphocytes respond normally to stimulation in an allogeneic MLC[78, 79], the auto-MLC response is markedly depressed in patients with active disease, but only slightly lower than normal controls in inactive disease[66, 78-80]. In active SLE the ability of both T_γ and $T_{non-\gamma}$ lymphocytes to respond[66, 78, 80] and of the non-T cells to stimulate[78-80] is reduced, whereas only the T_γ response remains abnormal when the disease is quiescent[66, 78, 80]. However, other studies of SLE patients and their MLC-identical siblings indicate that the depressed auto-MLC in the disease is due to a defect in the stimulating non-T cells[79]. This conflict may reflect methodological differences such as the use of nylon columns to remove adherent cells (mostly monocytes) which might lead to the loss of a regulatory subpopulation of T cells (JRA $^+$)[17]. Also, fractionation of the responding T lymphocytes is necessary in order to demonstrate abnormal reactivity of T_γ cells during inactive phases of the disease[66, 78, 80]. Those results showing defective T cell reactivity in the auto-MLC, a model of autologous immune regulation, may identify the same abnormality demonstrated in other studies as deficient Con A-inducible suppressor cells. It has been demonstrated recently that the T cell population activated in the auto-MLC has suppressor activity[81] and that elimination of these cells abolishes the capacity of Con A to induce suppressor cells[82]. Thus, a subset of T cells, either defective or eliminated by autoantibody and complement in SLE, would not be able to respond in the auto-MLC (or to Con A) to generate suppressor activity. This in turn would allow hyperactivity of B cells with the production of auto-antibodies, including more antilymphocyte antibodies.

The characterization of the suppressor cell precursor and its target has still to be completed. As shown above, the lack of potential suppressor activity appears to correlate with a lack of T_γ cells, but the identity of this 'lymphocyte' subset is currently uncertain[28]. The target for this suppressor activity is itself likely to be a T cell, since both the MLC[83] and PWM-induced immunoglobulin synthesis[84] are T-dependent reactions. Thus abnormal immunoregulation in SLE arises at the level of 'T'–T cell interaction.

Other T cell functions

Considerable evidence using various assays is available to show defective T cell function in SLE. Thus, SLE lymphocytes show depressed responses to PHA[85-88], PWM[58, 62, 64, 89] and to tetanus toxoid[90]. In vivo skin testing with a battery of antigens showed anergy in 25% SLE patients and impaired delayed hypersensitivity correlated to disease activity[91]. This may be related to the findings of reduced 'active' E rosettes in active SLE[92] since this test has been shown to correlate with reactivity on skin testing[93]. Recent reports also show reduced levels of NK cell activity in patients with SLE compared with matched controls[94, 95]. The involvement of humoral factors in the above systems is difficult to assess. Thus, the depressed response of SLE lymphocytes to PHA has, in one study, been correlated with hypocomplementaemia suggesting a possible role of immune complexes[86]. Reduction of PHA-induced cytotoxicity may be mediated, however, by a non-immunoglobulin factor found in active SLE serum[88], whereas in other studies of lymphocyte blasto-genesis, no evidence of humoral factor involvement has been obtained[87, 90].

Null lymphocytes (FcR-positive)

Reduced proportions of FcR-bearing lymphocytes have been detected in SLE peripheral blood using a human erythrocyte (Ripley) EA rosette assay[96]. This is in contrast to other work showing that SLE patients have normal levels of L lymphocytes[97], a subpopulation known to be included in those identified by the rosette system above[45]. Immune complexes blocking the FcR of some patients' cells may be responsible for these differences. However, reduced FcR-positive lymphocytes in SLE would be in agreement with the report[98] of reduced K cell activity in this disease. This reduction of ADCC was observed when Chang liver cells were used as target cells but not with chicken erythro-cytes (CRBC) as targets. The latter concurs with an earlier study[99] which found no difference between control and SLE K cell activity against CRBC. The Chang liver cell appears to act as a target in ADCC for small lymphocytes (K cells) only, whereas IgG-coated CRBC may be lysed by other cell types such as monocytes[100].

Concluding remarks

Many of the abnormal immune responses and aberrant lymphocyte functions in SLE, especially suppressor cells, have been correlated with disease activity. This in itself is fairly remarkable and similar correlations have yet to be realized in other rheumatic disorders. It is important to appreciate that the major aberrations of immune regulation observed in active SLE are reversible and cell function becomes almost normal as the disease activity subsides. This argues against a simple genetically determined malfunction of the immune system in SLE but supports a role for an environmental agent mediating the effects, perhaps in genetically susceptible hosts. The involvement of anti-lymphocyte antibodies in the regulation of autoimmune phenomena requires further exploration. There seems to be a chicken-and-egg problem of which comes first—the autoantibody or the failure of suppressor cells. If the anti-body mediates the loss of suppressor cells, why is this self-reactive antibody synthesized in the presence of functional suppressors? Alternatively, what makes the suppressor cells fail to switch off the antilymphocyte antibody-secreting clone? One hypothesis might be that the antilymphocyte antibody is not primarily self-reactive but is a response against a cell altered (and rendered non-functional) by viral infection.

RHEUMATOID ARTHRITIS (RA)

Introduction

Rheumatoid synovial tissue contains very large numbers of lymphocytes, plasma cells and monocytes[101]. There is considerable evidence of T and B lymphocyte activity within the joint with the finding of lymphokine in rheumatoid synovial fluid[102] and high levels of immunoglobulin synthesis by RA synovium[103]. These results have led to the concept of the rheumatoid synovium acting as an ectopic lymphoid organ capable of producing all the factors necessary to maintain the chronic inflammatory reaction in the synovial membrane. The pathogenetic role of the lymphoid cells in RA is emphasized by the achievement of significant clinical improvement following removal of circulating lymphocytes by thoracic duct drainage (TDD)[104]. TDD has demonstrated that the ectopic lymphoid nature of the synovium is not self-perpetuating but requires continual reinforcement by circulating cells. Removal of these cells by TDD leads to rapid clinical improvement[105]. These experiments illustrate the need for selective depletion of the damaging cells since, by removing essentially all circulating lymphocytes, TDD renders the patients susceptible to many environmental pathogens. The identity of the 'pathogenic lymphocyte' is still unknown, but several candidates are available, including regulatory T cells, rheumatoid-factor-secreting B cells, cytotoxic lymphocytes and activated cells. These subpopulations will be reviewed in the following sections.

T Lymphocytes

Since an earlier review of cell-mediated immunity in RA[106], many studies have provided some evidence of a mild degree of impaired T cell function in this disease. These have included skin-testing to six common antigens[107], mitogen-induced blastogenesis[85, 87, 108–114] and response to various viral antigens[115, 116]. Lymphocyte activation by PHA and Con A, but not PWM, was found to be depressed in a subgroup of RA patients with erosive disease[108] and in one study, PHA responses were lower in patients positive for antinuclear antibody[109]. Although the reduction in mitogen responsiveness is less marked in RA than in SLE[85], there is some evidence of association with disease activity. Thus, abnormal mitogen responses have been shown to return to normal values in those patients who improve clinically with gold treatment[114]. Studies comparing rheumatoid lymphocytes from the peripheral blood (PB) with those isolated from synovial fluid (SF) all show significantly reduced response to mitogens by the SF cells[110–113]. This effect is not due to humoral factors present in the fluid and may reflect preactivation of the SF lymphocytes *in vivo* as suggested by an increased spontaneous [³H]thymidine uptake[110]. The reduced activity of SF lymphocytes to mitogens compared with PB cells is not, however, specific for RA, since SF cells from other inflammatory diseases show similar effects[113]. This lack of specificity is supported by the detection of activated T cells in joint effusions from various arthritides[117] and of activated T cells expressing Ia antigens in the peripheral blood of rheumatoid and other patients[118]. Ia is a marker expressed on T lymphocytes only following activation of these cells[23]. Other evidence of lymphocyte activation in RA is discussed in the section on activated lymphocytes.

Lymphocytes extracted from synovial tissue are generally accepted to be mostly of T cell origin both in the adult[119] and juvenile[120] forms of RA. Studies of *in vitro* reactivity of these cells have yielded conflicting results. Synovial tissue lymphocytes respond poorly to T cell mitogens[121, 122] but response to the antigen PPD has been found by various authors to be either suppressed[122] or enhanced[121] when compared with PB cells. Stimulation of synovial fluid lymphocytes with PPD has also provided evidence of suppressed[122], normal[111] and enhanced[112] responses. On balance it appears that the PPD response of synovial lymphocytes is at least not suppressed to the same extent as the PHA response. This could be explained by an enrichment of reactive cells in the inflammatory site or by a local aberration of normal immunoregulatory mechanisms. Recent evidence has provided support for the latter possibility. Rheumatoid synovial lymphocytes are deficient in suppressor cell function, both in direct assays[123] and following incubation with Con A[124]. Some specificity of this observation for RA synovial tissue is suggested by finding normal suppressor activity in synovial lymphocytes from one patient with JRA and another with psoriatic arthritis[124]. The lack of suppressor cells in rheumatoid synovium appears to be a local phenomenon since these cells are reported to be normal in RA peripheral blood (noted in references 125 and 126). The significance of, and explanation for, this discovery are still uncertain. The effect of diminished suppressor activity on cells involved in rheumatoid factor production[127] is particularly relevant. The apparently local nature of this abnormality could arise from an effect induced by the passage of the cells through the vascular endothelium on their way into the inflamed synovium[128]. Alternatively, a humoral factor may be produced in the tissue which blocks suppressor cell function. Such factors could be immune complexes or an antilymphocyte antibody similar to that identified in the serum of patients with active JRA[20]. These antibodies are associated with the loss of a regulatory subset of T cells in active disease[33]. Further studies of this and similar antibody specificities and their association, if any, with the lack of suppressor activity in RA synovium are clearly required. It should be noted that, in one JRA patient, synovial suppressor cell function was normal[124].

Null lymphocytes (FcR-positive)

Receptors for IgG (FcR) on rheumatoid lymphocytes have received considerable attention in recent years. There is a slightly greater number of reports showing increased FcR expression on RA cells[129–134] than of those showing no differences between rheumatoid and control lymphocytes[97, 135, 136]. In addition, lymphocytes with 'intermediate' electrophoretic mobility are increased in RA blood and synovial fluid[137] and have been shown to express Fc receptors[138]. In parallel with the overall disagreement over FcR-positive lymphocytes in RA, a number of articles describe conflicting data on ADCC (K cell) activity in RA patients. In peripheral blood this has been shown to be increased[139], unchanged[95, 99, 140, 141] and reduced[136, 142] in comparison with healthy controls. Differences in methodology, for example the target cells used, may account for at least some of these discrepancies. Analysis of FcR-positive cells in rheumatoid synovial fluid shows reduced expression of FcR[96], reduced levels of T_γ cells[143] and reduced ADCC[99, 144]. Synovial tissue lymphocytes also display reduced K-cell activity compared with peripheral blood cells[145]. This may reflect blocking of FcR and hence inhibition of ADCC by antiglobulins and immune complexes present in RA serum and synovial fluid[96, 146]. One report indicates a lack of blocking factors responsible for reduced ADCC in synovial fluid[144]. However, modulation of FcR following interaction with immune complexes may account for this[11, 12].

Recently it has become apparent that FcR are expressed on several cell types and may be identified using a variety of techniques[147–149]. These assays

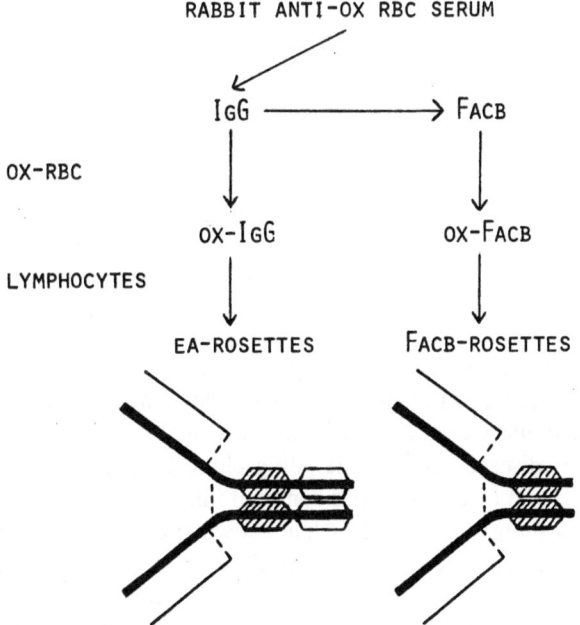

Figure 1.1 Detection of FcR-bearing lymphocytes by EA rosettes and Facb rosettes. The diagram illustrates the loss of the Cγ3 domains (open hexagon) and retention of the Cγ2 regions (hatched hexagons) in the structure of Facb compared with native IgG

generally detect FcR on more than one type of cell and so changes in a subset of cells may pass unnoticed. There is a need, therefore, for FcR assays with restricted specificity for separate subpopulations of lymphocytes or other FcR-positive cells. Since the Fc region of IgG contains two pairs of domains— $C\gamma2$ and $C\gamma3$, one way of restricting binding to FcR might be to look for receptors with specificity for one domain only. An assay has been developed which detects only those FcR with binding specificity for the $C\gamma2$ region of IgG. The technique involves rosette formation with rabbit Facb-sensitized calf erythrocytes (Figure 1.1). Rabbit Facb, prepared from IgG by plasmin digestion[150] lacks the terminal $C\gamma3$ domains of native IgG and so can only bind to FcR through the $C\gamma2$ region. This fragment does not interact with rheumatoid factor[150] and so cytophilic antiglobulins do not interfere with the Facb rosette assay as they might with rosetting red cells coated with intact IgG. The Facb rosette assay has been used to study FcR expression on rheumatoid mononuclear cells and control cells from patients with osteoarthritis (OA) or ankylosing spondylitis (AS) and healthy volunteers[134, 151]. These results are summarized in Table 1.2. There is a highly significant

Table 1.2 Facb-rosette formation by peripheral blood mononuclear cells from patients with rheumatoid arthritis, osteoarthritis, ankylosing spondylitis and from healthy controls

Subjects	No. tested	Percentage of Facb rosettes (mean $\pm$ 1 S.D.)
Healthy	18	6.6 ± 3.5*
RA	27	12.2 ± 3.4*
OA	18	5.9 ± 3.5†
AS	24	8.7 ± 3.8†

* p 0.001 compared with healthy controls
† Not significantly different from control values

increase in the proportion of Facb-rosetting cells in RA compared with the other groups. This is in agreement with an earlier finding that rabbit Facb caused specific inhibition of rheumatoid leukocyte migration[152]. The level of Facb rosettes in individual RA patients could not be correlated with various assessments of disease activity, including clinical examination, plasma viscosity, rheumatoid factor titre and synovial inflammation. Characterization of the cells forming Facb-rosettes has shown them to be non-phagocytic, E-rosette-negative, surface immunoglobulin-negative and C3 receptor-negative[153]. They thus appear to be similar to L cells[39], that is, to form part of the null lymphocyte population. In addition to peripheral blood lymphocytes, a number of cell lines have been studied for Facb rosette formation. So far, all have been negative, including numerous lines of B cell origin transformed by Epstein–Barr virus (EBV) and K562 cells, a myelomonocytic cell line, although the latter cells have been shown to express FcR detected by an EA-rosette assay (unpublished).

An unusual property of Facb-rosetting cells in RA but not in AS (or in healthy controls) is their ability to adhere to styrenedivinylbenzene beads (Table 1.3). Increased adherence of rheumatoid null cells has been observed previously[135]. This may explain the finding of normal levels of L lymphocytes in RA peripheral blood[97] since an adherence step (to remove monocytes) is included in the purification scheme for these cells[45].

Table 1.3 Fractionation of lymphocytes from RA and AS patients by adherence to styrenedivinylbenzene beads

	Percentage of Facb rosettes	
Patient	Unfractionated cells	Non-adherent cells
RA 1	9	1
2	9	2
3	13	0
4	13	3
AS 1	5	5
2	7	5
3	7	5
4	2	2

Table 1.4 Specificity of Facb receptor for human and rabbit IgG preparations

Addition (40 µg/ml)	Relative percentage of Facb rosettes (mean ± 1 SD)
None	100
Human native IgG	91 ± 27
Heat-aggregated IgG	23 ± 20
Heat-aggregated IgG1	36 ± 16
Heat-aggregated IgG2	94 ± 22
Heat-aggregated IgG3	24 ± 13
Heat-aggregated IgG4	78 ± 24
Rabbit native IgG	59 ± 18
Rabbit native Facb	72 ± 23
Rabbit native F(ab')$_2$	85 ± 11
Rabbit native Fab	99 ± 20
Rabbit native Fc	73 ± 28
Rabbit native pFc'	102 ± 34

Facb rosette formation was carried out in the absence or presence of various IgG preparations at final concentration of 40 µg/ml. The effect of these samples on rosette formation was calculated relative to the control percentage of rosettes in the absence of competitor (= 100%). Each figure represents the mean relative percentage of Facb rosettes ± 1 standard deviation of between eight and 14 experiments

The FcR detected by Facb rosettes has been characterized in terms of its binding specificity for human IgG myeloma proteins and rabbit IgG fragments (Table 1.4). The receptor is blocked much more effectively by heat-aggregated human IgG than by native IgG. IgG1 and IgG3 myeloma proteins inhibit rosette formation more strongly than IgG4 and IgG2. Rabbit IgG fragments also compete for the Facb-receptor. Thus, Facb and $F(ab')_2$ both cause significant inhibition of Facb-rosette formation, whereas Fab and pFc' are inactive. Fc fragment is able to block Facb rosettes but in molar terms is much less effective than native IgG. This result, together with the inhibitory effect of $F(ab')_2$, suggests that the hinge region of the IgG is involved in the binding to the Facb receptor. The overall pattern of inhibition of Facb rosettes by the various IgGs (Table 1.4) is very similar to their inhibitory effects on rheumatoid leukocyte migration[152]. It is therefore possible that cells expressing receptors detected by Facb rosettes are involved in the rheumatoid leukocyte response to IgG. The function of Facb-rosetting cells is still unknown. Preliminary results (unpublished) suggest a lack of K cell activity in this population. However, both negative[44] and positive[46] immunoregulatory functions have recently been ascribed to FcR-positive null lymphocytes and these and other assays are currently being applied to the lymphocyte subpopulation detected by Facb rosettes.

Activated lymphocytes

A number of techniques have been used to enumerate activated lymphocytes in patients with RA. These include morphological studies[154, 155], spontaneous DNA synthesis measured by $[^3H]$thymidine incorporation[117, 155] and expression of surface proteins associated with cell activation[118]. The above techniques do not allow the rapid separation of activated cells for further analysis. In order to achieve this, use has been made of the fact that lymphocytes become less dense upon activation. Thus, they may be fractionated by centrifugation in a density gradient either of bovine serum albumin[156] or Ficoll[157]. This causes the activated cells to be concentrated in the less dense area of the gradient where they are easily harvested for further studies of cell markers and function. Decreased density seems to be a more sensitive assay of lymphocyte activation[156] than the increased size used to identify immunoblasts[154, 155]. The technique of discontinuous Ficoll density gradient analysis has been considerably refined by Dr S. D. Carter in our department and applied to the study of circulating lymphocytes in patients with RA[158].

Lymphocytes are layered on to a discontinuous (16–23% w/v) Ficoll gradient and centrifuged at $3000\,g$ for $60\,min$ at $10°C$ (Figure 1.2). The cells distribute themselves at the interfaces A–G with cell debris forming a pellet (H) under the 30% Ficoll cushion. The layers are harvested sequentially using a Pasteur pipette and the cells washed for counting and further analysis. The low-density cells (fractions A–E) incorporate significantly more $[^3H]$thymidine into DNA than the small, dense cells in fraction G. The distribution of lymphocytes from healthy volunteers and from RA patients with clinically inactive or active disease is shown in Figure 1.3. Approximately 70% of normal lymphocytes are recovered from fraction G. Rheumatoid cells from patients with clinically inactive disease have a normal density pattern, but lymphocytes from active RA show a significant shift in distribution towards the less dense area (top) of the gradient. More recent studies have demonstrated that patients with active synovitis have increased numbers of activated

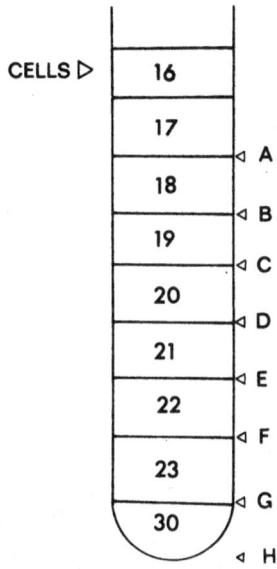

Figure 1.2   Lymphocyte separation on a discontinuous Ficoll gradient. Cells are layered on to the gradient in 16% Ficoll. After centrifugation (3000 g, 60 min, 10 °C) lymphocytes are recovered from the interfaces A–G and debris from the pellet H

lymphocytes in their circulation whereas patients with active extra-articular disease (e.g. vasculitis) have normal distribution patterns[159]. The association between circulating activated lymphocytes and active synovitis is emphasized by preliminary data of the sequential analysis of lymphocyte density distribution during treatment with gold[160]. These results show a close correlation between clinical response to the drug and reversion of the Ficoll gradient analysis pattern to normal.

Surface marker studies of the lymphocyte fractions from the Ficoll gradient reveal that the low-density cells are heterogeneous[161]. Activated T cells retain their ability to form E rosettes and B blasts still express surface immunoglobulin, although their receptors for IgG and C3 are lost[162]. As shown in Figure 1.4, there is a relative depletion of T cells and enrichment of B cells in the low-density fractions compared with unfractionated lymphocytes (similar to fraction G). The proportion of T and B cells in each fraction is the same for healthy controls and rheumatoid patients. The distribution of FcR-positive cells within the Ficoll gradient is illustrated in Figure 1.5. Both 'high-avidity' FcR and 'low-avidity' FcR (defined as total EA rosettes − 'high-avidity' EA rosettes) on healthy cells are detected fairly evenly throughout the gradient. In contrast, there is a significant increase in 'high-avidity' EA rosetting cells in RA in agreement with results using Facb-rosette formation (see Table 1.2 and the section on null lymphocytes). This is due to the increased number of small dense FcR-positive lymphocytes found in fractions

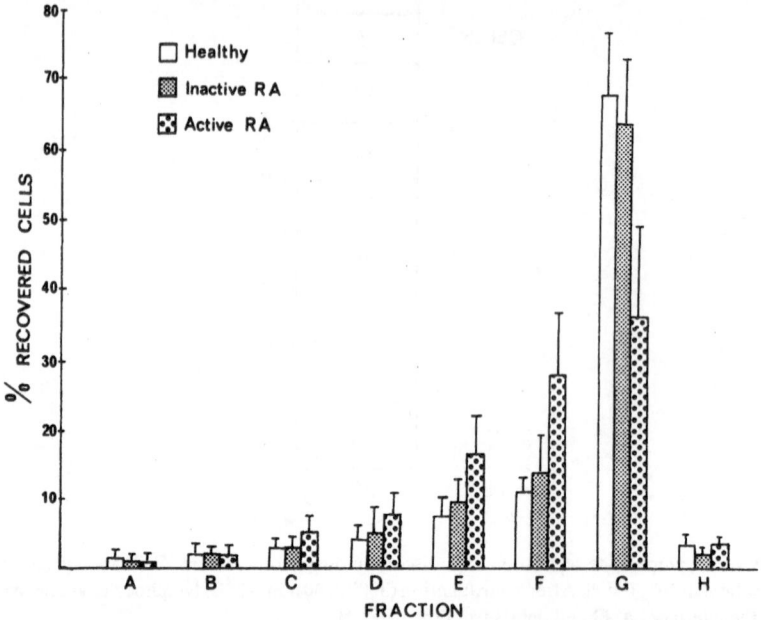

Figure 1.3 Lymphocyte density distribution in healthy and rheumatoid subjects. Results are expressed as the percentage of total recovered cells in each fraction. Fractions A–H are as illustrated in Figure 1.2. Each histogram and bar represents the mean and 1 standard deviation of n experiments (healthy $n = 23$; inactive RA $n = 12$; active RA $n = 11$). There are no significant differences between healthy controls and RA subjects with inactive disease, but highly significant differences between healthy subjects and patients with active RA in fractions C, D, E, F and G ($p < 0.001$)

E–G. No information is available as yet on specific functions of the low-density activated cells detected in RA peripheral blood. Most of these are of B cell origin and are therefore likely to be involved in immunoglobulin synthesis and possibly local rheumatoid factor production, although they do not correlate closely with serum rheumatoid factors. Cells synthesizing high-avidity rheumatoid factor have been detected in RA peripheral blood using a plaque-forming cell assay[163].

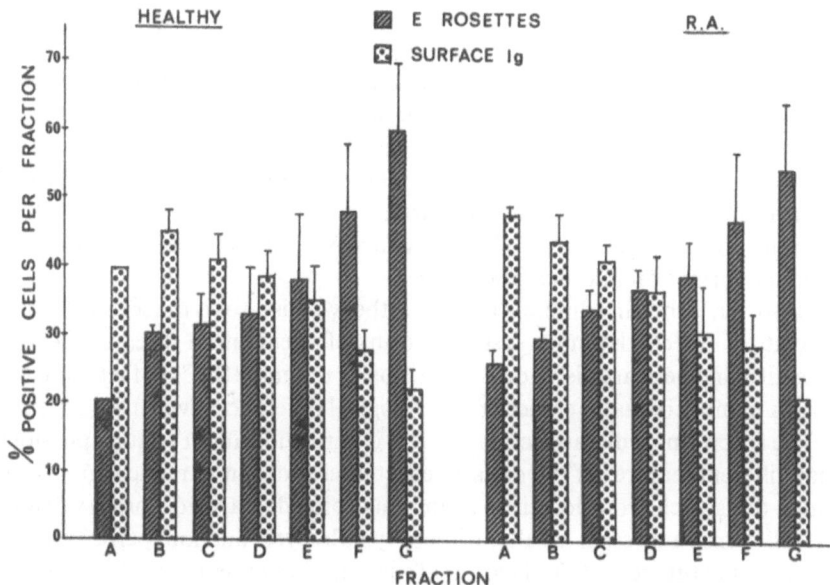

Figure 1.4 Density distribution of T cells (E rosettes) and B cells (surface immunoglobulin) in healthy and rheumatoid subjects. Results are expressed as percentages of positive cells in each fraction, and each column and bar represents the mean and standard deviation of nine experiments. There are no significant differences between the results from healthy and rheumatoid subjects

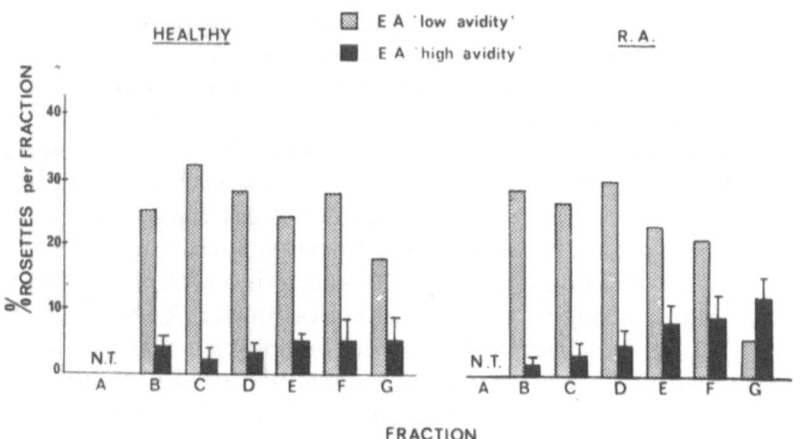

Figure 1.5 Density distribution of FcR-positive lymphocytes in healthy and rheumatoid subjects. EA rosette assays were set up with both heavy and light IgG sensitization (total EA and 'high-avidity' EA respectively). 'Low-avidity' EA rosettes were calculated as total EA minus 'high-avidity' EA. The results show a significantly increased percentage of 'high-avidity' EA-rosetting cells in RA samples compared with healthy controls in fraction G ($p < 0.01$)

Concluding remarks

There is clear evidence of abnormal immune function in patients with RA although the form that this takes is more subtle than in SLE and is less clearly associated with exacerbations and remissions of the disease. This may reflect the more generalized dysfunction of immune regulation detectable in the circulation of SLE patients in comparison with the apparently local intra-articular loss of suppressor cell activity in RA, an important finding which needs confirmation in other laboratories.

However, if the only difference between the two diseases is the severity of the regulatory defect, the more systemic forms of rheumatoid disease, such as vasculitis and pericarditis, should more closely resemble SLE. In fact there remain a number of major clinical and serological differences even in severe RA.

The spectrum of disease activity in RA is very wide and it is quite possible that different features of the disease reflect alterations in immune regulation. Thus, the switch from localized grumbling joint damage to florid systemic vasculitis may represent an alteration of lymphocyte function, perhaps analogous to the tuberculoid and lepromatous extremes of leprosy. The evidence suggests that RA is not simply a milder form of SLE but rather that the abnormal immune function in the two diseases is qualitatively, as well as quantitatively, different.

The specificity of the autoimmune reaction in RA — mostly antiglobulins — differs from the spectrum of antinuclear antibodies predominating in SLE. Changes in Fc receptor function on rheumatoid lymphocytes may play a part in this[164] although direct evidence to support such a hypothesis is lacking. Antibodies to IgG might be synthesized as a result of polyclonal activation of B cells in the disease. Evidence of increased levels of activated B lymphocytes in RA patients has been presented in the previous section. Much interest has arisen recently in a possible role of a 'natural' polyclonal B cell activator, Epstein–Barr virus (EBV), in the pathogenesis of RA[165]. Infection of healthy human B lymphocytes with EBV causes them to synthesize rheumatoid factor[166]. The establishment of EBV-transformed cell lines is more readily accomplished from RA lymphocytes than from healthy cells, suggesting some altered *in vivo* interaction with the virus[166]. A majority of RA patients have in their serum an antibody reacting against a nuclear antigen (RANA) present in EBV-transformed cell lines[167]. This has been proposed as a useful serological marker for RA[168] but may only reflect prior infection with EBV[169]. So far the argument has centred on the significance and specificity of anti-RANA antibodies. Any special role of the rheumatoid B cell as the potential host of the virus has not been evaluated. Similarly, activation of suppressor cells during EBV infection[170, 171] has not been studied in RA patients. It is possible that rheumatoid lymphocytes are genetically predisposed to respond abnormally to viral infection and thus trigger off reactions leading to antiglobulin production.

Acknowledgments

The projects detailed in the sections on null and activated lymphocytes were supported by the Arthritis and Rheumatism Council for Research and by Ciba–Geigy. Much of this work was carried out in collaboration with Dr S. D. Carter, Dr G. Papadimitriou and Miss V. R. Winrow.

References

1. Hobart, M. J. and McConnell, I. (1976). *The Immune System.* (Oxford: Blackwell Scientific Publications)
2. Loor, F. and Roelants, G. E. (eds.) (1977). *B and T Cells in Immune Recognition.* (London: John Wiley and Sons)
3. Frøland, S. S. and Natvig, J. B. (1973). Identification of three different human lymphocyte populations by surface markers. *Transplant. Rev.,* **16**, 114
4. Robbins, D. L. and Gershwin, M. E. (1978). Identification and characterization of lymphocyte subpopulations. *Sem. Arth. Rheum.,* **7**, 245
5. Cantor, H. and Boyse, E. A. (1977). Regulation of cellular and humoral immune responses by T cell subclasses. *Cold Spring Harbour Symp. Quant. Biol.,* **41**, 23
6. Moretta, L., Ferrarini, M., Durante, M. L. and Mingari, M. C. (1975). Expression of a receptor for IgM by human T cells *in vitro. Eur. J. Immunol.,* **5**, 565
7. Dickler, H. B., Adkinson, N. F. Jnr. and Terry, W. D. (1974). Evidence for individual human peripheral blood lymphocytes bearing both B and T cell markers. *Nature (London),* **247**, 213
8. Brown, G. and Greaves, M. F. (1974). Cell surface markers for human T and B lymphocytes. *Eur. J. Immunol.,* **4**, 302
9. Moretta, L., Webb, S. R., Grossi, C. E., Lydyard, P. M. and Cooper, M. D. (1977). Functional analysis of two human T-cell subpopulations: help and suppression of B-cell responses by T cells bearing receptors for IgM or IgG. *J. Exp. Med.,* **146**, 184
10. Shen, L., Lydyard, P. M., Penfold, P. and Roitt, I. M. (1979). Evidence for antibody-dependent cell-mediated cytotoxicity by T cells bearing receptors for IgG. *Clin. Exp. Immunol.,* **35**, 276
11. Moretta, L., Mingari, M. C. and Romanzi, C. A. (1978). Loss of Fc receptors for IgG from human T lymphocytes exposed to IgG immune complexes. *Nature (London),* **272**, 618
12. Mingari, M. C., Moretta, L., Moretta, A., Ferrarini, M. and Preud'homme, J. L. (1978). Fc-receptors for IgG and IgM immunoglobulins on human T lymphocytes: mode of re-expression after proteolysis or interaction with immune complexes. *J. Immunol.,* **121**, 767
13. Pichler, W. J., Lum, L. and Broder, S. (1978). Fc-receptors on human T lymphocytes. I. Transition of T_γ to T_μ cells. *J. Immunol.,* **121**, 1540
14. Hayward, A. R., Layward, L., Lydyard, P. M., Moretta, L., Dagg, M. and Lawton, A. R. (1978). Fc-receptor heterogeneity of human suppressor T cells. *J. Immunol.,* **121**, 1
15. Evans, R. L., Breard, J. M., Lazarus, H., Schlossman, S. F. and Chess, L. (1977). Detection, isolation and functional characterization of two human T cell subclasses bearing unique differentiation antigens. *J. Exp. Med.,* **145**, 221
16. Evans, R. L., Lazarus, H., Penta, A. C. and Schlossman, S. F. (1978). Two functionally distinct subpopulations of human T cells that collaborate in the generation of cytotoxic cells responsible for cell-mediated lympholysis. *J. Immunol.,* **120**, 1423
17. Reinherz, E. L., Strelkauskas, A. J., O'Brien, C. and Schlossman, S. F. (1979). Phenotypic and functional distinctions between the TH_2^+ and JRA^+ T cell subsets in man. *J. Immunol.,* **123**. 83

18. Reinherz, E. L. and Schlossman, S. F. (1979). Con-A inducible suppression of MLC: evidence for mediation by the TH_2^+ T cell subset in man. *J. Immunol.*, **122**, 1335

19. Reinherz, E. L., Kung, P. C., Goldstein, G. and Schlossman, S. F. (1980). A monoclonal antibody reactive with the human cytotoxic/suppressor T cell subset previously defined by a heteroantiserum termed TH_2. *J. Immunol.*, **124**, 1301

20. Strelkauskas, A. J., Schauf, V., Wilson, B. S., Chess, L. and Schlossman, S. F. (1978). Isolation and characterization of naturally occurring subclasses of human peripheral blood T cells with regulatory functions. *J. Immunol.*, **120**, 1278

21. Reinherz, E. L., Kung, P. C., Goldstein, G. and Schlossman, S. F. (1979). A monoclonal antibody with selective reactivity with functionally mature human thymocytes and all peripheral human T cells. *J. Immunol.*, **123**, 1312

22. Kung, P. C., Goldstein, G., Reinherz, E. L. and Schlossman, S. F. (1979). Monoclonal antibodies defining distinctive human T cell surface antigens. *Science*, **206**, 347

23. Reinherz, E. L., Kung, P. C., Pesando, J. M., Ritz, J., Goldstein, G. and Schlossman, S. F. (1979). Ia determinants on human T cell subsets defined by monoclonal antibody. Activation stimuli required for expression. *J. Exp. Med.*, **150**, 1472

24. Reinherz, E. L., Kung, P. C., Goldstein, G. and Schlossman, S. F. (1979). Separation of functional subsets of human T cells by a monoclonal antibody. *Proc. Natl. Acad. Sci. USA*. **76**, 4061

25. Reinherz, E. L., Kung, P. C., Goldstein, G. and Schlossman, S. F. (1979). Further characterization of the human inducer T cell subset defined by monoclonal antibody. *J. Immunol.*, **123**, 2894

26. Reinherz, E. L., Kung, P. C., Breard, J. M., Goldstein, G. and Schlossman, S. F. (1980). T cell requirements for generation of helper factor(s) in man: analysis of the subsets involved. *J. Immunol.*, **124**, 1883

27. Breard, J., Reinherz, E. L., Kung, P. C., Goldstein, G. and Schlossman, S. F. (1980). A monoclonal antibody reactive with human peripheral blood monocytes. *J. Immunol.*, **124**, 1943

28. Reinherz, E. L., Moretta, L., Roper, M., Breard, J. M., Mingari, M. C., Cooper, M. D. and Schlossman, S. F. (1980). Human T lymphocyte subpopulations defined by Fc receptors and monoclonal antibodies: a comparison. *J. Exp. Med.*, **151**, 969

29. Kaplan, J. and Callewaert, D. M. (1978). Expression of human T-lymphocyte antigens by natural killer cells. *J. Natl. Cancer Inst.*, **60**, 961

30. Herberman, R. B., Djeu, J. Y., Kay, H. D., Ortaldo, J. R., Riccardi, C., Bonnard, G. D., Holden, H. T., Fagnani, R., Santoni, A. and Puccetti, P. (1979). Natural killer cells: characteristics and regulation of activity. *Immunol. Rev.*, **44**, 43

31. Reinherz, E. L., Parkman, R., Rappeport, J., Rosen, F. S. and Schlossman, S. F. (1979). Aberrations of suppressor T cells in human graft-versus-host disease. *N. Engl. J. Med.*, **300**, 1061

32. Reinherz, E. L., Rubinstein, A., Geha, R. S., Strelkauskas, A. J., Rosen, F. S. and Schlossman, S. F. (1979). Abnormalities of immunoregulatory T cells in disorders of immune function. *N. Engl. J. Med.*, **301**, 1018

33. Strelkauskas, A. J., Callery, R. T., McDowell, J., Borel, Y. and Schlossman, S. F. (1978). Direct evidence for loss of human suppressor cells during active autoimmune disease. *Proc. Natl. Acad. Sci. USA*, **75**, 5150

34. Arbeit, R. D., Henkart, P. A. and Dickler, H. B. (1977). Differences between the Fc receptors of two lymphocyte subpopulations of human peripheral blood. *Scand. J. Immunol.*, **6**, 873

35. Frøland. S. S.. Wisløff. F. and Michaelsen, T. E. (1974). Human lymphocytes with receptors for IgG. A population of cells distinct from T and B lymphocytes. *Int. Arch. Allergy*, **47**, 124

36. Lobo, P. I. and Horwitz, D. A. (1976). An appraisal of Fc receptors on human peripheral blood B and L lymphocytes. *J. Immunol.*, **117**, 939

37. Alexander, E. L. and Henkart, P. A. (1978). Human peripheral lymphocytes bearing surface immunoglobulin do not have readily detectable Fc receptors. *Clin. Exp. Immunol.*, **33**, 332
38. Dickler, H. B. (1976). Lymphocyte receptors for immunoglobulin. *Adv. Immunol.*, **24**, 167
39. Horwitz, D. A. and Lobo, P. J. (1975). Characterization of two populations of human lymphocytes bearing easily detectable surface immunoglobulin. *J. Clin. Invest.*, **56**, 1464
40. Perlmann, P., Perlmann, H. and Wigzell, H. (1972). Lymphocyte-mediated cytotoxicity *in vitro*. Induction and inhibition by humoral antibody and nature of effector cells. *Transplant. Rev.*, **13**, 91
41. Wislǿff, F., Frǿland, S. S. and Michaelsen, T. E. (1974). Antibody-dependent cytotoxicity mediated by human Fc receptor-bearing cells lacking markers for B and T lymphocytes. *Int. Arch. Allergy*, **47**, 139
42. Brier, A. M., Chess, L. and Schlossman, S. F. (1975). Human antibody-dependent cellular cytotoxicity. Isolation and identification of a subpopulation of peripheral blood lymphocytes which kill antibody-coated autologous target cells. *J. Clin. Invest.*, **56**, 1580
43. Niaudet, P., Greaves, M. and Horwitz, D. (1979). Phenotypes of 'null' lymphoid cells in human blood. *Scand. J. Immunol.*, **9**, 387
44. Frǿland, S. S. and Abrahamsen, T. G. (1979). Lymphocyte populations in blood, synovial fluid and synovial tissue in rheumatoid arthritis. In Panayi, G. S. and Johnson, P. M. (eds.) *Immunopathogenesis of Rheumatoid Arthritis*, pp. 25–30. (Chertsey, Surrey: Reed Books)
45. Horwitz, D. A. and Garrett, M. A. (1977). Distinctive functional properties of human blood L lymphocytes: a comparison with T lymphocytes, B lymphocytes and monocytes. *J. Immunol.*, **118**, 1712
46. Carvalho, E. M. and Horwitz, D. A. (1980). Characterization of a non-T, non-B human blood lymphocyte that mediates the enhancing effects of immune complexes on lymphocyte blastogenesis. *J. Immunol.*, **124**, 1656
47. Chess, L., Levine, H., MacDermott, R. P. and Schlossman, S. F. (1975). Immunologic functions of isolated human lymphocyte subpopulations. VI. Further characterization of the surface Ig negative, E rosette negative (null cell) subset. *J. Immunol.*, **115**, 1483
48. Haegert, D. G. (1979). Demonstration of surface membrane immunoglobulin on L lymphocytes by the mixed antiglobulin rosetting reaction (MARR) and by the direct antiglobulin rosetting reaction (DARR). *Immunology*, **38**, 459
49. Balch, C. M., Ades, E. W., Loken, M. R. and Shore, S. L. (1980). Human 'null' cells mediating antibody-dependent cellular cytotoxicity express T lymphocyte differentiation anttigens. *J. Immunol.*, **124**, 1845
50. Huber, H., Polley, M. J., Linscott, W. D., Fudenberg, H. H. and Müller-Eberhard, H. J. (1968). Human monocytes: distinct receptor sites for the third component of complement and for immunoglobulin G. *Science*, **162**, 1281
51. Shaw, G. M., Levy, P. C. and LoBuglio, A. F. (1979). Re-examination of the EA rosette assay (Ripley) for Fc receptor leucocytes. *Clin. Exp. Immunol.*, **36**, 496
52. Horwitz, D. A., Kight, N., Temple, A. and Allison, A. C. (1979). Spontaneous and induced cytotoxic properties of human adherent mononuclear cells: killing of non-sensitized and antibody-coated non-erythroid cells. *Immunology*, **36**, 221
53. Gehrz, R. C. and Knorr, S. O. (1979). Characterization of the role of mononuclear cell subpopulations in the *in vitro* lymphocyte proliferation assay. *Clin. Exp. Immunol.*, **37**, 551
54. Markenson, J. A., Morgan, J. W., Lockshin, M. D., Joachim, C. and Winfield, J. B. (1978). Responses of fractionated cells from patients with systemic lupus erythematosus and normals to plant mitogen: evidence for a suppressor population of monocytes. *Proc. Soc. Exp. Biol. Med.*, **158**, 5
55. Klippel, J. H., Karsh, J., Stahl, N. I., Decker, J. L., Steinberg, A. D. and Schiffman, G. (1979). A controlled study of pneumococcal polysaccharide vaccine in systemic lupus erythematosus. *Arth. Rheum.*, **22**, 1321

56. Budman, D. R., Merchant, E. B., Steinberg, A. D., Doft, B., Gershwin, M. E., Lizzio, E. and Reeves, J. P. (1977). Increased spontaneous activity of antibody-forming cells in the peripheral blood of patients with active SLE. *Arth. Rheum.*, **20**, 829

57. Morimoto, C., Abe, T., Hara, M. and Homma, M. (1977). *In vitro* TNP-specific antibody formation by peripheral lymphocytes from patients with systemic lupus erythematosus. *Scand. J. Immunol.*, **6**, 575

58. Nies, K. M. and Louie, J. S. (1978). Impaired immunoglobulin synthesis by peripheral blood lymphocytes in systemic lupus erythematosus. *Arth. Rheum.*, **21**, 51

59. Morimoto, C. (1978). Loss of suppressor T lymphocyte function in patients with systemic lupus erythematosus (SLE). *Clin. Exp. Immunol.*, **32**, 125

60. Ginsburg, W. W., Finkelman, F. D. and Lipsky, P. E. (1979). Circulating and pokeweed mitogen-induced immunoglobulin-secreting cells in systemic lupus erythematosus. *Clin. Exp. Immunol.*, **35**, 76

61. Shou, L. S., Schwartz, A. and Good, R. A. (1976). Suppressor cell activity after concanavalin A treatment of lymphocytes from normal donors. *J. Exp. Med.*, **143**, 1100

62. Sakane, T., Steinberg, A. D. and Green, I. (1978). Studies of immune functions of patients with systemic lupus erythematosus. I. Dysfunction of suppressor T cell activity related to impaired generation of, rather than response to, suppressor cells. *Arth. Rheum.*, **21**, 657

63. Sagawa, A. and Abdou, N. I. (1978). Suppressor cell dysfunction in systemic lupus erythematosus. Cell involved and *in vitro* correction. *J. Clin. Invest.*, **62**, 789

64. Fauci, A. S., Steinberg, A. D., Haynes, B. F. and Whalen, G. (1978). Immunoregulatory aberrations in systemic lupus erythematosus. *J. Immunol.*, **121**, 1473

65. Sakane, T., Steinberg, A. D., Reeves, J. P. and Green, I. (1979). Studies of immune functions of patients with systemic lupus erythematosus. T cell subsets and antibodies to T cell subsets. *J. Clin. Invest.*, **64**, 1260

66. Sakane, T., Steinberg, A. D. and Green, I. (1980). Studies of immune functions of patients with systemic lupus erythematosus. V. T cell suppressor function and autologous mixed lymphocyte reaction during active and inactive phases of disease. *Arth. Rheum.*, **23**, 225

67. Hamilton, M. E. and Winfield, J. B. (1979). T_γ cells in systemic lupus erythematosus. Variation with disease activity. *Arth. Rheum.*, **22**, 1

68. Moretta, A., Mingari, M. C., Santoli, D., Perlmann, P. and Moretta, L. (1979). Human T-lymphocyte subpopulations: alterations in systemic lupus erythematosus. *Scand. J. Immunol.*, **10**, 223

69. Matsumoto, K., Osakabe, K., Ohi, H., Yoshizawa, N., Harada, M. and Hatano, M. (1980). Alteration of T lymphocyte subpopulations in patients with primary renal diseases and systemic lupus erythematosus. *Scand. J. Immunol.*, **11**, 187

70. Twomey, J. J., Laughter, A. H. and Steinberg, A. D. (1978). A serum inhibitor of immune regulation in patients with systemic lupus erythematosus. *J. Clin. Invest.*, **62**, 713

71. Morimoto, C., Abe, T., Toguchi, T., Kiyotaki, M. and Homma, M. (1979). Studies of anti-lymphocyte antibody of patients with active SLE. I. Cause of loss of suppressor T lymphocyte function. *Scand. J. Immunol.*, **10**, 213

72. Koike, T., Kobayashi, S., Yoshiki, T., Itoh, T. and Shirai, T. (1979). Differential sensitivity of functional subsets of T cells to the cytotoxicity of natural T-lymphocytotoxic auto-antibody of systemic lupus erythematosus. *Arth. Rheum.*, **22**, 123

73. Okudaira, K., Nakai, H., Hayakawa, T., Kashiwado, T., Tanimoto, K., Horiuchi, Y. and Juji, T. (1979). Detection of anti-lymphocyte antibody with two-color method in systemic lupus erythematosus and its heterogeneous specificities against human T cell subsets. *J. Clin. Invest.*, **64**, 1213

74. Edelson, R., Finkelman, F., Steinberg, A., Ahmed, A., Broder, S., Strong, D. M. and Green, I. (1978). Reactivity of lupus erythematosus antibodies with leukemic helper T cells. *J. Invest. Dermatol.*, **70**, 42

75. Haynes, B. F. and Fauci, A. S. (1978). Activation of human B lymphocytes. X. Hetero-

geneity of concanavalin A-generated suppressor cells of the pokeweed mitogen-induced plaque-forming cell response of human peripheral blood lymphocytes. *J. Immunol.*, **121**, 559

76. Lobo, P. I. and Spencer, C. E. (1979). Inhibition of humoral and cell-mediated immune responses in man by distinct suppressor cell systems. *J. Clin. Invest.*, **63**, 1157

77. Kuntz, M. M., Innes, J. B. and Weksler, M. E. (1976). Lymphocyte transformation induced by autologous cells. IV. Human T lymphocyte proliferation induced by autologous or allogeneic non-T lymphocytes. *J. Exp. Med.*, **143**, 1042

78. Sakane, T., Steonberg, A. D. and Green, I. (1978). Failure of autologous mixed lymphocyte reactions between T and non-T cells in patients with systemic lupus erythematosus. *Proc. Natl. Acad. Sci. USA*, **75**, 3464

79. Kuntz, M. M., Innes, J. B. and Weksler, M. E. (1979). The cellular basis of the impaired autologous mixed lymphocyte reaction in patients with systemic lupus erythematosus. *J. Clin. Invest.*, **63**, 151

80. Sakane, T., Steinberg, A. D., Arnett, F. C., Reinertsen, J. L. and Green, I. (1979). Studies of immune functions of patients with systemic lupus erythematosus. III. Characterization of lymphocyte subpopulations responsible for defective autologous mixed lymphocyte reactions. *Arth. Rheum.*, **22**, 770

81. Innes, J. B., Kuntz, M. M., Kim, Y. T. and Weksler, M. E. (1979). Induction of suppressor activity in the autologous mixed lymphocyte reaction and in cultures with concanavalin A. *J. Clin. Invest.*, **64**, 1608

82. Sakane, T. and Green, I. (1979). Specificity and suppressor function of human T cells responsive to autologous non-T cells. *J. Immunol.*, **123**, 584

83. Lohrmann, H.-P. and Whang-Peng, J. (1974). Human mixed leucocyte culture: identification of the proliferating lymphocyte subpopulation by sex chromosome markers. *J. Exp. Med.*, **140**, 54

84. Keightley, R. G., Cooper, M. D. and Lawton, A. R. (1976). The T cell dependence of B cell differentiation induced by pokeweed mitogen. *J. Immunol.*, **117**, 1538

85. Horwitz, D. A. and Garrett, M. A. (1977). Lymphocyte reactivity to mitogens in subjects with systemic lupus erythematosus, rheumatoid arthritis and scleroderma. *Clin. Exp. Immunol.*, **27**, 92

86. Utsinger, P. D. and Yount, W. J. (1977). Phytohaemagglutinin response in systemic lupus erythematosus. Reconstitution experiments using highly purified lymphocyte subpopulations and monocytes. *J. Clin. Invest.*, **60**, 626

87. Scheinberg, M. A., Santos, L., Mendes, N. F. and Musatti, C. (1978). Decreased lymphocyte response to PHA, Con A and calcium ionophore (A 23187) in patients with RA and SLE, and reversal with levamisole in rheumatoid arthritis. *Arth. Rheum.*, **21**, 326

88. Ruíz-Argüelles, A., Díaz-Jouanen, E. and Alarcón-Segovia, D. (1979). PHA-induced cellular cytotoxicity. Inhibition by a non-immunoglobulin factor present in sera from patients with active systemic lupus erythematosus. *Arth. Rheum.*, **22**, 59

89. Bobrove, A. M. and Miller, P. (1977). Depressed *in vitro* B lymphocyte differentiation in systemic lupus erythematosus. *Arth. Rheum.*, **20**, 1326

90. Gottlieb, A. B., Lahita, R. G., Chiorazzi, N. and Kunkel, H. G. (1979). Immune function in systemic lupus erythematosus. Impairment of *in vitro* T cell proliferation and *in vivo* antibody response to exogenous antigen. *J. Clin. Invest.*, **63**, 885

91. Andrianakos, A. A., Tsichlis, P. N., Merikas, E. G., Marketos, S. G., Sharp, J. T. and Merikas, G. E. (1977). Cell-mediated immunity in systemic lupus erythematosus. *Clin. Exp. Immunol.*, **30**, 89

92. Rivero, S. J., Llorente, L., Díaz-Jouanen, E. and Alarcón-Segovia, D. (1977). T lymphocyte subpopulation in untreated SLE. Variations with disease activity. *Arth. Rheum.*, **20**, 1169

93. Felsburg, P. J., Edelman, R. and Gilman, R. H. (1976). The active E rosette test: correlation with delayed cutaneous hypersensitivity. *J. Immunol.*. **116**. 1110

94. Oshimi, K., Sumiya, M., Gonda, N., Kano, S. and Takaku, F. (1979). Natural killer cell activity in systemic lupus erythematosus. *Lancet*, **2**, 1023

95. Penschow, J. and Mackay, I. R. (1980). NK and K cell activity of human blood: differences according to sex, age and disease. *Ann. Rheum. Dis.*, **39**, 82

96. Nakai, H., Morito, T., Tanimoto, K. and Horiuchi, Y. (1977). Reduced Fc receptor-bearing cells in peripheral bloods of patients with systemic lupus erythematosus and in rheumatoid synovial fluid. *J. Rheumatol.*, **4**, 405

97. Horwitz, D. A. and Juul-Nielsen, K. (1977). Human blood L lymphocytes in patients with active systemic lupus erythematosus, rheumatoid arthritis and scleroderma: a comparison with T and B cells. *Clin. Exp. Immunol.*, **30**, 370

98. Cooper, S. M., Harding, B., Mirick, G. R., Schneider, J., Quismorio, F. P. and Friou, G. J. (1978). Selective decrease in antibody-dependent cell-mediated cytotoxicity in systemic lupus erythematosus and progressive systemic sclerosis. *Clin. Exp. Immunol.*, **34**, 235

99. Díaz-Jouanen, E., Bankhurst, A. D. and Williams, R. C. Jnr. (1976). Antibody-mediated lymphocytotoxicity in rheumatoid arthritis and systemic lupus erythematosus. *Arth. Rheum.*, **19**, 133

100. Nelson, D. L., Bundy, B. M., Pitchon, H. E., Blaese, R. M. and Strober, W. (1976). The effector cells in human peripheral blood mediating mitogen-induced cellular cytotoxicity and antibody-dependent cellular cytotoxicity. *J. Immunol.*, **117**, 1472

101. Zvaifler, N. J. (1973). The immunopathology of joint inflammation in rheumatoid arthritis. *Adv. Immunol.*, **16**, 265

102. Stastny, P., Rosenthal, M., Andreis, M. and Ziff, M. (1975). Lymphokines in the rheumatoid joint. *Arth. Rheum.*, **18**, 237

103. Smiley, J. D., Sachs, C. and Ziff, M. (1968). *In vitro* synthesis of immunoglobulin by rheumatoid synovial membrane. *J. Clin. Invest.*, **47**, 624

104. Paulus, H. E., Machleder, H. I., Levine, S., Yu, D. T. Y. and MacDonald, N. S. (1977). Lymphocyte involvement in rheumatoid arthritis. Studies during thoracic duct drainage. *Arth. Rheum.*, **20**, 1249

105. Ueo, T., Tanaka, S., Tominaga, Y., Ogawa, H. and Sakurami, T. (1979). The effect of thoracic duct drainage on lymphocyte dynamics and clinical symptoms in patients with rheumatoid arthritis. *Arth. Rheum.*, **22**, 1405

106. Yu, D. T. Y. and Peter, J. B. (1974). Cellular immunological aspects of rheumatoid arthritis. *Sem. Arth. Rheum.*, **4**, 25

107. Andrianakos, A. A., Sharp, J. T., Person, D. A., Lidsky, M. D. and Duffy, J. (1977). Cell-mediated immunity in rheumatoid arthritis. *Ann. Rheum. Dis.*, **36**, 13

108. Silverman, H. A., Johnson, J. S., Vaughan, J. H. and McGlamory, J. C. (1976). Altered lymphocyte reactivity in rheumatoid arthritis. *Arth. Rheum.*, **19**, 509

109. Menard, H. A., Dion, J. and Richard, C. (1977). Antinuclear antibody: predictive of lymphocyte response in rheumatoid arthritis. *J. Rheumatol.*, **4**, 21

110. Stratton, J. A. and Peter, J. B. (1978). The responses of peripheral blood and synovial fluid lymphocytes of patients with rheumatoid arthritis to *in vitro* stimulation with mitogens. *Clin. Immunol. Immunopathol.*, **10**, 233

111. Burmester, G. R., Kalden, J. R., Peter, H. H., Schedel, I., Beck, P. and Wittenborg, A. (1978). Immunological and functional characteristics of peripheral blood and synovial fluid lymphocytes from patients with rheumatoid arthritis. *Scand. J. Immunol.*, **7**, 405

112. Abrahamsen, T. G., Frøland, S. S. and Natvig, J. B. (1978). *In vitro* mitogen stimulation of synovial fluid lymphocytes from rheumatoid arthritis and juvenile rheumatoid arthritis patients: dissociation between the response to antigens and polyclonal mitogens. *Scand. J. Immunol.*, **7**, 81

113. Corrigall, V., Panayi, G. S. and Laurent, R. (1979). Lymphocyte studies in rheumatoid arthritis. III. A comparative study of the responses of peripheral blood and synovial fluid lymphocytes to phytomitogens. *Scand. J. Rheumatol.*, **8**, 10

114. Percy, J. S., Davis, P., Russell, A. S. and Brisson, E. (1978). A longitudinal study of *in vitro* tests for lymphocyte function in rheumatoid arthritis. *Ann. Rheum. Dis.*, **37**, 416

115. Wolf, R. E. (1978). Hyporesponsiveness of lymphocytes to virus antigens in rheumatoid arthritis. *Arth. Rheum.*, **21**, 238

116. Chattopadhyay, H., Chattopadhyay, C. and Natvig, J. B. (1979). Hyporesponsiveness to virus antigens in rheumatoid synovial and blood lymphocytes using the indirect leucocyte migration inhibition test. *Scand. J. Immunol.*, **10**, 585

117. Galili, U., Rosenthal, L., Galili, N. and Klein, E. (1979). Activated T cells in the synovial fluid of arthritic patients: characterization and comparison with *in vitro* activated human and murine T cells in co-operation with monocytes in cytotoxicity. *J. Immunol.*, **122**, 878

118. Yu, D. T. Y., Winchester, R. J., Fu, S. M., Gibofsky, A., Ko, H. S. and Kunkel, H. G. (1980). Peripheral blood Ia-positive T cells. Increases in certain diseases and after immunization. *J. Exp. Med.*, **151**, 91

119. Abrahamsen, T. G., Frøland, S. S., Natvig, J. B. and Pahle, J. (1975). Elution and characterization of lymphocytes from rheumatoid inflammatory tissue. *Scand. J. Immunol.*, **4**, 823

120. Abrahamsen, T. G., Frøland, S. S., Natvig, J. B. and Pahle, J. (1977). Lymphocytes eluted from synovial tissue of juvenile rheumatoid arthritis patients. *Arth. Rheum.*, **20**, 772

121. Abrahamsen, T. G., Frøland, S. S., Natvig, J. B. and Pahle, J. (1976). Antigen and unspecific mitogen stimulation of lymphocytes eluted from rheumatoid inflammatory tissue. *Scand. J. Immunol.*, **5**, 1057

122. Meijer, C. J. L. M., van de Putte, L. B. A., Lafaber, G. J. M., de Haas, E. and Cats, A. (1980). Membrane and transformation characteristics of lymphocytes isolated from the synovial membrane and paired peripheral blood of patients with rheumatoid arthritis. *Ann. Rheum. Dis.*, **39**, 75

123. Chattopadhyay, C., Chattopadhyay, H., Natvig, J. B., Michaelsen, T. E. and Mellbye, O. J. (1979). Lack of suppressor cell activity in rheumatoid synovial lymphocytes. *Scand. J. Immunol.*, **10**, 309

124. Chattopadhyay, C., Chattopadhyay, H., Natvig, J. B. and Mellbye, O. J. (1979). Rheumatoid synovial lymphocytes lack concanavalin-A-activated suppressor cell activity. *Scand. J. Immunol.*, **10**, 479

125. Segond, P., Delfraissy, J. F., Galanaud, P., Wallon, C., Massias, P. and Dormont, J. (1979). Depressed primary *in vitro* antibody response in rheumatoid arthritis. *Clin. Exp. Immunol.*, **37**, 196

126. Chattopadhyay, C., Natvig, J. B. and Chattopadhyay, H. (1980). Excessive suppressor T cell activity of the rheumatoid synovial tissue in X-linked hypogammaglobulinaemia. *Scand. J. Immunol.*, **11**, 455

127. Dobloug, J. H., Førre, Ø, Natvig, J. B. and Michaelsen, T. E. (1979). Demonstration of rheumatoid factor idiotypic antigens on peripheral blood B and T lymphocytes from patients with rheumatoid arthritis. *Scand. J. Immunol.*, **9**, 273

128. Dumonde, D. C., Kelly, R. H. and Morley, J. (1976). Lymphoid and microvascular dysfunction in experimental models of rheumatoid inflammation. In Dumonde, D. C. (ed.) *Infection and Immunology in the Rheumatic Diseases*, pp. 375–403. (Oxford: Blackwell Scientific Publications)

129. Bach, J.-F., Delrieu, F. and Delbarre, F. (1970). The rheumatoid rosette. A diagnostic test unifying seropositive and seronegative rheumatoid arthritis. *Am. J. Med.*, **49**, 213

130. Scherak, O., Sitko, C., Eibl, M. and Kolarz, G. (1976). EA-rosetten bei Patienten mit progredient Chronischer Polyarthritis (in German). *Z. Rheumatol.*, **35**, 103

131. Sharpin, R. K. C. and Wilson, J. D. (1977). Increased EA-rosette formation by lymphocytes from patients with rheumatoid arthritis. *Clin. Exp. Immunol.*, **29**, 205

132. Wooley, P. H. and Panayi, G. S. (1978). Studies of lymphocytes in rheumatoid arthritis. I. Uptake of ^{125}I-heat aggregated human IgG by Fc-receptor bearing lymphocytes. *Ann. Rheum. Dis.*, **37**, 343

133. Warnatz, H. and Thommes, M. (1979). *In vitro* studies on lymphocytotoxicity to synovial cells and Chang cells in rheumatoid arthritis patients and healthy controls. *Z. Rheumatol.*, **38**, 129

134. Hall, N. D. and Winrow, V. R. (1979). A new approach to the study of high avidity Fc receptors on rheumatoid lymphocytes. *Ann. Rheum. Dis.*, **38**, 485

135. Frøland, S. S., Natvig, J. B. and Wisløff, F. (1975). Lymphocyte subpopulations in rheumatoid arthritis. *Rheumatology*, **6**, 231

136. Froebel, K., Sturrock, R. D., Reynolds, P., Grennan, A., Roxburgh, A. and MacSween, R. N. M. (1979). *In vitro* reactions of lymphocytes in rheumatoid arthritis and other rheumatic diseases. *Ann. Rheum. Dis.* **38**, 535

137. Brown, K. A., Embling, P. H. F., Perry, J. D. and Holborow, E. J. (1979). Electrophoretic behaviour of blood and synovial fluid lymphocytes in rheumatoid arthritis. *Clin. Exp. Immunol.*, **36**, 272

138. Brown, K. A., Perry, J. D. and Holborow, E. J. (1979). Lymphocyte subpopulations from synovial fluid and peripheral blood of rheumatoid arthritis patients. In Preece, A. W. and Sabolovic, D. (eds.) *Cell Electrophoresis: Clinical Applications and Methodology*, pp. 55–68. (Amsterdam: North Holland)

139. Sany, J., Clot, J., Freitas, M., Charmasson, E. and Serre, H. (1976). Antibody-dependent cell cytotoxicity (ADCC) of rheumatoid arthritis blood lymphocytes. *Rev. Rheum.*, **43**, 333

140. Panayi, G. S. and Corrigall, V. (1977). Functional assay of cytotoxic lymphocytes involved in antibody-mediated cytotoxicity in normal and rheumatoid subjects. *Ann. Rheum. Dis.*, **36**, 257

141. Rosenberg, J. N. and Currey, H. L. F. (1979). Antibody-dependent and PHA-induced cellular cytotoxicity in rheumatoid arthritis. *Ann. Rheum. Dis.*, **38**, 347

142. McGill, P. E. and Twinn, I. (1977). Antibody-mediated cytotoxicity in rheumatoid arthritis. *Ann. Rheum. Dis.*, **36**, 268

143. Biberfeld, G., Nilsson, E. and Biberfeld, P. (1979). T lymphocyte subpopulations in synovial fluid of patients with rheumatic disease. *Arth. Rheum.*, **22**, 978

144. Corrigall, V. M. and Panayi, G. S. (1978). Lymphocyte studies in rheumatoid arthritis. II. Antibody-mediated and mitogen-induced lymphocyte cytotoxicity in synovial fluid and peripheral blood. *Ann. Rheum. Dis.*, **37**, 410

145. Abrahamsen, T. G., Frøland, S. S., Natvig, J. B. and Pahle, J. (1977). Antibody-dependent cytotoxicity mediated by cells eluted from synovial tissues of patients with rheumatoid arthritis and juvenile rheumatoid arthritis. *Scand. J. Immunol.*, **6**, 1251

146. Fink, P. C., Schedel, I., Peter, H. H. and Deicher, H. (1977). Inhibition of spontaneous and antibody-dependent cellular cytotoxicity by sera and isolated antiglobulin preparations from rheumatoid arthritis patients. *Scand. J. Immunol.*, **6**, 173

147. Pang, G. and Wilson, J. D. (1978). Different rosette assays for detecting Fc receptor-bearing lymphocytes measure different subpopulations. *Immunology*, **35**, 407

148. Clements, P. J. and Levy, J. (1978). Receptors for IgG (Fc receptors) on human lymphocytes: re-evaluation by multiple techniques. *Clin. Exp. Immunol.*, **34**, 281

149. Winchester, R. J., Hoffman, T., Ferrarini, M., Ross, G. D. and Kunkel, H. G. (1979). Comparison of various tests for Fc receptors on different human lymphocyte subpopulations. *Clin. Exp. Immunol.*, **37**, 126

150. Stewart, G. A., Smith, A. K. and Stanworth, D. R. (1973). Biological activities associated with the Facb fragment of rabbit IgG. *Immunochemistry*, **10**, 755

151. Hall, N. D., Winrow, V. R. and Bacon, P. A. (1980). Lymphocytes bearing Fcγ receptors in rheumatoid arthritis. I. An increased subpopulation of cells in RA detected with Facb rosettes. *Ann. Rheum. Dis.*, **39**, 554

152. Hall, N. D. (1978). Leucocyte migration inhibition with IgG-IgG complexes and rabbit IgG fragments in patients with rheumatoid arthritis. *Clin. Exp. Immunol.*, **34**, 219

153. Hall, N. D. and Winrow, V. R. (1981). Lymphocytes bearing Fcγ receptors in rheumatoid

arthritis. III. Increased subpopulation of 'null' lymphocytes in RA detected by Facb rosettes. (In preparation)

154. Delbarre, F., Le Gô, A. and Kahan, A. (1975). Hyperbasophilic immunoblasts in circulating blood in chronic inflammatory rheumatic and collagen diseases. *Ann. Rheum. Dis.*, **34**, 422

155. Bacon, P. A., Sewell, R. L. and Crowther, D. (1975). Reactive lymphoid cells ('immunoblasts') in autoimmune and haematological disorders. *Clin. Exp. Immunol.*, **19**, 201

156. Steinman, R. M., Machtinger, B. G., Fried, J. and Cohn, Z. A. (1978). Mouse spleen lymphoblasts generated *in vitro*. Recovery in high yield and purity after flotation in dense bovine plasma albumin solutions. *J. Exp. Med.*, **147**, 279

157. Glinski, W., Gershwin, M. E., Budman, D. R. and Steinberg, A. D. (1976). Study of lymphocyte subpopulations in normal humans and patients with systemic lupus erythematosus by fractionation of peripheral blood lymphocytes on a discontinuous Ficoll gradient. *Clin. Exp. Immunol.*, **26**, 228

158. Carter, S. D. (1979). Density distribution of peripheral blood lymphocytes in health and rheumatoid disease. *PhD Thesis*. University of Bath

159. Papadimitriou, G., Hall, N. D. and Bacon, P. A. (1981). Lymphocyte subpopulations isolated by Ficoll density gradient in rheumatoid synovitis and rheumatoid disease. (In preparation)

160. Papadimitriou, G., Bacon, P. A., Carter, S. D. and Hall, N. D. (1981). Rheumatoid immunoblasts and the effect of gold and cytotoxic drugs. In Willoughby, D. A. and Giroud, J. P. (eds.) *Inflammation: Mechanisms and Treatment*, pp. 555–560. (Lancaster: MTP Press)

161. Carter, S. D., Bacon, P. A. and Hall, N. D. (1981). The characterization of activated lymphocytes in the peripheral blood of patients with rheumatoid arthritis. *Ann. Rheum. Dis.* (In press)

162. Jondal, M. (1974). Surface markers on human B and T lymphocytes. IV. Distribution of surface markers on resting and blast-transformed lymphocytes. *Scand. J. Immunol.*, **3**, 739

163. Robbins, D. L., Moore, T. L., Carson, D. A. and Vaughan, J. H. (1978). Relative reactivities of rheumatoid factors in serum and cells. Evidence for a selective deficiency in serum rheumatoid factor. *Arth. Rheum.*, **21**, 820

164. Johnson, P. M., Watkins, J. and Holborow, E. J. (1975). Antiglobulin production to altered IgG in rheumatoid arthritis. *Lancet*, **1**, 611

165. Vaughan, J. H. (1979). Rheumatoid arthritis, rheumatoid factor and the Epstein–Barr virus. *J. Rheumatol.*, **6**, 381

166. Slaughter, L., Carson, D. A., Jensen, F., Holbrook, T. L. and Vaughan, J. H. (1978). *In vitro* effects of Epstein–Barr virus on peripheral blood mononuclear cells from patients with rheumatoid arthritis and normal subjects. *J. Exp. Med.*, **148**, 1429

167. Alspaugh, M. A., Jensen, F. C., Rabin, H. and Tan, E. M. (1978). Lymphocytes transformed by Epstein–Barr virus. Induction of nuclear antigen reactive with antibody in rheumatoid arthritis. *J. Exp. Med.*, **147**, 1018

168. Ng, K. C., Brown, K. A., Perry, J. D. and Holborow, E. J. (1980). Anti-RANA antibody: a marker for seronegative and seropositive rheumatoid arthritis. *Lancet*, **1**, 447

169. Catalano, M. A., Carson, D. A., Niederman, J. C., Feorino, P. and Vaughan, J. H. (1980). Antibody to the rheumatoid arthritis nuclear antigen. Its relationship to *in vivo* Epstein–Barr virus infection. *J. Clin. Invest.*, **65**, 1238

170. Johnsen, H. E., Madsen, M. and Kristensen, T. (1979). Lymphocyte subpopulations in man: suppression of PWM-induced B cell proliferation by infectious mononucleosis T cells. *Scand. J. Immunol.*, **10**, 251

171. Tosato, G., Magrath, I., Koski, I., Dooley, N. and Blaese, M. (1979). Activation of suppressor T cells during Epstein–Barr virus-induced infectious mononucleosis. *N. Engl. J. Med.*, **301**, 1133

2
Lymphocyte Traffic through Chronic Inflammatory Lesions: Relevance to Rheumatic Disease

J. B. HAY, T. B. ISSEKUTZ and W. G. CHIN

INTRODUCTION

The visual, immunopathological description of the lesions found in rheumatic diseases underestimates the complexity and the multitude of immune and inflammatory processes which occur. Nevertheless, even in the various animal models there are common features which emphasize similarities between these diseases and implicate the mechanisms of cell-mediated immunity and delayed hypersensitivity. For example, the adjuvant arthritis model in the rat depends upon intact regional lymph nodes for the ultimate expression of mononuclear cell infiltration beyond the site of stimulation in the footpad[1]. Furthermore, there is a critical time following which the removal of these lymph nodes does not prevent lesions in the ears, tail and other connective tissue sites. It would seem that lymph node products are directly responsible and from what is known about the output of both cellular and humoral node products in efferent lymph draining adjuvant lesions[2], taken together with the capacity to transfer pathology in a variety of models with thymus-derived (T) lymphocytes[3], a role for sensitized lymphocytes is strongly implicated. The nature of the sensitizing antigens in rheumatic diseases is still unclear.

One of the most fundamental features of these lesions is their mononuclear cell nature. Although this is described on histopathological grounds as infiltration, accumulation, or by some other static description, there is compelling evidence, at least in the animal system described here, that these are likely to be

29

true lymphocyte traffic sites. In fact, the evidence indicates that the traffic in chronically inflamed skin is as extensive as it is in lymph nodes. Although secondary lymphoid tissue is well designed to accommodate this traffic as part of its normal function what are the consequences of comparable traffic through non-lymphoid tissues? Does extensive traffic beyond the confines of established traffic pathways represent a significant pathological process in itself, regardless of whether cytotoxic lymphocytes, antibodies, lymphokines or inflammatory cell products participate? This question is particularly relevant in an articulating joint where even minor disruption can compromise its efficiency. It is likely that this traffic would have less consequence in a rheumatoid nodule or a skin lesion than is the case with synovitis. Nevertheless, the stimulus and the mechanisms are probably the same, regardless of the tissue site. Lymphocyte traffic has never been measured in natural or induced synovitis. However, based on the data showing that a wide variety of mononuclear inflammatory sites have a substantial increase in the output of lymphocytes in the regional, afferent lymph, it seems likely to us that rheumatoid joints would be similar. It is well documented that lymphocyte traffic normally occurs in secondary lymphoid tissue[4-6]. However, it is equally clear that we can experimentally manipulate the conditions so as to induce probable traffic sites in a variety of other tissues. Lymphocyte output in afferent lymph is increased as much as 30-fold or even higher from lymphocyte allografts[7], renal allografts[8], heart allografts (Simpson-Morgan, unpublished observations), tuberculin reactions[9] and adjuvant granulomas[10]. Moreover, based upon physiological and quantitative data, it is clear that there is as much traffic through granulomatous lesions as there is through lymph nodes[11]. Some of these and other experimental results are summarized in the following synopsis.

The bases of the experiments outlined here have arisen from exploitation of the chronic lymphatic drainage techniques described by Morris and his colleagues in sheep[12]. The physiological integrity of this approach means that this is more than a convenient model of these biological processes in that it represents a description and quantitation of these processes as they occur *in vivo*.

Our utilization of these techniques has focused on an attempt to define and quantitate properties of various lymphocyte compartments and we have made an attempt to measure the extent and the rates of lymphocyte movement between them. A desirable end would be a quantitative analysis of the blood vascular compartment at the site of a lesion, the rate of replication and other behaviour of cells within the lesion and the rate of exit of cells from the lesion. It would be helpful to have a qualitative description of the cells, based on cell marker analysis, superimposed on this scheme. The addition of such data to our present knowledge of quantitative lymphatic physiology may be enlightening with respect to collagen vascular diseases. The lymphocyte traffic aspect of rheumatic diseases is part of a broader question. How and why do lymphocytes preferentially leave the blood at these inflammatory sites? Do certain lymphocyte subpopulations more effectively or preferentially leave at one site rather than another?

Our present experimental approach is to induce chronic inflammatory lesions in the skin with Freund's adjuvant, BCG, allogeneic lymphocytes or tuberculin in appropriately sensitized animals. Under anaesthetic, catheters are positioned (as shown in Figure 2.1) in:

(A) the arterial and/or venous blood;
(B) the efferent lymphatic of one or more subcutaneous lymph nodes;
(C) the efferent lymphatic of the regional node draining the lesion;
(D) an afferent lymphatic vessel leaving the lesion; and
(E) a normal, usually contralateral afferent lymphatic.

In some experiments intestinal lymph (F) is collected and analysed. A usual animal preparation would have about four such catheters patent during the experimental period of a few days. On occasion, however, lymph has been continuously collected from some individual catheters for periods greater than 3 months. Sheep are free to stand or lie in metabolism cages for this time without ill effects. Furthermore, a series of skin lesions of various age and type can be induced in a shaved area of the flank or in the hair-free skin of the groin region. Radiolabelled microspheres introduced to the left heart have been used to quantitate blood flow and thereby deduce lymphocyte delivery to lesions, normal skin and lymph nodes[7]. Recent protocols involve the labelling of certain lymphocytes with ^{111}In and other lymphocytes with ^{51}Cr and their

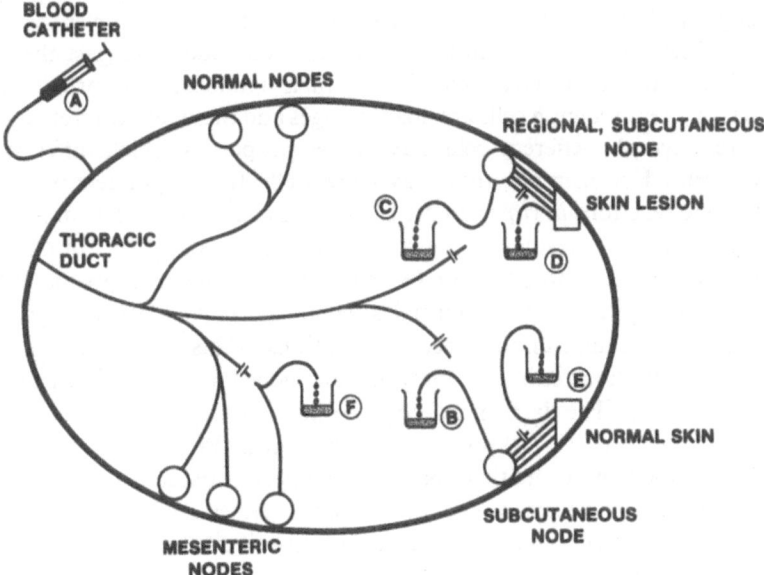

Figure 2.1 Sites for the analysis of lymphocyte traffic in sheep (see text for explanation)

simultaneous injection into the blood. The specific activity of labelled cells is thereafter monitored in various of the six compartments described in Figure 2.1. Furthermore, the ratio of one isotope-labelled population to the other isotope-labelled population can be analysed. A comparison of the labelling and detection characteristics, as well as the kinetics and recovery of the blood to lymph migration of both [111]In- and ^{51}Cr-labelled cells, has been described[13]. Finally, if the animal is sacrificed after some period of time the radioactivity and the ratio of labels can be analysed in the lesions and some comparisons can be made between the lymph, blood, node and lesion compartments. A review of some present concepts of lymphocyte migration is briefly considered before considering some of this more recent data.

THE EXTENT OF LYMPHOCYTE TRAFFIC THROUGH RESTING LYMPH NODES AND CONNECTIVE TISSUE SPACES

The demonstration in sheep and in man that significant migration of lymphocytes and, to a lesser degree, monocyte macrophages occurs in connective tissue spaces[14, 15] is of fundamental significance. Smith et al.[16] and others have collected normal afferent lymph from kidneys, livers, thyroid, skin, ovaries, uterus and testes. Most of the plasma and cells probably leave the blood in the connective tissue in these organs probably associated with the framework and, if present, the capsule. It seems likely that the cells normally found in the pleural and peritoneal cavities are analogous to those of afferent lymph. Although the hourly output of cells in afferent lymph is much lower than the output of cells in efferent lymph from nodes these studies suggest that the normal migration of cells from blood to lymph is significant[15]. Approximately 10–20% of afferent lymph cells are macrophages and these cells cannot be seen in efferent lymph. Afferent cells have other properties which differ from efferent cells. For example, they may be less effective responders in mixed lymphocyte reactions *in vitro* and are clearly less effective inducers of normal lymphocyte transfer lesions in the skin of allogeneic sheep[16, 17]. In animals previously injected with either BCG or Freund's complete adjuvant, PPD-sensitive cells appear in both normal afferent and normal efferent lymph[18] (als Hay and Cahill, unpublished observations). This would suggest that som of the lymphocytes in afferent lymph are indeed part of the recirculating lymphocyte pool. The data on isotope labelling and migration of these cells would support this[11, 29]. The presence of recirculating PPD-sensitive lymphocytes in afferent lymph, and therefore in the connective tissue spaces, probably indicates that the principal trigger of delayed-hypersensitivity phenomena — the interaction of sensitized lymphocytes with specific antigen — occurs in the extravascular tissues.

Differences in the proportions of T and B lymphocytes in blood, efferent lymph and afferent lymph have been described in sheep and man[19, 20]. In general, the proportion of B cells is less in afferent lymph than in blood, efferent lymph and probably also in so-called fixed, secondary lymphoid tissue. The gut-associated lymphoid tissue may be fundamentally different in this respect[21].

The hourly cell output of a popliteal afferent lymphatic in a sheep is approximately 1 million cells[5,11]. The hourly cell output in efferent lymph from the same node is 30 million[5,11]. It has been calculated that approximately 90% of the efferent lymphocyte output is derived from the blood within the lymph node[22]. Calculations based on blood flow measurements have suggested that 25% of the blood-borne lymphocytes which enter a normal node cross the endothelium, traverse the node and enter the efferent lymph[23]. Antigenic challenge leads to an increase in both the blood flow and the lymphocyte output of a lymph node. When such a node is heavily irradiated the cell output in the lymph falls but rapidly recovers due to repopulation from the blood[24]. Such studies emphasize the dynamic nature of lymph node lymphocytes. It is a reasonable working hypothesis that the vast majority of small lymphocytes in secondary lymphoid tissue and in chronic inflammatory lesions are migrating cells and are always in the process of migration. Significant numbers of sessile, small lymphocyte may not even exist in such regions. Therefore, the use of such terms as trapping and accumulation to describe small lymphocyte behaviour may be misleading and erroneous, as Cahill *et al.* have argued[25]. The issue concerning the possible retention of the small but crucial number of antigen-reactive cells (in this discussion including sensitized cells) at sites of antigen deposition remains unclear and controversial[18,26,27].

THE EXTENT OF LYMPHOCYTE TRAFFIC THROUGH STIMULATED LYMPH NODES AND THE GENERATION OF SENSITIZED CELLS

There are descriptions of the changes in lymphocyte output in efferent lymph following the stimulation of a node with a variety of soluble, viral, bacterial or mammalian cellular antigens[5,9,25]. Perhaps of more relevance in the present discussion is the change in traffic in a regional node challenged by the injection of Freund's adjuvant in the drainage area. Such a response has been represented in Figure 2.2 based on previously published data. At the time of these experiments it was suggested that PPD-sensitive cells were generated in the node (the early peak) and in the granuloma itself. The latter conclusion was based upon the observation that the maximum cell output in the afferent lymph from such a lesion occurs after the cellular events in the node have subsided (see Figure 2.3). However, there was no direct demonstration that sensitized cells were produced in the lesion. Other variations in the lymph output of PPD-sensitive cells following the injection of BCG have been described elsewhere[18].

Some studies have been done with the intravenous injection of ^{51}Cr-labelled normal lymphocytes during the early stages following antigenic challenge of a node. Although the output of lymphocytes was enhanced, the specific activity (counts min^{-1} 10^{-7} cells) was similar to that seen in a normal node[25]. However, systematic studies have not been done in sheep by labelling small lymphocytes at a time when there are substantial numbers of sensitized cells in the lymph. In the rat adjuvant disease model no difference was found between

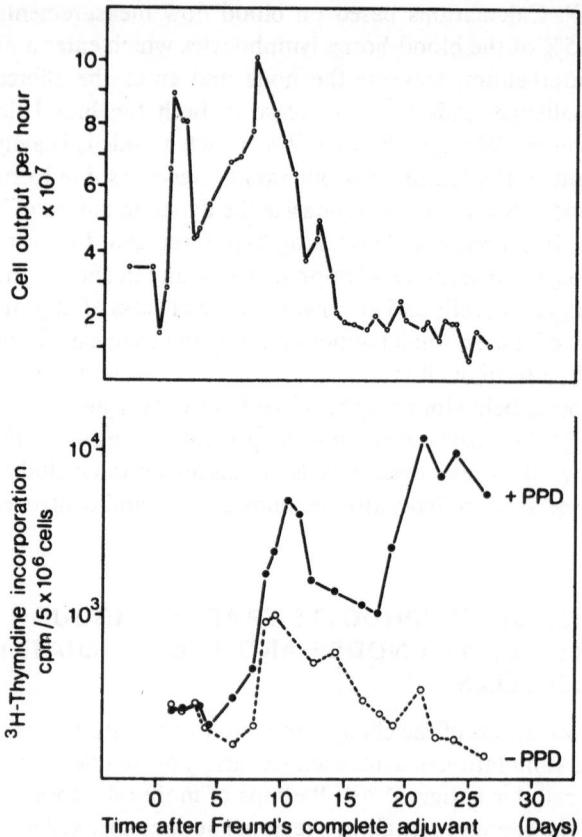

Figure 2.2 Description of total cell output and appearance of tuberculin-sensitive cells in efferent lymph from an adjuvant stimulated node. Data from reference 2 (with permission of Academic Press)

the migration of thoracic duct cells from animals with adjuvant disease compared with normal rats when cell transfers were made to arthritic recipients[28]. These investigators thought that a role for the vascular endothelium in arthritic lesions was more relevant than the nature or source of the migratory lymphocytes themselves. If the rat data can be compared with the sheep data it would be our contention that lymph cells other than thoracic duct cells might

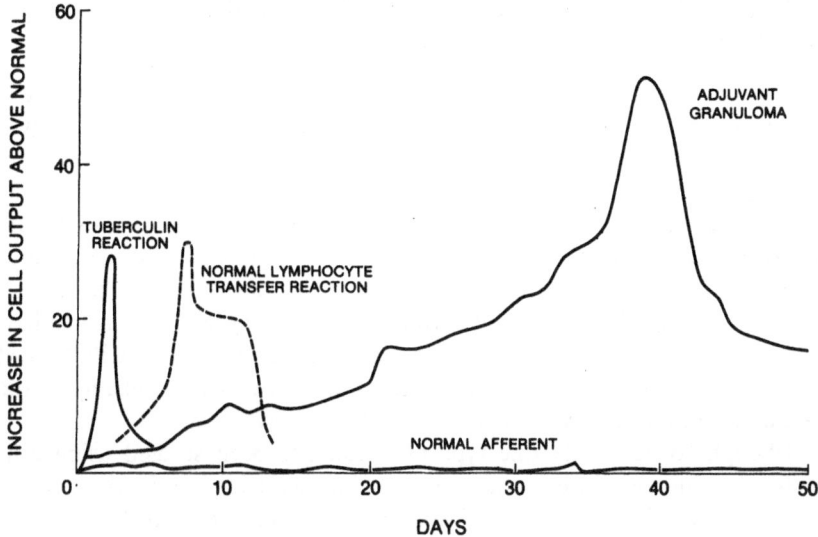

Figure 2.3   Cell output in afferent lymph from chronic inflammatory lesions. Data re-expressed from reference 9 (tuberculin reaction), 7 (normal lymphocyte transfer reaction), 10 (adjuvant granuloma) and unpublished observations (normal afferent)

be more relevant. In sheep, cells from intestinal lymph are poorer than efferent lymph cells from subcutaneous nodes at migrating through adjuvant inflammatory sites[11,29]. The thoracic duct contains a predominance of intestinal lymph[30]. Afferent lymph cells exhibit the most extensive traffic through chronic inflammatory sites induced by Freund's adjuvant[11] (see Figure 2.4).

Another feature of the efferent lymph from stimulated nodes is the transient appearance of lymphokines in the lymph plasma. Migration inhibition factor and a lymphocyte mitogen were detected following stimulation with tuberculin in appropriately sensitized animals[9]. More recently a significant burst in the output of interferon has been demonstrated in the efferent lymph from stimulated nodes[31]. The possible involvement of lymphokines in rheumatic disease pathology has been discussed by Dumonde[32]. Although these factors have not been studied in afferent lymph there are other inflammatory products and potential inflammatory mediators which have been assayed in cells of afferent lymph draining adjuvant granulomas. These include a vasoactive substance and plasminogen activator[33] and a thromboplastin-like material[34]. The vasoactive material is probably[35] phospholipase A_2. These factors appear to be released by the macrophages in the stimulated afferent lymph. Insignificant activity was found in normal afferent lymph cells and no activity was found in efferent lymph cells. Although significant E and F type prostaglandin has also been detected in afferent lymph from such chronic lesions[36] much greater levels of prostaglandin were found in acute inflammatory lymph containing large numbers of polymorphonuclear leukocytes[37].

THE EXTENT OF LYMPHOCYTE TRAFFIC THROUGH CHRONIC INFLAMMATORY SITES IN SHEEP

The afferent lymph draining a variety of chronic inflammatory sites has been examined (see below). The output of mononuclear cells from such lesions was found to be many times greater than normal in all cases. Although it seemed reasonable at the time of these experiments to conclude that many of the cells in this afferent lymph were recently derived from the blood and that they were not solely a consequence of local proliferation, a more conclusive demonstration that this indeed represented a traffic site is more recent[11]. The kinetics of the cell output of three types of chronic inflammatory lesions characterized by mononuclear cells is shown in Figure 2.3. These are compared with the cell output of a normal afferent lymphatic. In all three of these examples the maximum cell output was greater than 20 times normal.

Although to date only one type of lesion has been studied using cell-labelling techniques, the evidence indicates that the lesion is a site of extensive lymphocyte traffic. When normal efferent lymph cells are labelled and returned to the blood, labelled cells subsequently appeared in the afferent

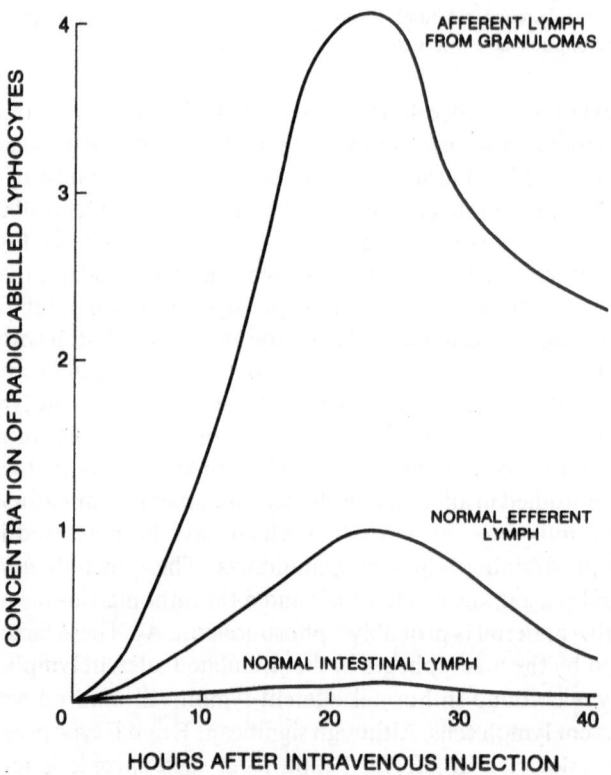

Figure 2.4 Appearance of intraveneously injected, labelled afferent lymph cells from granulomas in different lymphatics. Data from references 11 and 12

lymph[11]. Similarly, when cells in afferent lymph draining a granuloma are labelled and injected into the blood, cells reappeared in the afferent lymph. We concluded from this analysis that both normal efferent cells and afferent granuloma cells migrate into and through such lesions. When quantitative comparisons were made on 13 such experiments with respect to the recovery of labelled cells over 40 h, it was concluded that the lesions were as significant a site for lymphocyte traffic as were lymph nodes. However, different patterns of traffic were apparent and these are described in the subsequent section. It would seem very likely that tuberculin lesions and normal lymphocyte transfer lesions are also sites of lymphocyte traffic, although such experiments using labelled cells have not been done.

DIFFERENT PATTERNS OF LYMPHOCYTE TRAFFIC THROUGH NORMAL NODES, ADJUVANT GRANULOMAS AND MESENTERIC NODES

Although there is extensive migration of either afferent or efferent lymphocytes through granulomas there are some interesting differences in the migratory pattern depending on the lymph compartment that is analysed. The results shown in Figure 2.4 represent a composite of data described in detail elsewhere[11,12,29]. When afferent cells from an adjuvant granuloma are labelled and injected into the blood they reappear in the lymph compartment of origin in concentrations greater than in the efferent lymph. The lowest concentration of labelled cells is found in intestinal lymph. When efferent, intestinal cells are labelled they reappear in the highest concentration in intestinal lymph as described originally by Cahill et al.[29] and the concentration in afferent lymph from granulomas is even lower than in normal efferent lymph from subcutaneous nodes. These results suggest several interesting and testable questions. What is the situation with normal, afferent cells? What happens in a granuloma produced in the bowel rather than the skin? What is the pattern of traffic through a chronically inflamed joint?

The functional significance of these patterns is not clear. However, some characterization of the cells has been done. Velocity sedimentation separation of cells in afferent lymph from granulomas demonstrated that radioactivity correlated best with small lymphocytes but not with macrophages. Depletion of at least 90% of the macrophages in afferent lymph by Sephadex G-10 columns did not significantly alter the specific activity of labelled lymphocytes in the afferent lymph. Specific activities did not change significantly when afferent lymph was depleted of surface immunoglobulin-positive cells by nylon wool columns. These data are consistent with the conclusion that these patterns are due to small, recirculating, T lymphocytes. Using a double-label approach attempts are being made to further investigate lymphocyte traffic and retention in these various compartments.

Acknowledgment

This work was supported by a grant from MRC (Canada).

References

1. Pearson, C. M. and Chang, T.-Y. (1978). The contribution of adjuvant arthritis to the recognition of anti-rheumatic drugs. In Dumonde, D. C. and Jasani, M. K. (eds.) *The Recognition of Anti-Rheumatic Drugs*. (Lancaster: MTP Press)
2. Hay, J. B., Lachmann, P. J. and Trnka, Z. (1973). Kinetic studies on the production of sensitized lymphocytes and soluble lymph node factors. In Daguillard, F. (ed.) *Proc. Seventh Leucocyte Culture Conference.* (New York: Academic Press)
3. Hay, J. B. (1979). Delayed (cellular) hypersensitivity. In Movat, H. Z. (ed.) *Inflammation, Immunity and Hypersensitivity. Molecular and Cellular Mechanisms*, 2nd Edn (Hagerstown, Maryland: Harper and Row)
4. Gowans, J. L. (1959). The recirculation of lymphocytes from blood to lymph in the rat. *J. Physiol. (London)*, **146**, 54
5. Hall, J. G. and Morris, B. (1962). The output of cells in lymph from the popliteal node of sheep. *QJ Exp. Physiol.*, **47**, 360
6. Cahill, R. N. P., Hay, J. B., Frost, H. and Trnka, Z. (1974). Changes in lymphocyte circulation after administration of antigen. *Haematologia*, **8**, 321
7. Hay, J. B., Hobbs, B. B., Johnston, M. G. and Movat, H. Z. (1977). The role of hyperemia in cellular hypersensitivity reactions. *Int. Arch. Allergy Appl. Immunol.*, **55**, 324
8. Pedersen, N. C. and Morris, B. (1970). The role of the lymphatic system in the rejection of homografts: a study of lymph from renal transplants. *J. Exp. Med.*, **131**, 936
9. Hay, J. B., Lachmann, P. J. and Trnka, Z. (1973). The appearance of migration inhibition factor and a mitogen in lymph draining tuberculin reactions. *Eur. J. Immunol.*, **3**, 127
10. Smith, J. B., McIntosh, G. H. and Morris, B. (1970). The migration of cells through chronically inflamed tissues. *J. Pathol. Bacteriol.*, **100**, 21
11. Issekutz, T. B., Chin, W. G. and Hay, J. B. (1980). Lymphocyte traffic through granulomas: differences in the recovery of Indium-111 labelled lymphocytes in afferent and efferent lymph. *Cell. Immunol.*, **54**, 79
12. Lascelles, A. K. and Morris, B. (1961). Surgical techniques for the collection of lymph from unanaesthetized sheep. *QJ Exp. Physiol.*, **46**, 199
13. Issekutz, T. B., Chin, W. G. and Hay, J. B. (1980). Measurement of lymphocyte traffic with Indium-111. *Clin. Exp. Immunol.*, **39**, 215
14. Smith, J. B., McIntosh, G. H. and Morris, B. (1970). The traffic of cells through tissues: a study of peripheral lymph in sheep. *J. Anat.*, **107**, 87
15. Engeset, A., Hager, B., Nesheim, A. and Kilbenstnedt, A. (1973). Studies on human peripheral lymph. I. Sampling method. *Lymphology*, **6**, 1
16. Lafferty, K. J., Walter, K. Z., Scollay, R. G. and Killby, V. A. A. (1972). Allogeneic interactions provide evidence for a novel class of immunological reactivity. *Transplant. Rev.*, **12**, 198
17. Scollay, R. G. and Lafferty, K. J. (1975). Differences in the graft-versus-host reactivity of cells migrating through nonlymphoid tissue or lymph nodes. *Transplantation*, **19**, 170
18. Hay, J. B. and Morris, B. (1976). Generation and selection of specific reactive cells by antigen. *Br. Med. Bull.*, **32**, 135
19. Miller, H. R. P. and Adams, E. P. (1977). Reassortment of lymphocytes in lymph from normal and allografted sheep. *Am. J. Pathol.*, **87**, 59
20. Godal, T. and Engeset, A. (1978). A preliminary note on the composition of lymphocytes in human peripheral lymph. *Lymphology*, **11**, 208

21. Reynolds, J. (1980). Gut-associated lymphoid tissues in lambs before and after birth. In Trnka, Z. and Cahill, R. N. P. (eds.) *Essays on the Anatomy and Physiology of Lymphoid Tissues. Monographs in Allergy*, 16, p. 187 (Basel: Karger)

22. Hall, J. G. and Morris, B. (1965). The origin of the cells in the efferent lymph from a single lymph node. *J. Exp. Med.*, **121**, 901

23. Hay, J. B. and Hobbs, B. B. (1977). The flow of blood to lymph nodes and its relation to lymphocyte traffic and the immune response. *J. Exp. Med.*, **145**, 31

24. Hall, J. G. and Morris, B. (1964). Effect of X-irradiation of the popliteal lymph node on its output of lymphocytes and immunological responsiveness. *Lancet*, **1**, 1077

25. Cahill, R. N. P., Frost, H. and Trnka, Z. (1976). The effects of antigen on the migration of recirculating lymphocytes through single lymph nodes. *J. Exp. Med.*, **143**, 870

26. McCullagh, P. (1980). Unresponsiveness of recirculating lymphocytes after antigenic challenge. In Trnka, Z. and Cahill, R. N. P. (eds.) *Essays on the Anatomy and Physiology of Lymphoid Tissues. Monographs in Allergy*, 16, p. 143. (Basel: Karger)

27. Sprent, J. (1980). Antigen-induced selective sequestration of T lymphocytes: role of the major histocompatibility complex. In Trnka, Z. and Cahill, R. N. P. (eds.) *Essays on the Anatomy and Physiology of Lymphoid Tissues. Monographs in Allergy*, 16, p. 187. (Basel: Karger)

28. Kelly, R. H. and Harvey, V. S. (1978). Lymphocyte migratory pathways in adjuvant disease. I. Distribution of ^{51}Cr-labeled thoracic duct lymph-borne cells. *Am. J. Pathol.*, **91**, 345

29. Chin, W. G. and Hay, J. B. (1980). A comparison of lymphocyte migration through intestinal lymph nodes, subcutaneous lymph nodes and chronic inflammatory sites of sheep. *Gastroenterology*, **79**, 1231

30. Morris, B. (1956). The hepatic and intestinal contributions to the thoracic duct lymph. *QJ Exp. Physiol.*, **41**, 318

31. Trnka, Z. and Cahill, R. N. P. (1980). Aspects of the immune response in single lymph nodes. In Trnka, Z. and Cahill, R. N. P. (eds.) *Essays on the Anatomy and Physiology of Lymphoid Tissues. Monographs in Allergy*, 16, p. 245 (Basel: Karger)

32. Dumonde, D. C. (1978). The rheumatological significance of lymphokines. In Dumonde, D. C. and Jasani, M. K. (eds.) *The Recognition of Anti-Rheumatic Drugs.* (Lancaster: MTP Press)

33. Vadas, P., Wasi, S., Movat, H. Z. and Hay, J. B. (1979). A novel vasoactive product and plasminogen activator from afferent lymph cells draining chronic inflammatory lesions. *Proc. Soc. Exp. Biol. Med.*, **161**, 82

34. Burrowes, C. E., Wasi, S., Chin, G. W., Hay, J. B. and Movat, H. Z. (1981). Tissue thromboplastin-like activity from sheep alveolar macrophages. (Abstract submitted)

35. Vadas, P. and Hay, J. B. (1980). The secretion of a hyperemia-inducing moiety by mitogen or glycogen-stimulated mononuclear inflammatory cells of sheep and rabbit. *Int. Arch. Allergy Appl. Immunol.*, **62**, 142

36. Johnston, M. G. (1979). The distribution and significance of prostaglandins in lymph draining inflammatory lesions. *PhD Thesis*, University of Toronto

37. Johnston, M. G., Hay, J. B. and Movat, H. Z. (1979). Kinetics of prostaglandin production in lymph draining various inflammatory lesions. *Am. J. Pathol.*, **95**, 225

38. Chin, W. G., Issekutz, T. B. and Hay, J. B. (1981). Characterization of migratory cells from lymph. (Abstract submitted)

3
Autoantibodies in the Rheumatic Diseases

I. D. GRIFFITHS

INTRODUCTION

The detection of circulating non-organ-specific 'autoantibodies' in the connective tissue disorders has permitted a more rational classification of these groups of often confusing and overlapping disorders. At present no single autoantibody can be considered to be pathognomonic for a clinical disorder; and knowing how the clinical spectrum of these disorders may merge into one another, it is unlikely that these diseases will ever be defined satisfactorily on serological grounds alone. However, the detection of certain autoantibodies is undoubtedly useful at a purely diagnostic level, particularly in the early stages of disease, and as the quantitation of these antibodies has become increasingly reproducible their levels have often been shown to have both prognostic significance and value in monitoring response to therapy.

The demonstration that some of these autoantibodies may induce tissue damage, usually by virtue of forming immune complexes with subsequent complement activation either in circulation (e.g. DNA–anti-DNA) or synovial fluid (e.g. RF–IgG), lends further support to their importance. Other autoantibodies (e.g. lymphocytotoxic antibodies) appear to have dual activities, reacting with cell surface antigens on a variety of organs and also exerting an effect on the immunoregulation system by virtue of their anti-T cell activity. Yet other autoantibodies, while having clinical diagnostic value, have not as yet been shown to have any pathogenic activity (e.g. various components of extractable nuclear antigen).

Assuming the importance of these antibodies in inducing tissue damage, then what is the impetus to their synthesis? It cannot be argued that antibody production is stimulated by exposure of otherwise hidden antigens, as this is

41

patently not the situation with rheumatoid factor (RF), and nuclear antigens are repetitively released into the circulation following tissue injury. Moreover, low titres of many of these antibodies are present in normal subjects.

It seems increasingly probable that external factors, either in the form of bacterial or viral pathogens or physicochemical agents, are important. In some disorders the link has been demonstrated: RF production in subacute bacterial endocarditis and industrial lung disease, antinuclear antibody production in procainamide and hydrallazine-treated patients. However, in these situations the antibody production usually ceases when the inciting agents are removed. The role of viral agents has still to be established in human disease but they remain attractive contenders, either by modifying the autologous antigens to render them immunogenic or by inducing non-specific stimulation of B cells or loss of immunoregulation mechanisms. Other factors, though, have to be considered and these include possible immunogenetic predisposition and the effect of sex hormones. Probably several of these factors are working in concert in the development of a disease as reflected in the induction of a lupus-like illness following hydrallazine therapy which has been shown to depend upon the patient being female, of slow acetylator status and usually possession of HLA DrW4[1].

RHEUMATOID FACTORS

Introduction

The detection and quantitation of circulating antibody which is capable of agglutinating cells or particles coated with γ-globulin remains an important factor in both diagnosing and monitoring the course of patients with rheumatoid arthritis. Although the recognition of a serum factor capable of agglutinating sensitized sheep red cells, coated with rabbit anti-sheep immunoglobulin, occurred as early as 1922[2], it was not until 1940 that Waaler[3] drew attention to its association with rheumatoid arthritis. Rose and colleagues rediscovered and reconfirmed Waaler's findings in 1958[4] and the sheep cell agglutination test which bears their names still remains a diagnostic test for recognition of rheumatoid factor (RF) in many laboratories. Low titres of antibody are present in many normals and quantitation of the antibody is therefore necessary. To avoid the possibility that heterophile antibodies directed against the sheep red blood cells may also be detected and give rise to 'false-positive results', it is practice to react the test sera in parallel with both coated and uncoated sheep cells, and express the result as the difference in titres between the two assays; the differential agglutination titre (DAT). Alternatively, the test serum may be incubated with untreated sheep red blood cells to remove heterophile antibodies prior to testing with coated red blood cells (SCAT)[5].

A popular modification of the agglutination reaction is the latex test, in which polystyrene latex particles are coated with heat-denatured human Cohn fraction II γ-globulin[6], and a modification of this method is the bentonite flocculation test, where bentonite silicate particles are coated with human γ-globulin[7].

Assays using human red blood cells—either group O Rh-negative coated with rabbit/anti-human red blood cell antibody[8] or group O Rh-positive cells coated with incomplete human anti-CD antibody[9]—have not been widely adopted for routine clinical screenings, although they have the theoretical advantage of not detecting heterophile antibodies in test sera.

IMMUNOLOGY

Rheumatoid factor predominantly reacts with the Fc region of IgG and the antigenic sites appear to reside mainly in the CH_2 or CH_3 regions of the Fc fragment[10]; it is therefore unique as an antibody, in that it may self-aggregate, and even IgG RF may form large complexes, without the need of repeating antigenic sequences on the same molecule. This is particularly true if the concentration of non-RF IgG is low, as in synovial fluid, and hence favouring IgG RF–IgG RF complex formation. At one period it was felt the antigenic sites on the IgG molecule were exposed only when a structural alteration occurred, e.g. during heat-denaturation or on combining with an antigen[11, 12]. However, evidence now exists that the antibody-combining site on rheumatoid factor has a similar affinity for both monomeric and aggregated IgG[13, 14]. The overall avidity of rheumatoid factor for aggregated γ-globulin would be expected to be higher than for monomeric IgG because of the increased antigenic sites available, which may explain the observation that RF will only precipitate *in vitro* with aggregated γ-globulin[15]. The finding of 22S complexes in rheumatoid sera which may be dissociated into IgM RF and monomeric IgG[16] suggests that *in vivo* complexes of RF and monomeric IgG may be formed.

The observation that RF activity against Group O Rh-positive cells coated with incomplete anti-Rh CD sera could only be inhibited by certain human IgG preparations led to the recognition of the various Gm antigens on the Fc fragment[17], which have subsequently been shown to be genetically determined allotypes[18]. However, considerable heterogeneity in terms of Gm reactivity has been demonstrated in the rheumatoid factors obtained from individual patients[19–22] and also reactivity with Gm allotypes not possessed by the individual[23]. The recent interest in a possible immunogenetic predisposition to rheumatoid arthritis, as reflected by the increased incidence of HLA DrW4 B cell alloantigens[24] in patients with rheumatoid arthritis suggests that further studies on Gm allotyping of RA patients may be worthwhile, particularly as the loci for these antigens are also carried on chromosome 6[25]. The patterns of inheritance of another autoimmune disorder, myasthenia gravis, has been shown to be linked to a specific Gm haplotype[26].

Rheumatoid factor activity has been detected in all the major classes of immunoglobulin (IgG, A and M)[27,28]. However, IgM appears to be the predominant immunoglobulin class of RF activity in serum and is preferentially detected in agglutination reactions because of its pentavalent binding sites. In certain patients, however, the RF activity may be 'hidden' by virtue of its complexing with circulating γ-globulin. In this situation acid dissociation of the IgM serum fraction may then reveal IgM RF[29,30]. This phenomenon has been clearly demonstrated in the seronegative nodular rheumatoid[31] and in juvenile chronic polyarthritis[32,33]. Assays for other classes of rheumatoid factor have, until recently, been too laborious for routine clinical use, depending on the elution of RF from columns (e.g. cyanogen bromide-activated Sepharose) to which some form of IgG is linked as an immunoadsorbent[34]. The immunoglobulins eluted from the columns are assumed to have rheumatoid factor activity and can be quantitated in radial immunodiffusion assays. A variation of this method, depending upon the inherent 'stickiness' of aggregated γ-globulin for polystyrene tubes, has recently been introduced and may prove more suitable for routine use[35]. RF will adhere to the γ-globulin and may be detected and quantitated by subsequent incubation with radiolabelled anti-human Ig directed at the various classes of immunoglobulin. Close correlation was found between the technique using anti-IgM and the sheep cell agglutination titre, supporting the validity of the method, and in this group of patients IgG RF is also nearly always present. The majority of sera from patients classified as seronegative RA were found to have elevated IgG RF. However, with the exception of juvenile chronic polyarthritis, IgG RF has not been found in the sera of patients with other seronegative polyarthritides (e.g. psoriasis, Reiter's, ankylosing spondylitis, inflammatory bowel disease)[36]. To avoid the possibility that IgM RF may bind the Fc fragment of the second radiolabelled antibody, radiolabelled Fab^2 fragments with class specificity have been used[37].

Although IgM RF is detectable in the synovial fluid of patients with seropositive RA and in some synovial fluids from the seronegative RA group, it seems probable that IgG RF in synovial fluid may have a more important role in the formation of intra-articular complexes as judged by ultracentrifugation analysis[38,39]. Considerable heterogeneity of IgG complex sizes in synovial fluids exists, the smaller (7S to 14S) complexes inhibiting *in vitro* IgM RF agglutination, the intermediate (15S to 16S) precipitating with *in vitro* IgM RF and larger (> 16S) complexes precipitating with C1q[40,41]. Dissociation of the complexes reveals IgG RF which is selectively concentrated in comparison with IgG RF in the whole synovial fluid[42]. IgG–anti-IgG complexes detected in serum of patients are of lower molecular size and exist as dimers or trimers, whereas the IgG–anti-IgG complexes eluted from rheumatoid synovium are generally of higher molecular size (22S)[43]. This may be related to antigen–

antibody ratios that exist (low in serum, favouring small complexes; high in synovial tissue, favouring large lattice complexes) or the relative avidities of locally formed versus circulating rheumatoid factors. The recent demonstration of macrophage-like cells in synovial membranes of RA patients with receptors for IgG and C3 strongly suggests the presence of a synovial mechanism for reacting with complexes[44]. In addition, self-associating IgG RF has been shown to be the major response of plasma cells to stimulation in rheumatoid inflammatory tissue[45].

There is now little doubt that RF is capable of activating the complement system via the classical pathway[46, 47]. This has been demonstrated for purified IgM RF and has shown to involve the entire classical complement pathway and produce lysis of sensitized sheep red blood cells[48]. The subsequent development of a haemolytic assay for RFs has also provided a means of developing a plaque-forming assay, where sensitized sheep red blood cells are mixed in an agarose gel, to investigate RF synthesis by lymphocytes from RA patients[49, 50]. Using this assay it has been shown that the percentage of RF-synthesizing lymphocytes is consistently higher in both bone marrow and synovial fluid than in peripheral blood. Inhibition studies with a plaque-forming assay system have shown human monomeric IgG to be a more effective inhibitor of lysis than rabbit IgG and the apparent affinity of locally synthesized RF for IgG is considerably greater than that of RA detected in serum[51]. The relative importance of the locally synthesized high-avidity RF, which presumably complexes with available IgG and may then be rapidly cleared by the reticuloendothelial system, compared with the circulating low-avidity RF, is not known but, as with the interpretation of other autoantibody phenomenon (e.g. DNA Ab) demonstrates the pitfalls of extrapolating back from the biological activity of circulating unbound antibody.

Sites of synthesis of RF have been studied using immunofluorescent techniques, tissue culture, and the plaque-forming assay, and have shown synthesis in peripheral blood, bone marrow, synovium, synovial fluid, lymph nodes, and subcutaneous nodules. The production of immunoglobulins by rheumatoid synovial tissue has been shown to be predominantly IgG (80%) with IgM and IgA representing a further 10% each[52]. Initially, only 1% of the total immunoglobulin production could be shown to have RF activity. However, the assays were directed towards detecting IgM RF and the more recent recognition of the importance of IgG RF, and that locally synthesized RF is of high avidity and therefore forms complexes readily, probably resulted in an underestimation of total RF synthesis. Rheumatoid synovium in tissue culture is unlike most other antibody-forming tissue, in that it appears to be immortalized and continues to produce RF even after several years. These synovial B cell lines continue to synthesize predominantly IgG, and 74% of this has been shown to have IgG RF activity[53]. Although these cell lines show evidence of Epstein–Barr virus infection, it has been shown that lymphocytes from six out of ten RA patients, compared to two out of ten normal subjects, developed into permanent B cell lines without *in vitro* infection with EB virus[54].

The stimulus for the production of RFs is unknown. They are certainly not limited just to rheumatoid arthritis (RA), and have been detected in various chronic infectious states, including tuberculosis, syphilis, leprosy and sub-acute bacterial endocarditis, as well as the other chronic inflammatory diseases of connective tissue: Sjögren's syndrome, systemic lupus erythematosus and scleroderma. The occurrence of RF in subacute bacterial endocarditis (SBE) has attracted much attention and certain interesting contrasts have emerged when comparing it to the RFs present in RA. The SBE RF activity peaks after the detection of maximum levels of circulating complexes, suggesting that immune complexes may, in themselves, induce the production of RF[55]. However, in SBE the RF light chain composition was similar to that in total IgG and IgM whereas the RF detected in RA is more homogeneous, with a greater percentage of κ-light chains present than in the total Ig[56]. Finally, and probably most significant, the RF activity in SBE disappears after successful treatment with antibiotics.

The clinical recognition that polyarthritis may follow a variety of viral illnesses and, particularly in rubella, may have a pattern and chronicity identical with RA[57], has prompted study into a variety of viral inducers of RF synthesis. So far, the ubiquitous Epstein–Barr virus (EBV), which has been demonstrated to be a non-specific B cell mitogen[58], is the most clearly implicated inducer of RF activity *in vitro*. *In vitro*, EBV infection has been shown to be capable of stimulating IgM synthesis in both normal and rheumatoid lymphocytes, and about 10% of the IgM obtained from normal lymphocytes has RF activity and 20% when obtained from rheumatoid lymphocytes[59].

It has been recognized for many years that patients with RA, as well as possessing RF, also may have detectable circulating antinuclear antibodies, the incidence of these antibodies depending upon substrates and methods used. More recently, it has become apparent that RFs and antinuclear antibodies may cross-react[60]. A recent study has shown that half of the isolated RFs from patients with RA possessed antinuclear antibody activity and this was shown not to be dependent upon the formation of RF–ANA complexes as acid-disassociated IgM RF still had antinuclear antibody activity[61]. Whether this cross-reactivity is the result of a structural component common to both IgG and certain nuclear antigens or a reflection of multi-specificity of certain antibodies remained uncertain, but further studies have shown that isolated monoclonal IgM RF reacts with both IgG and DNA nucleoprotein, the affinity for IgG being slightly greater than for DNA nucleoprotein[62]. These findings, therefore, suggest that nucleic antigens may act as the immunogens for the development of RFs.

The recognition that patients with RA have a higher incidence of HLA D4 and DrW4 suggests an immunogenetic predisposition to the disease[24, 63] and a further study has shown that, within groups clinically defined as RA, an increased incidence of DrW4 is detectable only in the group with circulating RF[64].

ANTINUCLEAR ANTIBODIES

Introduction

The detection of the *in vitro* LE cell phenomenon in 1948[65] was the first indication of circulating factors with activity directed against nuclear antigens. The LE cell test is now known to be dependent upon complement-fixing antinuclear antibodies[66, 67] and the presence of nuclear material from *in vitro* disrupted white cells. Its close clinical association with systemic lupus erythematosus (SLE), which until then had been a bewildering array of multisystem disorders with a uniformly poor prognosis, allowed a unifying concept of SLE to develop as an autoimmune disorder, characterized by the presence of antinuclear antibodies which may have some bearing on the aetiology and pathogenesis of the disease. With the development of laboratory tests for LE cells the existence of mild forms of SLE with a good prognosis were recognized; the range of clinical features recognized became increasingly varied; it was also appreciated that the LE phenomenon was not confined to SLE, and certain clinically classifiable SLE patients did not demonstrate the LE cell phenomenon.

Immunology

The laborious and qualitative LE cell test has been replaced by semiquantitative immunofluorescent tests for antinuclear factors or antibodies[68, 69]. The incidence of antinuclear antibodies in various diseases was found to be dependent upon the substrate used and the pattern of fluorescence seen within the nuclei varied with the substrate, pointing towards the need for standardization within the assays[70, 71]. However, the observation that different sera, even when using the same substrate (most commonly rat liver), could produce varying immunofluorescent patterns suggested heterogeneity of ANA specificity[72]. The homogeneous staining pattern seen most commonly in SLE correlates best with antibodies to deoxynucleoprotein and is probably responsible for the LE cell phenomena[73]. The membranous, or rim, or shaggy peripheral staining occasionally seen appears to correlate with DNA antibodies[74], whereas the speckled staining pattern is usually due to antibodies to one or other component of extractable nuclear antigen[75] and the nucleolar pattern appears to be due to antibodies to 7S RNA[76] and is often seen in scleroderma sera[77]. However, the interpretation of nuclear fluorescent patterns is complicated by the observation that the pattern may vary with serum dilution and undue significance cannot be placed on the immunofluorescent patterns. Because of these inherent difficulties in interpreting immunofluorescent ANA tests it is wisest at this stage to consider them as relatively sensitive and invaluable assays for detecting the presence of antinuclear antibodies, but the presence of a positive reaction should prompt further investigation and classification of the antibody specificity using more purified and chemically defined nuclear antigens.

Some of these antigens are well defined and detection of circulating antibodies directed against them are clinically valuable (e.g. DNA). Others, while being well defined, have not, as yet, provided much additional information in a clinical context (e.g. histone). Others are still extremely heterogeneous (e.g. extractable nuclear antigen) but appear to be clinically valuable, while yet others are still at an early stage of assessment (e.g. RA nuclear antigen).

The variety of cellular, nuclear and cytoplasmic antigens to which antibodies have been detected continues to increase with amazing pace. Detailed studies on the specificity of these antibodies in terms of diagnostic precision is often lacking, as is the variation in antibody levels during the relapses and remissions of the disease, and the demonstration that complexes of the more recently described antigen–antibody systems may be detectable in either sera or tissue of patients. However, the detection of these varied autoantibodies in the connective tissue disorders suggests the heterogeneity of B cell activation.

As many of the methods available for detecting these antigen–antibody reactions are relatively insensitive it is not possible at this stage to determine whether these antibodies are detectable in low concentrations in normal sera, but the emerging evidence from more sensitive radioimmune assays with DNA suggest that low titres of antibody may be present in normal subjects and the development of a disease state may be more a reflection of a quantitative rather than absolute 'autoantibody' response[78].

ANTIBODIES TO DNA

Introduction

Circulating antibodies to DNA in patients with SLE were recognized virtually simultaneously in three centres in 1957[79–81]. Soon after this it was appreciated that these antibodies, as well as offering diagnostic specificity, were also of prognostic value in SLE, especially if viewed in context of the serum complement values[82, 83], elevated DNA binding and hypocomplementaemia being associated with an exacerbation of disease activity. Studies have, however, shown that the presence of high titres of DNA antibody are by no means inevitably associated with disease flares[84], and both DNA binding and complement values may be normal during CNS manifestations of SLE[85].

Immunology

Assays for the detection of DNA antibodies have become more sensitive since the original descriptions, when precipitation in agar gel using a double-diffusion technique was most commonly employed. Currently, the most favoured assays are:

(1) Immunoelectroprecipitation[86], which depends upon the negatively charged DNA antigen migrating towards the positively charged γ-globulin when an electric field is placed across an agarose gel. While this assay has the advantage of simplicity, it appears to lack some sensitivity and is only semiquantitative.

(2) Complement fixation[87] which, as well as being quantitative, also provides information about the biological activity of the DNA binding antibodies, but is time-consuming and may suffer the disadvantage of failing to detect any non-complement-fixing DNA antibodies.

(3) Radioimmunoassays, which have become technically simple yet sensitive and are in common use at present. The assay depends upon using a radiolabelled DNA preparation which may be externally (in vitro) labelled with ^{3}H using either actinomycin D or dimethyl sulphate[88] or with ^{125}I using thallium chloride[89]. Alternatively it may be internally labelled (in vivo) by the addition of radiolabelled nucleotide ([^{14}C]thymidine[90]) or nucleotide analogue ([^{125}I]iodeodeoxyuridine[91]) to the incubation media of growing cells. Despite the increased technical problems of in vivo labelling systems, the quality and homogeneity of radiolabelled DNA appears better, in that less single-stranded breaks occur and less single-stranded regions are radiolabelled. The separation of the radiolabelled DNA bound to DNA antibody from unbound radiolabelled DNA is usually achieved by the Farr[92, 93] method, which depends upon the observation that DNA–DNA antibody complexes are precipitated in half-saturated ammonium sulphate whereas free DNA remains in solution. Although such an assay has the advantage of detecting primary antigen–antibody binding[94], it is not a functional assay of DNA antibody and is open to criticism that low-avidity DNA antibody may be dissociated from its antigen in the high salt concentration used in the assay[95]. In practice, however, the results obtained using either half-saturated ammonium sulphate or second antibody to separate free from antibody-bound DNA are similar[96, 97].

Much consideration has been given to the state of the DNA antigen and whether it exists in a native double-stranded (ds) form or denatured single-stranded (ss) form. Native DNA can be converted to ss DNA either by boiling and rapid cooling or treatment with alkali. However, it is extremely difficult to obtain either ds or ss DNA in a pure form because ds DNA often develops breaks in the molecule, usually towards the ends of the chain[98] and ss DNA readily reforms into a double helix unless sonicated. Clinically, however, antibodies to ds DNA appear to offer the greatest specificity for SLE and a robust yet homogeneous ds DNA antigen is therefore required. Circular ds DNA extracted from PM_2 bacteriophages[99] appears an attractive contender because of its stability and lack of ss regions, but comparative clinical studies have not, as yet, shown that it offers greater specificity when compared with conventional internally labelled DNA antigens from other sources[100].

Different sources of DNA may show minor variations in reaction kinetics, but of greater importance is the molecular weight of the DNA, and it has been shown that the percentage binding of sera is linearly dependent on the molecular weight of DNA up to 10^7 Daltons[101]. The minimal size of the DNA antigen required for the formation of an antigen–antibody complex is variable, again reflecting the heterogeneity of DNA antibodies, some sera requiring as few as 20 base pairs on the DNA antigen while others required more than 180 base pairs[102].

These observations, coupled to inherent susceptibility of the DNA binding assay to variations in hydrogen ion content, molarity, temperature, incubation periods and age of antigen[103], all suggest the need for increased standardization of the assay if meaningful sequential studies and interlaboratory studies are to be performed. The incorporation of internal standard reference sera to the assay and expression of results in relationship to the primary standards goes some way to achieving this reproducibility[104].

While antibodies to ds DNA, particularly when present in high concentration, continue to provide the greatest specificity for the diagnosis of SLE, they are detectable, usually, in lower titre and lower frequency in other conditions, such as discoid lupus, Sjögren's syndrome, chronic active hepatitis[104] and occasionally RA[105]. Undue concentration on the quantitative aspect of DNA binding may, however, divert attention from other characteristics of the antibody which are of equal importance in determining the pattern of organ involvement; for example, immunoglobulin class of antibody and avidity of binding. DNA binding usually resides predominantly in the IgG fraction, but occasionally is seen mainly in the IgM component and then appears to be associated with low incidence of renal involvement[96, 106]. A switch from IgM to IgG DNA antibody production has also been observed in sequential studies of some lupus patients[107]. The observation that low-avidity circulating DNA antibody in NZB/W mice was associated with increased renal involvement[108] prompted studies on DNA antibody avidity in man and its relationship to end disease, with conflicting results[109, 110]. However, the finding that avidity of circulating DNA antibody in renal lupus patients was low but the avidity of DNA antibody obtained from renal elutes in the same patients was high[111] points strongly to the pitfalls of extrapolating serological findings to tissue pathology. The recent observation that complement-fixing DNA antibody and total DNA antibody, as measured using a *Crithidia luciliae* immunofluorescent assay, may vary independently of each other[112], and that complement-fixing DNA correlated best with renal involvement, again suggests the importance of qualitative as well as quantitative aspects of DNA antibody.

The hypothesis that DNA–DNA antibody complexes of varying composition, molecular size and biological activity circulate in the sera of patients with SLE is supported by the observation that both antibody and antigen are selectively enriched in the cryoprecipitates of lupus sera[113] and that DNA-binding activity may be enhanced by DNAse digestion of sera[114]. Evidence has been provided, however, that DNA may be selectively bound to glomerular basement membrane and local factors may, therefore, be of importance in trapping either antigen or antigen–antibody complexes[115]. An alternative explanation for the persistence of circulating immune complexes is a defect in clearance by the reticuloendothelial system, and experimental evidence for such an abnormality exists in several disorders, including SLE and primary biliary cirrhosis. Whether this is a primary abnormality or secondary to chronic immune complex load remains to be established.

ANTIBODIES TO RNA

Antibodies to RNA have been detected in the sera of up to 50% of lupus patients; the incidence depending on the sensitivity of the assay system employed[116, 117]. The description of antibodies to ds RNA which is not a constituent of mammalian cells and which could not be inhibited by prior incubation of sera with ss RNA raised the possibility that these antibodies were directed at viral RNA. The antibodies also showed a stronger reaction with ds RNA extracted from viruses[117]. However, some cross-reactivity of these antibodies with ss RNA and ss DNA has been shown subsequently[118, 119] and ds RNA has also been detected in normal mammalian liver[120]. Antibodies to ds RNA have also been detected in RA sera, in varying incidence[121]. Unlike antibodies to DNA, RNA antibodies appear to be most commonly of the IgM class[122].

One study showed the presence of antibodies to ss RNA in all patients with scleroderma and 50% of SLE sera. These antibodies appeared to be specific for the uracil base, which is not present in DNA[123].

ANTIBODIES TO EXTRACTABLE NUCLEAR ANTIGENS (ENA)

Introduction

Initially, it was observed that antibodies could be detected in the sera of patients with a variety of connective tissue disorders which reacted with saline extracts of calf thymus cell nuclei and that these sera commonly showed a speckled antinuclear antibody fluorescence[124, 125]. It soon became apparent that several antigens were present in these crude saline extracts. Some of these could be identified by virtue of their sensitivity to temperature changes or ability to be digested by RNAse or trypsin. Subsequently, other antigens have been identified as a result of Ouchterlony double-diffusion experiments which have allowed the identification of precipitin lines which show identity with lines obtained from reference sera.

At present, assay systems for detecting these antibody–antigen reactions are limited because of the difficulty in separating the antigens into purer components. Most favoured assays are precipitation in gel, either by immuno-electrophoresis[126] or double-diffusion[127], and haemagglutination[124] assays. In practice, the assay systems provide similar results but the RNP component of ENA may not always adhere to tanned red cells[128]. Often antibodies can be detected to several of the ENA constituents in any one serum[129].

One study has shown that the addition of ENA reduces anti-DNA–DNA haemagglutination *in vitro* and appears to lessen the severity of nephritis in the NZB/W mouse, suggesting a possible protective role in the prevention of DNA–anti-DNA immune complex disease[130]. This may be the result of DNA–ENA interaction which has been demonstrated *in vitro*[131].

IMMUNOLOGY

Ribonucleoprotein (RNP)

Antibodies to this component, which is sensitive to both RNAse and trypsin digestion, were identified in the haemagglutination assay (where the titre falls after enzyme digestion[124]) and the Ouchterlony assay[132]. In the latter assay the antigen was initially termed Mo but it appears increasingly probable that the same antigen–antibody system was being detected in both assays[133].

The importance of antibodies to RNP is the fact that they appear to be associated clinically with either a milder form of non-renal SLE or a possibly distinct clinical entity overlapping SLE, scleroderma and polymyositis, termed mixed connective tissue disease (MCTD)[134], which has a good prognosis and is responsive to steroid therapy. In the latter condition, high titres of RNP antibodies are a prerequisite for the diagnosis. Although debate continues about the clinical identity of MCTD[135,136], the detection of antibodies to RNP in SLE does appear to be clinically valuable in the identification of patients who have a lower incidence of renal involvement, but the antibodies are also detectable in a variety of other rheumatological disorders[137].

Sm

Antibodies to this thermolabile glycoprotein constituent of ENA were initially detected in precipitin reactions[127]. The antibodies are predominantly detected in sera of SLE patients[127,136]. These antibodies appear to be associated with a higher incidence of Raynaud's phenomenon and a lower incidence of renal and CNS disease[138]. As with many of these antibodies, they are not, however, confined to any one diagnostic group and may be present in other disorders, such as scleroderma, RA[139], and primary biliary cirrhosis[140].

PM₁

An apparently distinct antibody–antigen precipitin line in double-diffusion gel was detected against saline calf thymus extract in 61% of patients with polymyositis and not observed in any control sera[141]. The antigen is resistant to both RNAse, DNAse and trypsin digestion but destroyed by incubation at 56 °C. Antibodies to this antigen were also detected in the scleroderma–polymyositis overlap group.

ANTIBODIES TO SS ANTIGEN

These antigens were originally extracted from Wil_2 human B lymphocyte lines. They were of cellular origin, soluble in saline, resistant to both DNAse and RNAse digestion but sensitive to trypsin digestion. On the basis of Ouchterlony double-diffusion experiments with sera from various sources, it appeared that three distinct antigens existed: SS-A, SS-B and SS-C[142]. SS-A behaved immunologically identically to a previously described cytoplasmic antigen (Ro)[143] and SS-B appeared similar to a nucleic antigen, termed Ha[144], and a cytoplasmic antigen (La)[145].

The initial studies suggested that antibodies to these antigens were restricted to patients with either the sicca complex, who possessed anti-SS-A and/or anti-SS-B or the sicca syndrome and RA, who possessed anti-SS-C[146].

Further studies, however, have detected these antibodies in patients with SLE who did not have any features of the sicca syndrome and their diagnostic specificity appears, therefore, to be limited[147]. Although their role in the pathogenesis of disease has still to be established, they do provide additional information about the wide range of autoantibodies produced in these disorders.

ANTIBODIES TO RHEUMATOID ARTHRITIS-ASSOCIATED ANTIGEN (RANA)

Antibodies to this antigen were originally described in patients with rheumatoid arthritis in 1976[148]. The antigen appears to be located predominantly in the nucleus of human B lymphocytes which have been infected with EBV and has not been found in non-EBV-infected cells[149]. It was initially extracted from Wil_2 continuous lines of B lymphocytes. The antigen is not detectable in non-human cell lines, with the exception of primates which have been infected with EBV *in vitro*. The antigen, however, does not appear to be related to the EBV, in that EBV antibodies do not react with RANA and elevated titres of RANA antibody are not detectable in patients during an EBV infection or in patients with Burkitt's lymphoma[150].

RANA is resistant to both RNAse and DNAse digestion, but sensitive to trypsin digestion. Antibodies to RANA are detectable in about 70% of RA patients and 10% of the normal population[148] and are not, therefore, an absolute marker for RA, but the nature of the antigen and the high incidence of antibodies directed against it in patients with RA does suggest that environmental viral agents may induce the expression of restricted antigens which are of non-viral origin and which can induce antibody production in certain disorders. EBV infection, however, is extremely common and serological evidence of previous infection is detectable in approximately 90% of adults and the apparent specificity of RANA antibodies for rheumatoid arthritis may, in part, reflect the insensitivity of the Ouchterlony assay for detecting antibody–antigen reactions and be a quantitative rather than qualitative difference between the RA group and normals, reflecting increased polyclonal antibody production occurring in RA patients. More sensitive immunofluorescent assays, using Raji cells as a substrate, while confirming the high incidence of RANA antibodies in seropositive and seronegative RA, still only found a 16% incidence in normals. RANA antibodies did not, however, correlate with disease activity[149].

LYMPHOCYTOTOXIC ANTIBODIES

Introduction

Cold-reacting lymphocytotoxic antibodies (LCA) occur in the majority of SLE patients[151–153] and are associated with a variety of clinical manifestations, including CNS involvement, renal and cutaneous[154] disease, spontaneous abortions[155] and lymphopenia. Like most other antibodies found in SLE, they have a heterogeneous specificity reacting with brain tissue[156], trophoblast antigens[155], chronic lymphatic leukaemic cells, i antigens of cord red blood cells[157], as well as T and B lymphocytes[158, 159].

Immunology

The accumulating evidence suggests that an alteration in T cell immunoregulation of antibody response[160, 161] is present in SLE. Lymphocytotoxic antibodies may therefore exert their influence at a more fundamental level of the immune response. It has been shown that polyclonal antibody synthesis and DNA antibody production of SLE B lymphocytes, while not being suppressed by the addition of autologous T lymphocytes, is suppressed by the addition of homologous T lymphocytes from normal individuals and these also cause a switch from predominantly IgM DNA antibody to IgG DNA antibody[161]. Further studies have demonstrated a defect in circulating T_γ (suppressor) lymphocytes in lupus[162] and the finding that IgM anti-T cell lymphocytotoxic antibody, which is detectable in the active phases of SLE, may block the conversion of ConA-induced normal T cells to T suppressor cells[163], suggests that lymphocytotoxic antibodies may, in part, be responsible for the loss of suppressor T cell function.

Studies of cell surface reactions of the lymphocytotoxic antibodies have suggested that these, in part, are linked to the HLA A, B and C major histocompatibility locus and can be partially inhibited by preincubation of the target lymphocytes with $F(ab)_2$ antisera specific to the HLA loci present[164]. Antisera to HLA Dr loci failed to inhibit cell lysis, suggesting that the Dr MHC alloantigens are not contributing to any autoimmune lymphocyte lysis. However, no preferential MHC alloantigen specificity was found either in the lupus group or in members of the families, and the observation that only 50% of the cellular lysis could be blocked by pretreatment with MHC antisera suggests that these autoantibodies are only a subset of the lymphocytotoxic antibodies. The correlation of lymphocytotoxic antibodies and antibodies to the HLA-linked B_2 microglobulin[165, 166], whose genetic locus resides on chromosome 15 (rather than 6 for the MHC loci) also suggests that the lymphocytotoxic antibodies are not necessarily reacting with the heavy-chain glycoproteins of the HLA complex, and also raises the possibility that B_2 microglobulin–lymphocytotoxic antibody complex formation may play a part in the production of circulating immune complexes.

References

1. Batchelor, J. R., Welsh, K. I., Inoco, R. M., Dollery, C. T., Hughes, G. R. V., Bernstein, R., Ryan, P., Naish, P. F., Aber, G. M., Bing, R. F. and Russel, G. I. (1980). Hydralazine induced systemic lupus erythematosus: influence of HLA DR and sex on susceptibility. *Lancet*, 1, 1107

2. Meyer, K. (1972). Veber hamagglutininvermerung und hamagglutination forderride wirkung bei nienschlichen seren. *Z. Immunitatsforsch. Exp. Ther.*, 34, 229

3. Waaler, E. (1940). On the occurrence of a factor in human serum activating the specific agglutination of sheep blood corpuscles. *Acta Pathol. Microbiol. Scand.*, 16, 172

4. Rose, H. M., Ragan, C., Pearce, E. and Lipman, M. O. (1948). Differential agglutination of normal and sensitized sheep erythrocytes by sera of patients with rheumatoid arthritis. *Proc. Soc. Exp. Biol. Med. (NY)*, 68, 1

5. Ball, J. (1950). A serum factor in Ra agglutinating sensitized sheep cells. *Lancet*, 2, 520

6. Singer, J. M. and Plotz, C. M. (1956). Latex fixation test. 1. Application to serologic diagnosis of rheumatoid arthritis. *Am. J. Med.*, 21, 888

7. Bozicevich, J., Bunim, J. J., Freund, J. and Ward, S. B. (1958). Benotite flocculation test for rheumatoid arthritis. *Proc. Soc. Exp. Biol. Med. (NY)*, 97, 180

8. Podliachon, R. L., Eyquem, A. and Jacqueline, F. (1958). Le diagnostic de la polyarthrite chronique evolutive par agglutination des globules rouge humans sensibilises. *Ann. Inst. Pasteur*, 94, 659

9. Waller, M. V. and Vaughan, J. H. (1956). Use of anti-Rh sera for demonstrating agglutination activating factor in rheumatoid arthritis. *Proc. Soc. Exp. Biol. Med. (NY)*, 92, 198

10. Natvig, J. B., Gaarder, P. L. and Turner, M. W. (1972). IgG antigens of Cγ2 and Cγ3 homology regions interacting with rheumatoid factor. *Clin. Exp. Immunol.*, 12, 177

11. Edelman, G. M., Kunkel, H. G. and Franklin, E. C. (1958). Interaction of rheumatoid factor with antigen–antibody complex and aggregated gamma globulin. *J. Exp. Med.*, 108, 105

12. Glynn, L. E., Holborow, E. J. and Johnson, G. D. (1957). The nature of the Rose–Waaler factor. *Proc. R. Soc. Med.*, **50**, 469

13. Normansell, D. E. (1971). Anti-γ-globulins in rheumatoid arthritis sera. 11. The reactivity anti-γ-globulin rheumatoid factors with altered γ-globulin. *Immunochemistry*, **8**, 593

14. Eisenberg, R. (1976). The specificity and polyvalency of binding of monoclonal rheumatoid factor. *Immunochemistry*, **13**, 358

15. Christian, C. L. (1958). Characterization of the 'reactant' (gammaglobulin factor) in the F-11 precipitation reaction and the F-11 tanned sheep cell agglutination test. *J. Exp. Med.*, **108**, 139

16. Franklin, E. C., Holman, H. R., Müller-Eberhard, H. J. and Kunkel, H. G. (1957). An unusual protein compound of high molecular weight in the serum of certain patients with rheumatoid arthritis. *J. Exp. Med.*, **105**, 425

17. Grubb, R. (1956). Agglutination of erythrocytes coated with incomplete anti-Rh by certain rheumatoid arthritis sera and some other sera. The existence of human serum groups. *Acta Pathol. Microbiol. Scand.*, **39**, 195

18. Grubb, R. and Laurell, A. B. (1956). Hereditary serological human serum groups. *Acta Pathol. Microbiol. Scand.*, **39**, 390

19. Harboe, M. and Lundevall, J. (1959). A new type of Gm system. *Acta Pathol. Microbiol. Scand.*, **45**, 357

20. Harboe, M. (1959). A new haemagglutinating substance in the Gm system, anti-Gm^b. *Acta Pathol. Microbiol. Scand.*, **47**, 191

21. Natvig, J. B. (1966). Gm(g)–A 'new' gamma globulin factor. *Nature (London)*, **211**, 318

22. Allen, J. C. and Kunkel, H. G. (1966). Hidden rheumatoid factors with specificity for native γ-globulins. *Arth. Rheum.*, **9**, 758

23. Natvig, J. B., Munthe, E. and Gaarder, P. L. (1971). Molecular specificity and possible biological significance of rheumatoid factors. In Muller, W., Herwerth, H. G. and Fehr, K. (eds.) *Rheumatoid Arthritis.* (London and New York: Academic Press)

24. Panayi, G. S., Wooley, P. H. and Batchelor, J. R. (1978). Genetic basis of rheumatoid arthritis. HLA antigens, disease manifestations and toxic reactions to drugs. *Br. Med. J.*, **2**, 1326

25. Smith, M. and Hirschhom, K. (1978). Location of the genes of human heavy chain immunoglobulin to chromosome 6. *Proc. Natl. Acad. Sci. USA*, **75**, 3367

26. Nakao, Y., Matsumato, H., Miyazaki, T., Nishitami, H., Ota, K., Fujita, T. and Tsuji, K. (1980). Gm allotypes in myasthenia gravis. *Lancet*, **1**, 677

27. Torrigiani, G. and Roitt, I. M. (1967). Antiglobulin factors in sera from patients with rheumatoid arthritis and normal subjects. *Ann. Rheum. Dis.*, **26**, 334

28. Panush, R. S., Bianco, N. E. and Schur, P. H. (1971). Serum and synovial fluid IgG, IgA and IgM antigammaglobulin in rheumatoid arthritis. *Arth. Rheum.*, **14**, 737

29. Allen, J. C. and Kunkel, H. G. (1966). Hidden rheumatoid factors with specificity for native gamma globulins. *Arth. Rheum.*, **9**, 758

30. Cracchiolo, A., Bluestone, R. and Goldberg, L. S. (1970). Hidden antiglobulins in rheumatic disorders. *Clin. Exp. Immunol.*, **7**, 651

31. Bluestone, R., Goldberg, L. S. and Cracchiolo, A. (1969). Hidden rheumatoid factors in seronegative nodular rheumatoid arthritis. *Lancet*, **2**, 878

32. Moore, T. L., Domer, R. W. and Zuckner, J. (1974). Hidden rheumatoid factors in seronegative juvenile rheumatoid arthritis. *Ann. Rheum. Dis.*, **3**, 255

33. Moore, T. L., Suckner, J., Baldassare, A. R., Weiss, T. D. and Domer, R. W. (1978). Complement fixing hidden rheumatoid factor in juvenile rheumatoid arthritis. *Arth. Rheum.*, **21**, 935

34. Torrigiani, G., Roitt, I. M., Lloyd, K. N. and Corbett, M. (1970). Elevated IgG anti-globulins in patients with seronegative RA. *Lancet*, **1**, 14

35. Hay, F. C., Nineham, L. J. and Roitt, I. M. (1975). Routine assay for detection of IgG and IgM antiglobulins in seronegative and seropositive rheumatoid arthritis. *Br. Med. J.*, **3**, 203

36. Pope, R. M. and McDuffy, S. T. (1979). IgG rheumatoid factor: relation to clinical activity in seropositive rheumatoid arthritis and absence in seronegative arthropathies. *Arth. Rheum.*, **22**, 648

37. Carson, D. A., Lawrence, S., Catalano, M. and Vaughan, J. H. (1977). Radioimmunoassay for IgG and IgM rheumatoid factors reacting with human IgG. *J. Immunol.*, **119**, 295

38. Winchester, R. J., Agnello, V. and Kunkel, H. G. (1969). The joint fluid gamma globulin complexes and their relationship to intra-articular complement diminution. *Ann. NY Acad. Sci.*, **168**, 195

39. Winchester, R. J., Agnello, V. and Kunkel, H. G. (1970). Gamma globulin complexes in synovial fluid of patients with rheumatoid arthritis. Partial characterization and relationship to lowered complement levels. *Clin. Exp. Immunol.*, **6**, 689

40. Winchester, R. J., Agnello, V. and Kunkel, H. G. (1971). Occurrence of gamma complexes in serum and synovial fluid of rheumatoid arthritis patients. Use of monoclonal rheumatoid factors as reagents for their demonstration. *J. Exp. Med.*, **134**, 2865

41. Agnello, V., Winchester, R. J. and Kunkel, H. G. (1970). Precipitin reactions of Ciq component of complement with γ-globulin and complexes in gel diffusion. *Immunology*, **119**, 909

42. Carson, D. A., Lawrence, S., Slaughter, L. and Vaughan, J. H. (1979). Immunochemical properties of anti-IgG antibodies. In Panayi, G. and Johnson, P. (eds.) *Immunopathogenesis of Rheumatoid Arthritis*, p. 51. (Chertsey, Surrey: Reed Books Ltd.)

43. Munthe, E. and Natvig, J. B. (1971). Characterization of IgG complexes in eluates from rheumatoid tissue. *Clin. Exp. Immunol.*, **8**, 249

44. Theofilopoulos, A. N., Carson, D. A., Tavassoli, M., Slovin, S. F., Speers, W. C., Jensen, F. B. and Vaughan, J. H. (1980). Evidence for the presence of receptors for C_3 and IgG Fc on human synovial cells. *Arth. Rheum.*, **23**, 1

45. Gilliland, B. C., Ford, D. K. and Mannik, M. (1978). Synthesis by an established lymphocyte cell line from a rheumatoid synovium. *Arth. Rheum.*, **21**, 330

46. Zvaifler, N. J. and Schur, P. H. (1968). Reactions of aggregated mercaptoethanol treated gamma globulin with rheumatoid factor, precipitin and complement fixation studies. *Arth. Rheum.*, **11**, 523

47. Tesar, J. T. and Schmid, F. R. (1970). Conversion of soluble immune complexes into complement fixing aggregates by IgM rheumatoid factor. *J. Immunol.*, **105**, 1206

48. Tanimoto, K., Cooper, W. R., Johnson, J. S. and Vaughan, J. H. (1975). Complement fixation by rheumatoid factor. *J. Clin. Invest.*, **55**, 437

49. Taylor-Upsahl, M. M., Abrahamsen, T. G. and Natvig, J. B. (1977). Rheumatoid factor plaque-forming cells in rheumatoid synovial tissue. *Clin. Exp. Immunol.*, **38**, 197

50. Vaughan, J. H., Chihara, T., Moone, T. L., Robbins, D. Z., Tanimoto, K., Johnson, J. and McMillan, R. (1976). Rheumatoid factor producing cells detected by direct haemolytic plaque assay. *J. Clin. Invest.*, **58**, 933

51. Robbins, D. L., Moore, T. L., Carson, D. A. and Vaughan, J. H. (1978). Relative reactivities of rheumatoid factors in serum and cells. Evidence for a selective deficiency in serum rheumatoid factor. *Arth. Rheum.*, **21**, 820

52. Smiley, J. D., Sachs, C. and Ziff, M. (1968). *In vitro* synthesis of immunoglobulin by rheumatoid synovial membrane. *J. Clin. Invest.*, **47**, 624

53. Gilliland, B. C., Ford, D. K. and Mannik, M. (1978). Synthesis by an established cell line from a rheumatoid synovium. *Arth. Rheum.*, **21**, 330

54. Carson, D. A., Lawrance, S., Slaughter, L. and Vaughan, J. H. (1979). Immunochemical properties of anti-IgG antibodies. In Panayi, G. and Johnson, P. (eds.) *Immunopathogenesis of Rheumatoid Arthritis*, p. 51 (Chertsey, Surrey: Reed Books Ltd.)

55. Carson, D. A., Bayer, A. S., Eisenberg, R. A., Lawrance, S. and Theofilopoulos, A. (1978).

IgG rheumatoid factor in subacute bacterial endocarditis: relationship to IgM rheumatoid factor and circulating immune complexes. *Clin. Exp. Immunol.*, **31**, 100

56. Carson, D. A. and Lawrance, S. (1978). Light chain heterogeneity of 19S and 7S anti-γ-globulin in rheumatoid arthritis and subacute bacterial endocarditis. *Arth. Rheum.*, **21**, 438

57. Hart, H. and Marion, B. P. (1977). Rubella virus and rheumatoid arthritis. *Ann. Rheum. Dis.*, **36**, 3

58. Rosen, A., Gergely, T., Jondal, M., Klein, G. and Britton, S. (1977). Polyclonal IgG production after Epstein–Barr virus infection of human lymphocytes *in vitro. Nature (London)*, **267**, 52

59. Slaughter, L., Carson, D. A., Jensen, F. C., Holbrook, T. L. and Vaughan, J. H. (1978). *In vitro* effects of Epstein–Barr virus on peripheral blood mononuclear cells from patients with rheumatoid arthritis and normal subjects. *J. Exp. Med.*, **148**, 1429

60. Hannestad, K. and Johannessen, A. (1976). Polyclonal human antibodies to IgG (rheumatoid factor) which cross reacts with cell nuclei. *Scand. J. Immunol.*, **5**, 541

61. Aitcheson, C. T., Peebles, C., Joslin, F. and Tan, E. M. (1980). Characteristics of antinuclear antibodies in rheumatoid arthritis. *Arth. Rheum.*, **23**, 528

62. Agnello, V., Arbetter, A., Ibanez, G., Powell, R., Tan, E. M. and Joslin, F. (1980). Evidence for a subset of rheumatoid factors that cross react with DNA histone and have distinct idiotype. *J. Exp. Med.*, **151**, 1514

63. Stastny, P. (1978). Association of B-cell alloantigen DrW4 with rheumatoid arthritis. *N. Engl. J. Med.*, **298**, 868

64. Doblong, J. H., Forre, O., Kass, E. and Thornaby, E. (1980). HLA antigens and rheumatoid arthritis. Association between HLA DrW4 positivity and IgM rheumatoid factor production. *Arth. Rheum.*, **23**, 309

65. Hargreaves, M. M., Richmond, H. and Morton, R. (1948). Presentation of two bone marrow elements: the tart cell and LE cell. *Proc. Staff Meet., Mayo Clin.*, **23**, 25

66. Hasserick, J. R. and Lewis, L. A. (1950). Blood factor in acute SLE: induction of specific antibodies against LE factor. *Blood*, **5**, 718

67. Scalettar, R., Marcus, D. M., Simonton, L. A. and Muschel, L. H. (1960). The nucleoprotein complement fixation test in the diagnosis of SLE. *N. Engl. J. Med.*, **263**, 226

68. Friou, G. J. (1957). Clinical application of lupus serum–nucleoprotein reaction using fluorescent antibody technique. *J. Clin. Invest.*, **36**, 890

69. Friou, G. J. (1964). Immunofluorescence and antinuclear antibodies. *Arth. Rheum.*, **7**, 161

70. Beck, J. S. (1961). Variations in the morophological patterns of autoimmune nuclear fluorescence. *Lancet*, **1**, 1203

71. Quismorio, F. P. and Frion, G. J. (1976). Immunological phenomena in patients with SLE. In Dubois, E. L. (ed.) *Lupus Erythematosus*, 2nd Edn., chap. 65. (University of South California Press)

72. Johnson, G. D., Chantler, S., Batty, I. and Holborrow, E. J. (1979). Use and abuse of international reference preparations in immunofluorescence. In Dumonde, E. C. and Stewart, M. W. (eds.) *Laboratory Tests in Rheumatic Diseases*, chap. 11. (Lancaster: MTP Press)

73. Bonomo, L., Tursi, A. and Dammaco, F. (1965). Characterization of antibodies producing the homogeneous and speckled fluorescence patterns of cell nuclei. *J. Lab. Clin. Med.*, **66**, 42

74. Casals, S. P., Frion, G. J. and Teague, P. O. (1963). Specific nuclear reaction pattern of antibody to DNA in LE sera. *J. Lab. Clin. Med.*, **62**, 625

75. Lachmann, P. J. and Kunkel, H. G. (1961). Correlation of antinuclear antibodies and nuclear staining patterns. *Lancet*, **2**, 436

76. Schur, P. H. (1970). Antinuclear antibodies. *N. Engl. J. Med.*, **282**, 1205

77. Ritchie, R. F. (1970). Antinuclear antibodies: their frequency and diagnostic associations. *N. Engl. J. Med.*, **282**, 1174

78. Maini, R. N., Holian, J. and Griffiths, I. D. (1979). Circulating anti-DNA antibodies:

aspects of clinical application. In Dumonde, E. C. and Stewart, M. W. (eds.) *Laboratory Tests in Rheumatic Diseases*, chap. 17. (Lancaster: MTP Press)

79. Ceppellini, R., Polli, E. and Celeda, F. (1957). DNA reacting factor in serum of a patient with lupus erythematosus diffusus. *Proc. Soc. Exp. Biol. Med.*, **96**, 572

80. Robbins, W. C., Holman, H. R., Deider, H. and Kunkel, H. G. (1957). Complement fixation with cell nuclei and DNA in LE. *Proc. Soc. Exp. Biol. Med.*, **96**, 575

81. Seligman, M. (1957). Evidence in the serum of patients with SLE of a substance producing a precipitation reaction with DNA. *CR Soc. Biol. (Paris)*, **245**, 243

82. Pincus, T., Schur, P. H., Rose, M. D., Decker, J. L. and Talal, N. (1969). Measurement of DNA binding activity in SLE. *N. Engl. J. Med.*, **281**, 701

83. Schur, P. H. and Sandson, J. (1968). Immunologic factors and clinical activity in LE. *N. Engl. J. Med.*, **278**, 533

84. Lightfoot, R. W. and Hughes, G. R. (1976). Significance of persisting serological abnormalities in SLE. *Arth. Rheum.*, **19**, 837

85. Winfield, T. B., Brunner, C. M. and Koffler, D. (1978). Serologic studies in patients with systemic lupus erythematosus and central nervous system dysfunction. *Arth. Rheum.*, **21**, 289

86. Johnson, G. D., Edmonds, J. P. and Holborrow, E. J. (1973). Precipitating antibody to DNA detected by two stage electrophoresis. *Lancet*, **2**, 883

87. Seligman, M., Arana, R. and Cannat, A. (1968). Heterogeneity of DNA antibodies in SLE and their clinical significance. In Duthie, J. J. R. and Alexander, W. R. M. (eds.) *Rheumatic Diseases*, pp. 211–224. (Baltimore: Williams and Wilkins Co.)

88. Carr, R. I., Koffler, D., Agnello, V. and Kunkel, H. G. (1969). Studies on DNA antibodies using DNA labelled with actinomycin-D (H^3) or dimethyl (H^3) sulphate. *Clin. Exp. Immunol.*, **4**, 527

89. Commerford, S. L. (1971). Radioiodination of nucleic acids *in vitro. Biochemistry*, **10**, 1993

90. Pincus, T., Schur, P. H. and Talal, N. (1968). A diagnostic test for SLE using a DNA binding assay. *Arth. Rheum.*, **11**, 837

91. Glass, D. N., Caffin, J., Maini, R. N. and Scott, J. T. (1973). Measurement of DNA antibodies by double antibody precipitation. *Ann. Rheum. Dis.*, **32**, 343

92. Farr, R. S. (1952). A quantitative immunochemical measure of primary interaction between I* BSA and antibody. *J. Infect. Dis.*, **103**, 239

93. Wold, R. T., Young, F. E., Tan, E. M. and Farr, R. S. (1968). DNA antibody method to detect its primary interaction with DNA. *Science*, **161**, 806

94. Minden, P., Anthony, B. F. and Farr, R. S. (1969). A comparison of seven procedures to detect primary binding of antigen by antibody. *J. Immunol.*, **102**, 832

95. Aarden, L. A. (1977). Measurement of anti-DNA antibodies. *Ann. Rheum. Dis.*, **365**, 91

96. Griffiths, I. D., Holian, J., Maini, R. N., Glass, D. N. and Scott, J. T. (1977). Anti-DNA antibodies: quantitative and qualitative aspects of measurement using ^{125}I labelled DNA. *Ann. Rheum. Dis.*, **365**, 122

97. Rubin, R. L., Lafferty, J. and Carr, R. I. (1978). Re-evaluation of the ammonium sulphate assay for DNA antibody. *Arth. Rheum.*, **21**, 950

98. Samaha, R. J. and Irvin, W. S. (1975). DNA strandedness. Partial characterization of antigenic regions using antibodies in lupus erythematosus sera. *J. Clin. Invest.*, **56**, 446

99. Aarden, L. A., Lakmaker, F., De Groot, E. R., Swaak, A. J. G. and Feltkamp, T. E. W. (1975). Detection of antibodies to DNA by radioimmunoassay and immunofluorescence. *Scand. J. Rheumatol.*, **115**, 12

100. Griffiths, I. D., Maini, R. N. and Holian, J. (1977). Measurement of anti-DNA antibodies: report on the organization and results of an ARC Workshop Study (1976). *Ann. Rheum. Dis.*, **365**, 67

101. Aarden, L. A., Ladmakar, F. and Feltkamp, T. E. W. (1976). Immunology of DNA: the effect of size and structure of the antigen on the Farr assay. *J. Immunol. Methods*, **10**, 39

102. Geibert, M., Heicke, B., Metzmann, E. and Zahn, R. (1975). Influence of molecular weight of DNA on the determination of anti-DNA antibodies in systemic lupus erythematosus sera by radioimmunoassay. *Nucleic Acid Res.*, **2**, 521

103. Pincus, T. (1971). Immunochemical conditions affecting the measurement of DNA antibodies using ammonium sulphate. *Arth. Rheum.*, **14**, 623

104. Holian, J., Griffiths, I. D., Glass, N. D., Maini, R. N. and Scott, J. T. (1975). Human anti-DNA antibody. Reference standards for diagnosis and management of SLE. *Ann. Rheum. Dis.*, **34**, 438

105. Hasselbecher, P. and Le Roy, E. C. (1974). Serum DNA binding activity in healthy subjects and in rheumatic disease. *Arth. Rheum.*, **17**, 63

106. Pennebaker, J. B., Gilliam, J. N. and Ziff, M. (1977). Immunoglobulin class of DNA binding activity in serum and skin in systemic lupus erythematosus. *J. Clin. Invest.*, **60**, 1331

107. Talal, N. and Pillarisetty, R. (1975). IgM and IgG antibodies to DNA, RNA and DNA–RNA in SLE. *Clin. Immunol.*, **4**, 24

108. Soothill, J. R. and Steward, M. W. (1971). The immunological significance of the heterogeneity of antibody affinity. *Clin. Exp. Immunol.*, **9**, 193

109. Steward, M. W., Glass, D. N., Maini, R. N. and Scott, J. T. (1974). Role of low avidity antibody to native DNA in human and murine lupus syndromes. *J. Rheumatol.*, **1**, 41

110. Gershwin, M. E. and Steinberg, A. D. (1974). Qualitative characteristics of anti-DNA antibodies in lupus nephritis. *Arth. Rheum.*, **17**, 947

111. Winfield, J. B., Faiferman, I. and Koffer, D. (1977). Avidity of anti-DNA antibodies in serum and IgG glomerular eluates from patients with SLE. Association of high avidity anti-native DNA antibody with glomerulonephritis. *J. Clin. Invest.*, **59**, 90

112. Beaulieu, A., Quismorio, F. P., Frion, G. J., Vayavegula, B. and Mirick, G. (1979). IgG antibodies to double-stranded DNA in SLE sera. Independent variation of complement fixing activity and total antibody content. *Arth. Rheum.*, **22**, 565

113. Winfield, J. B., Koffler, D. and Kinkel, H. G. (1975). Specific concentration of polynucleotide immune complexes in the cryoprecipitates of patients with SLE. *J. Clin. Invest.*, **56**, 399

114. Harbeck, R. J., Bardana, E. J., Kohler, P. F. and Carr, R. I. (1973). DNA: anti-DNA complexes, their detection in SLE sera. *J. Clin. Invest.*, **52**, 789

115. Izui, S., Lambert, P. H. and Meischer, P. A. (1976). *In vitro* demonstration of a particular affinity of glomerular basement membrane and collagen for DNA. *J. Exp. Med.*. **144**, 428

116. Schur, P. H. and Monroe, M. (1969). Antibodies to ribonucleic acid in systemic lupus erythematosus. *Proc. Natl. Acad. Sci. USA*, **63**, 1108

117. Schur, P. H., Stollar, B. D., Steinberg, A. and Talal, N. (1971). Incidence of antibodies to double-stranded RNA in systemic lupus erythematosus and related diseases. *Arth. Rheum.*, **14**, 342

118. Koffler, D., Carr, R., Agnello, V., Thobum, R. and Kunkel, H. G. (1971). Antibodies to polynucleotides in human sera: antigenic specificity and relation to disease. *J. Exp. Med.*, **134**, 294

119. Natali, P. G. and Tan, E. M. (1972). Precipitin reactions between polyribonucleotides and heat labile serum factors. *J. Immunol.*, **108**, 318

120. De Maeyer, E., De Maeyer Guiguard, J. and Montagnier, L. (1971). Double-stranded RNA from rat liver induces interferon. *Nature (London)*, **229**, 109

121. Tan, E. M. and Epstein, W. V. (1973). A solid phase immunoassay for antibody to DNA and RNA. *J. Lab. Clin. Med.*, **81**, 122

122. Talal, N. and Pillarisetty, R. (1977). IgM and IgG antibodies to DNA, RNA and DNA: RNA in systemic lupus erythematosus. *Clin. Immunol. Immunopathol.*, **4**, 24

123. Alacron-Segovia, D., Fishbein, E., Garcia-Ortigoza, E. and Estrada-Porra, S. (1975). Uracil specific anti-DNA antibodies in scleroderma. *Lancet*, **1**, 363

124. Sharp, G. C., Irvin, W. S.. La Roque, R. L., Velez, C., Daly, V., Kaiser, A. D. and Holman,

H. R. (1971). Association of auto-antibodies to different nuclear antigens with clinical patterns of rheumatic disease and responsiveness to therapy. *J. Clin. Invest.*, **50**, 350

125. Northway, J. D. and Tan, E. M. (1972). Differentiation of antinuclear antibodies giving speckled staining patterns in immunofluorescence. *Clin. Immunol. Immunopathol.*, **1**, 140

126. Tan, E. M. and Kurata, N. (1976). Identification of antibodies to nuclear acidic antigens by counter immunoelectrophoresis. *Arth. Rheum.*, **19**, 574

127. Tan, E. M. and Kunkel, H. G. (1966). Characteristics of a soluble nuclear antigen precipitating with sera of patients with systemic lupus erythematosus. *J. Immunol.*, **96**, 464

128. Jonsson, J., Steiner, M. and Klein, E. (1976). An extractable nuclear antigen not attaching to tannic acid treated erythrocytes. *Clin. Exp. Immunol.*, **25**, 144

129. Mattioli, M. and Reichlin, M. (1973). Physical association of two nuclear antigens and the mutual occurrence of their antibodies. The relationship of the Sm and RNA protein (Mo) systems in SLE sera. *J. Immunol.*, **110**, 1318

130. Morris, A. D., Littleton, C., Sharp, G. C., Corman, L. C. and Esterly, J. (1975). Extractable nuclear antigen effect on the DNA–anti-DNA reaction and NZB/NZW mouse nephritis. *J. Clin. Invest.*, **55**, 903

131. Hamburger, M., Friedlander, L. and Barland, P. (1974). Interactions of extractable nuclear antigen (ENA) and double-stranded DNA. *Arth. Rheum.*, **17**, 469

132. Mattioli, M. and Reichlin, M. (1971). Characterization of a soluble nuclear ribonucleoprotein antigen reactive with SLE sera. *J. Immunol.*, **107**, 128

133. Reichlin, M. and Mattioli, M. (1972). Correlation of a precipitin reaction to a RNA protein antigen and a low prevalence of nephritis in patients with systemic lupus erythematosus. *N. Engl. J. Med.*, **286**, 908

134. Sharp, G. C., Irvin, W. S., Tan, E. M., Gould, R. C. and Holman, H. R. (1972). Mixed connective tissue disease—an apparent distinct rheumatic disease syndrome associated with a specific antibody to an extractable nuclear antigen. *Am. J. Med.*, **52**, 148

135. Reichlin, M. (1976). Problems in differentiating SLE and mixed connective tissue disease. *N. Engl. J. Med.*, **295**, 1194

136. Sharp, G. C., Irvin, W. S., May, C. M., Holman, M. D., McDuffie, F. C., Hess, E. V. and Schmid, F. R. (1976). Association of antibodies to ribonucleoprotein and Sm antigens with mixed connective tissue disease, systemic lupus erythematosus and other rheumatic diseases. *N. Engl. J. Med.*, **295**, 1149

137. Notman, D. D., Kurata, N. and Tan, E. M. (1975). Profiles of antinuclear antibodies in systemic rheumatic diseases. *Ann. Intern. Med.*, **83**, 464

138. Winn, D. M., Wolfe, J. F., Lindberg, D. A., Fristoe, F. H., Kingsland, L. and Sharp, G. C. (1979). Identification of a clinical subset of systemic lupus erythematosus by antibodies to the Sm antigen. *Arth. Rheum.*, **22**, 1334

139. Griffiths, I. D., Mumford, P., Maini, R. N. and Scott, J. T. (1977). Clinical significance of antibodies to extractable nuclear antigens. *Ann. Rheum. Dis.*, **36**, 479

140. Clarke, A. K., Galbraith, R. M., Hamilton, E. B. D. and Williams, R. (1978). Rheumatic disorders in primary biliary cirrhosis. *Ann. Rheum. Dis.*, **37**, 42

141. Wolfe, J. F., Adelstein, E. and Sharp, G. C. (1977). Antinuclear antibody with distinct specificity for polymyositis. *J. Clin. Invest.*, **59**, 176

142. Alspaugh, M. A. and Tan, E. M. (1975). Antibodies to cellular antigens in Sjögren's syndrome. *J. Clin. Invest.*, **55**, 1067

143. Clark, G., Reichlin, M. and Thomasi, T. B. (1969). Characterization of a soluble cytoplasmic antigen reactive with sera from patients with SLE (Ro). *J. Immunol.*, **102**, 117

144. Akizuki, M., Powers, R. and Holman, H. R. (1977). A soluble acidic protein of the cell nucleus which reacts with serum from patients with SLE and Sjögren's syndrome. *J. Clin. Invest.*, **264**, 264

145. Alspaugh, M. and Maddison, P. (1979). Resolution of the identity of certain antigen–antibody systems in SLE and Sjögren's syndrome: an interlaboratory collaboration. *Arth. Rheum.*, **22**, 769

146. Alspaugh, M. A., Talal, N. and Tan, E. M. (1976). Differentiation and characterization of auto-antibodies and their antigen in Sjögren's syndrome. *Arth. Rheum.*, **216**, 11

147. Scopelitis, E., Biundo, J. J. and Alspaugh, M. A. (1980). Anti-SS-A antibody and other antinuclear antibodies in SLE. *Arth. Rheum.*, **23**, 287

148. Alspaugh, M. A. and Tan, E. M. (1976). Serum antibody in rheumatoid arthritis reactive with a cell associated antigen. Demonstration by precipitation and immunofluorescence. *Arth. Rheum.*, **19**, 711

149. Ng, K. C., Brown, K. A., Perry, J. D. and Holborow, E. J. (1980). Anti-RNA antibody: a marker for seronegative and seropositive rheumatoid arthritis. *Lancet*, **1**, 447

150. Alspaugh, M. A., Jensen, F. C., Rabin, H. and Tan, E. M. (1978). Lymphocytes transformed by Epstein–Barr virus. Induction of nuclear antigen reactive with antibody in rheumatoid arthritis. *J. Exp. Med.*, **147**, 1018

151. Mittal, K. K., Rosen, R. D., Sharp, J. T., Lidsky, M. D. and Butler, W. T. (1970). Lymphocyte cytotoxic antibodies in systemic lupus erythematosus. *Nature (London)*, **225**, 1255

152. Teraski, P. I., Mottironi, V. D. and Barrett, E. V. (1970). Cytotoxins in disease: auto-cytotoxins in lupus. *N. Engl. J. Med.*, **283**, 724

153. Schocket, A. L. and Kohler, P. F. (1979). Lymphocytotoxic antibodies in systemic lupus erythematosus and clinically related conditions. *Arth. Rheum.*, **22**, 1060

154. Butler, W. T., Sharp, J. T., Roseen, R. D., Lidsky, M. D., Mittall, K. K. and Gard, D. A. (1972). Relationship of the clinical cause of systemic lupus erythematosus to the presence of circulating lymphocytotoxic antibodies. *Arth. Rheum.*, **15**, 231

155. Bresnihan, B., Grigor, R. P., Oliver, M., Leukonia, R. M. and Hughes, G. R. V. (1977). Immunological mechanism for spontaneous abortion in systemic lupus erythematosus. *Lancet*, **2**, 1205

156. Bluestein, H. G. and Zvaifler, N. J. (1976). Brain-reactive lymphocytotoxic antibodies in the serum of patients with SLE. *J. Clin. Invest.*, **57**, 509

157. Goldberg, L. S., Bresnihan, B. and Hughes, G. R. V. (1978). Lymphocytotoxic antibodies in systemic lupus erythematosus: evidence for reactivity with i antigen. *Clin. Exp. Immunol.*, **31**, 443

158. Winfield, J. B., Winchester, R. J., Wernet, P., Fu, S. M. and Kunkel, H. G. (1975). Nature of cold reactive antibodies to lymphocyte surface determinants in SLE. *Arth. Rheum.*, **18**, 1

159. Koike, T., Kabayashi, S., Yoshilei, T., Hoh, T. and Shirai, T. (1979). Erythrocyte rosette inhibition as an assay for naturally occurring T lymphocytotoxicity antibody in SLE. *Arth. Rheum.*, **22**, 1064

160. Twomey, J. J., Laughter, A. H. and Steinberg, A. D. (1978). A serum inhibitor of immune regulation in patients with SLE. *J. Clin. Invest.*, **62**, 713

161. Clough, J. D., Frank, S. A. and Calabrase, L. H. (1980). Deficiency of T cell mediated regulation of anti-DNA production in SLE. *Arth. Rheum.*, **23**, 24

162. Alacron-Segovia, D. and Ruiz-Arguelles, A. (1978). Decreased circulating thymus derived cells with receptors for the Fc portion of immunoglobulin G in SLE. *J. Clin. Invest.*, **62**, 1390

163. Sakane, T., Steinberg, A., Reeves, J. and Green, I. (1979). Studies of immune functions in patients with SLE. Complement dependent immunoglobulin M anti-thymus cell antibodies preferentially inactive suppressor cells. *J. Clin. Invest.*, **63**, 954

164. Messner, R. P., Deltoratwis, R. and Ferrone, S. (1980). Lymphocytotoxic antibodies in SLE patients and their relatives. Reactivity with the HLA antigenic molecular complex. *Arth. Rheum.*, **23**, 265

165. Ooi, B. S., Ooi, Y. M., Pesce, A. J. and Pollak, J. E. (1977). Antibodies to B_2 microglobulins in sera of patients with SLE. *Immunology*, **33**, 535

166. Revilland, J. P., Vincent, C. and Rivera, S. (1979). Anti-B_2 microglobulin lymphocytotoxic auto-antibodies in SLE. *J. Immunol.*, **122**, 613

4
Antigen–Antibody Complexes: Their Nature and Role in Animal Models of Antigen–Antibody Complex Disease

M. W. STEWARD and M. E. DEVEY

INTRODUCTION

The most casual observer of the current literature on experimental and clinical immunology will find that there is an enormous interest in 'immune complexes' or, more accurately, antigen–antibody complexes. Such complexes have been detected, by a variety of laboratory tests, in a host of disease states (and also in healthy individuals) and their presence in the circulation and tissues of patients has led to speculation as to their role in disease processes. This interest in the pathogenicity of antigen–antibody complexes in human disease has developed directly as a result of extensive laboratory work on animal models, particularly of glomerulonephritis.

The early work on animal models has been comprehensively reviewed by Weigle[1], Unanue and Dixon[2], and more recently by Cochrane and Koffler[3] and Germuth and Rodriguez[4]. We do not propose to cover the same ground in detail. The purpose of this chapter is to review, in general terms, the nature of antigen–antibody complexes and to discuss their role in animal models of human disease with particular reference to chronic antigen–antibody complex disease. These models are of particular importance for our understanding of rheumatic disease since there is little doubt that antigen–antibody complex formation is a critical factor in the development of rheumatoid synovitis[5] and, in addition, in the extra-articular manifestations of the disease[6].

THE NATURE OF ANTIGEN–ANTIBODY COMPLEXES

A basic feature of the host immune response is the ability to eliminate foreign antigens and infective agents from the circulation. Antibodies are clearly involved in this process and under normal circumstances they combine with the antigen to form antigen–antibody complexes. The interaction of an antibody-combining site (Ab) with an antigenic determinant (Ag) is reversible and can be expressed as:

$$Ab + Ag \underset{k_d}{\overset{k_a}{\rightleftharpoons}} Ab - Ag$$

where k_a and k_d are the association and dissociation constants, respectively. The equilibrium constant or affinity (K) can be calculated from the relationship:

$$\frac{k_a}{k_d} = K = \frac{[Ab - Ag]}{[Ab][Ag]}$$

Antibody affinity is the summation of attractive and repulsive non-covalent intermolecular forces resulting from the interaction of an antibody-combining site with its homologous antigenic determinant. Low-affinity antibodies have a greater tendency to dissociate than higher affinity antibodies, and thus antigen–antibody complexes formed with low-affinity antibody are less stable than those formed with higher affinity antibody.

At this point, however, it is necessary to point out that antibodies are multivalent with antigen-binding valencies of two for IgG, IgA, IgD and IgE and a potential valence of 10 for IgM, and therefore the strength of interaction of a multivalent antibody with a multivalent antigen will be considerably in excess of the monovalent situation. This has been described as the *avidity* of an antibody–antigen reaction. Antibodies in serum are heterogeneous in both structural (e.g. isotypic, allotypic and idiotypic variation) and antigen-binding terms (i.e. affinity heterogeneity). This affinity heterogeneity may have important implications in antibody–antigen complex formation and, in particular, in determining the subsequent immunopathogenicity of complexes. Affinity heterogeneity has been defined by a continuous Gaussian or Sipsian distribution function[7,8] although this assumption has been challenged by several workers (see Steensgaard *et al.* for references[9]). Nevertheless, however it is defined, the affinity of an antibody population is heterogeneous and even in a 'low' average affinity population of antibody molecules there will also be some antibody molecules which bind antigen with high affinity.

The presence of antigen–antibody complexes in the host response to antigen can be demonstrated by physicochemical or immunochemical methods[10] and, under certain circumstances, can be visualized in the electron microscope, as in the case of the response to hepatitis B virus infection[11]. Following their formation, the complexes activate the complement system, and are phagocytosed by cells of the mononuclear phagocyte system and eliminated.

However, under certain circumstances soluble complexes can be deposited in blood vessels and tissues and become involved in tissue-damaging reactions. The nature and fate of circulating complexes produced *in vivo* depends upon the properties of the antigen and antibody components involved.

Antigen

A number of antigenic substances are soluble or can disperse freely in solution and are thus potentially able to form soluble complexes with antibody. Among this group of molecules are bacterial toxins and toxoids, carbohydrates, glycoproteins, proteins and lipoproteins. In addition, the antigenic determinants on the surface of bacteria, viruses or fungi and mammalian cells can also interact with antibody to produce complexes. Recent work has shown that common food antigens can also form antigen–antibody complexes in

Table 4.1 Antigens implicated in antigen–antibody complex disease in man

Antigen	*Disease example*
EXOGENOUS ANTIGENS	
Foreign serum, drugs	'serum sickness', drug allergy
Bacterial antigens:	
Streptococcus, Staphylococcus,	post-streptococcal glomerulonephritis,
Enterococcus, S. typhosa, C. bovis	leprosy
T. pallidum, M. leprae	
Viral antigens:	
Hepatitis B, dengue, measles,	hepatitis, dengue haemorrhagic fever,
E–B virus, leucovirus	infectious mononucleosis
Parasitic antigens:	
P. malariae, P. falciparum	malarial nephrotic syndrome
Schistosoma	schistosomiasis
Trypanosoma	trypanosomiasis
Onchocerca	onchocerciasis
Environmental antigens:	
Inhaled—spores	allergic alveolitis, gluten-sensitive
Ingested—gluten	enteropathy, dermatitis herpeteformis
ENDOGENOUS ANTIGENS	
Immunoglobulins	rheumatoid arthritis, cryoglobulinaemia
Nuclear antigens	lupus erythematosus
Thyroglobulin	thyroiditis–nephritis
Cellular antigens	tumours, autoimmune diseases
Renal tubular antigen	nephritis

healthy individuals. Complexes containing milk antigens have been demonstrated in the sera of healthy subjects following the ingestion of cows' milk[12]. Clearly, the fate of complexes involving these antigens will depend in part at least on the properties of the antigen such as composition, size, charge, optical configuration and the number and localization of antigenic determinants. Table 4.1 represents the antigens which have been implicated in human antigen–antibody complex disease in man and gives examples of the diseases concerned.

Antibody

In addition to the properties of the antigen, the nature of antigen–antibody complexes depends upon the ratio of antigen to antibody in the complex and upon the characteristics of the antibody involved, including the immuno-globulin class, subclass, ability to activate complement, physical form (i.e. polymeric or monomeric) and the affinity of the antibody for the corre-sponding antigen. Much of our understanding of the complexing of antigen with antibody and the subsequent insolubilization of the complex derives from the early work of Heidelberger and his colleagues[13].

As increasing amounts of antigen are added to a fixed amount of antibody, the quantity of antibody precipitated increases. Three zones have been de-scribed for this reaction:

(1) *The antibody excess zone*, where antibody is still detectable in the super-natant, and in the precipitate the ratio of antigen to antibody depends upon the valence of the antigen.

(2) *The equivalence zone*, where no free antibody or antigen can be detected in the supernatant. Marrack[14] suggested that at this point, antibody and antigen form a continuous stable 'lattice' which precipitates. More recently, it has been shown that immune-specific lattice formation is not solely responsible for the precipitation of antigen–antibody complexes and that the generation of hydrophobic regions on the complex is of great importance[15, 16].

(3) *The antigen excess zone*, where the addition of excess antigen results in the appearance of free antigen in the supernatant and solubilization of the antigen–antibody complex resulting from the competition by free antigen for the antibody sites in the precipitate leading to the formation of soluble complexes. It is clear that in this type of reaction, quantity of antibody and quality of antibody (affinity) are important in determining whether an insoluble precipitate will be formed. Furthermore, antigen valence is a critical parameter since a monovalent antigen will be totally unable to form a 'lattice' structure with the antibody, whatever its affinity.

The importance of these considerations to antigen–antibody complex disease lies in the fact that it appears from experimental studies that complexes in slight to moderate antigen excess are more likely to persist in the circulation and to be subsequently deposited in the tissues[17] than are complexes at other antigen–antibody ratios.

In addition to the characteristics of the antigen, the antibody and the antigen–antibody ratio in determining the nature of antigen–antibody complexes, consideration should also be given to other biologically active molecules which interact with, and alter the properties of, the complexes. These include the complement component C1q which interacts with complexed IgG via a receptor in the C_H2 domain and results in the activation of the complement pathway and subsequent production of activated C3 on the complex; antiglobulins (including rheumatoid factors) and antibodies to activated complement components (immunoconglutinins). The reaction of these molecules with antigen–antibody complexes may result in an alteration of the properties of the complexes; e.g. it has been postulated that small, non-complement-fixing complexes are converted to larger, complement-fixing complexes following the interaction with rheumatoid factors[18].

IN VIVO SITES OF FORMATION OF ANTIGEN–ANTIBODY COMPLEXES

In addition to the factors described above, the *in vivo* site of formation of antigen–antibody complexes is important. Whilst much of what has been discussed so far relates to intravascular complexes with soluble antigens, the

Table 4.2   Sites of formation of antigen–antibody complexes *in vivo*

Antigen	Site of formation of antigen–antibody complexes	Fate of complexes
A. *Cell-free antigens* e.g. from bacterial, viral parasitic infections	intravascular compartment	clearance via MPS, or persistence with potential for tissue deposition
	extravascular compartment	slow clearance, potential for local inflammation and pathology
B. *Cell-bound antigens* (i) Ag from infectious agents expressed on cell surface	cell-bound	complement-mediated lysis; adherence reactions, phagocytosis and Type II hypersensitivity reactions
(ii) New Ag expressed on surface of infected cells		? some release of complexes into extravascular compartment

formation of complexes with antigens on the surface of cells or antigens within extravascular spaces must also be considered. These possible sites of *in vivo* antigen–antibody complex formation are shown in Table 4.2.

BIOLOGICAL ACTIVITIES OF ANTIGEN–ANTIBODY COMPLEXES

Immunoglobulins in their native monomeric form, unreacted with antigen, do not activate complement or trigger cells. However, when aggregated, e.g. by denaturation, they do acquire biological activities. More specifically, when an antigen–antibody complex forms, various biological activities become very apparent. These activities are tabulated in Table 4.3.

Table 4.3   Biological activities of antigen–antibody complexes

Activity	*Effect*	*Cells involved*
Complement activation	(a) immune adherence to C3b	leukocytes, neutrophils, platelets
	(b) chemotaxis by C567 and C5a, C3a	leukocytes
	(c) degranulation (via C3b)	neutrophils
	(d) anaphylatoxin activity via C3a, C5a	basophils, mast cells
	(e) lysis of cells	cells with complex on surface, 'bystander' cells
Activation of cells	(a) clumping, release of vasoactive amines	platelets
	(b) release of proteolytic enzymes and basic peptides	neutrophils
	(c) cytotoxicity and phagocytic activity	eosinophils
	(d) release of vasoactive amines SRSA, PAF and ECF	basophils, mast cells
	(e) phagocytosis, lysis, release of enzymes	mononuclear phagocytes
	(f) inhibition of T-helper function; T-cytolytic activity; activation of T suppressors; inactivation of B cells; generation of B-memory cells	lymphocytes

Antigen–antibody complex disease has been defined as a state in which circulating antigen–antibody complexes, formed by coexisting immune reactants, induce vascular injury[19]. It is, however, important to recognize that although complexes have been implicated in several diseases (see below), their detection in a disease state does not necessarily mean that the complexes play any role in the pathology of the disease. The possibility also exists that a disease may be caused by complexes even though circulating complexes cannot be demonstrated. It is likely that in many situations, injurious complexes never enter the circulation or, if they do, their stay in the blood is very short. This raises the possibility that the antigen–antibody complexes which are detectable in the circulation in many diseases are not those which are causing tissue damage at all, and highlights the fact that we just do not know what type of complex (i.e. size, antigen–antibody ratio, immunoglobulin class, etc.) *actually* induces tissue damage. The answer to this question awaits the immunochemical characterization of complexes isolated from tissue lesions.

At the present time, there are no generally accepted criteria for the classification of a disease as being caused by antigen–antibody complexes. However, attempts have been made at such a classification by:

(1) the demonstration of the presence of circulating complexes of antibody, complement and antigen (where possible) by a variety of tests[10];
(2) evidence for complement activation; and
(3) demonstration of immunoglobulin, complement and antigen in the lesions by immunofluorescence and electron microscopy.

Table 4.4 presents a list of diseases in which antigen–antibody complexes have been implicated according to the above criteria and, in addition to the

Table 4.4 Some diseases in which antigen–antibody complexes are considered to play a pathogenetic role

Disease	Circulating complexes	Vasculitis*	Nephritis*	Other tissues involved
Systemic lupus erythematosus	yes	yes	yes	skin, joints, brain
Rheumatoid arthritis	yes	yes		joints
Polymyositis, dermatomyositis	–	yes		muscle, skin
Polyarteritis	yes	yes	yes	muscle, liver
Cutaneous vasculitis	yes	yes		skin
Fibrosing alveolitis	yes			lungs
Behçet's syndrome	yes	yes		mucosa, skin, joints
Diabetes	yes	yes	yes	
Wegener's granulomatosus	yes	yes	yes	respiratory tract
Thyroid disease	yes		yes	thyroid
Henoch–Schoenlein purpura			yes	skin, gastrointestinal tract, joints
Cryoglobulinaemia	yes	yes	yes	joints
Leprosy	yes		yes	joints, eyes, skin
Post-streptococcal nephritis	yes		yes	
Bacterial endocarditis	yes	yes	yes	heart
Shunt nephritis		yes	yes	
Malaria	yes		yes	
Trypanosomiasis (African)	yes	yes	yes	heart, brain
Schistosomiasis	yes		yes	
Onchocerciasis	yes	yes		skin, eyes
Syphilis			yes	
SSPE			yes	
Hepatitis	yes	yes	yes	liver, joints
Dengue haemorrhagic fever	yes		yes	skin
Infectious mononucleosis	yes			skin, joints
Multiple sclerosis	yes			
Guillian–Barré	yes			
Amyotrophic lateral sclerosis	yes			
Malignancies	yes		yes	
Drug-induced diseases	yes		yes	

* Immunoglobulin and complement shown by immunofluorescence in the lesions

presence of circulating complexes, vasculitis and nephritis, lists other tissues in which antigen–antibody complex-mediated lesions are thought to be involved. The table does not claim to cover all the diseases implicated in this way but simply serves to illustrate the wide variety of conditions in which complexes are thought to play a pathogenetic role. With reference to the overall subject of this book, it will be noted that the joints are often involved in the 'antigen–antibody complex diseases' listed in the table.

EXPERIMENTALLY DETERMINED PROPERTIES OF ANTIGEN–ANTIBODY COMPLEXES AND MODELS OF ANTIGEN–ANTIBODY COMPLEX DISEASE

The development of our understanding of the nature of antigen–antibody complexes and experimental models of diseases induced by complexes has been extensively discussed and reviewed over the last 20 years[1–3]. A brief outline of this development is given in Table 4.5, which for clarity has been divided into sections: (a) properties of antigen–antibody complexes; (b) experimental induction of acute antigen–antibody complex-mediated disease; (c) induction of chronic disease; and (d) the induction of disease by passive transfer of complexes.

The experimentally determined properties of *in vitro* produced antigen–antibody complexes are listed in chronological order in Table 4.5a. It can be seen that it has been appreciated for some considerable time that such complexes have potent biological properties. However, in pathogenetic terms, the simplest lesion which can be induced by antigen–antibody complexes is the reaction described by Arthus nearly 80 years ago[20, 21]. The *Arthus reaction* is a localized acute vasculitis with necrosis which develops 3–8 h after the intradermal injection of antigen into immunized animals. Antigen–antibody complexes precipitate in the vessel walls, fix complement and inflammation is induced by polymorphonuclear leukocytes which infiltrate the lesion and phagocytose the complexes. However, the understanding of the role of antigen–antibody complexes in human disease began with clinical observations in subjects receiving serum therapy in whom it was noted that 'serum disease' developed when antigen was being eliminated from the circulation just prior to the appearance of free antibody[22, 23] (Table 4.5b). 'Toxic bodies' arising as a result of the interaction of antigen and antibody were considered to be responsible for the disease symptoms. Serum sickness was induced in animals with similar results to those seen in man and it was clearly demonstrated that the 'toxic bodies' of von Pirquet were in fact antigen–antibody complexes. The lesions of serum sickness resolve following the eventual elimination of complexes but, as much human disease in which antigen–antibody complexes are involved is of a chronic nature, this model is of limited value. Of more interest is the induction of chronic antigen–antibody complex disease (Table

Table 4.5 Some historical aspects of experimental approaches to the study of the properties of antigen–antibody and models of antigen–antibody complex disease

4.5a Properties of antigen–antibody complexes

Experimental procedure	Observations	Reference
Injection of antigen and antibody mixtures into guinea-pigs	complexes induce anaphylaxis	79, 80
Intradermal injection of preformed complexes	complexes induce inflammatory reactions in skin	81
Intravenous injection of horse serum in rabbits	complexes induce diffuse periarteritis nodosa	25
Treatment of isolated uterine and intestinal muscle with complexes	complexes induce smooth muscle contraction	82
Treatment of buffy coat with antigen–antibody mixture	complexes release histamine from platelets and increase vascular permeability	83
Cutaneous reaction to injected antigen–antibody complexes	complexes can eventually produce vascular necrosis	84
Effect of preformed complexes on human complement	complexes activate complement	85

4.5b Induction of acute antigen–antibody complex-mediated disease

Experimental procedure	Observations	Reference
ARTHUS REACTION		
Intradermal injection of antigen in hyperimmunized rabbits	local antigen–antibody complex formation in venules produces erythema, oedema, vasculitis and necrosis	20
ACUTE SERUM SICKNESS		
'Serum disease' in rabbits	'toxic bodies associated with disease eruptions when antibody rises and antigen disappears'	22
'Serum disease' in man following injections of horse serum	recovery from serum sickness associated with appearance of free antibody in serum and disappearance of antigen; relationship between the precipitin response and the severity of the disease	23 86
Acute serum sickness in animals following injection of purified protein antigens	circulating complexes of antigen and antibody in antigen excess activate complement, initiate anaphylaxis and inflammatory lesions in the arteries, glomeruli and joints	31, 87, 88, 89, 90, 128
Renal artery injections of heat-killed bacteria into rabbits	acute glomerulonephritis	91, 92

4.5c   Induction of chronic antigen–antibody complex-mediated disease

Experimental procedure	Observations	Reference
Repeated 'anaphylactic shocks' following injections of foreign serum and egg white in dogs, cats, rabbits and guinea-pigs	inflammatory reactions in various organs; acute and chronic nephritis 'analogous to the local Arthus reaction'	24
Repeated injections of killed bacteria into experimental animals	glomerulonephritis	93, 94
Small repeated injections of horse serum into rabbits	diffuse glomerulonephritis	95
Repeated daily injections of protein in rabbits: amount adjusted to 'neutralize' amount of antibody produced	development of disease related to the relative amounts of antigen and antibody present in the circulation	26
Repeated injections of a fixed dose of antigen into rabbits	type of glomerulonephritis correlated with pattern of antibody response and dose of antigen	27
Repeated injections of a fixed dose of antigen into rabbits	disease related to the quality of antibody produced, i.e. non-precipitating antibodies associated with disease	28, 29
Chronic disease induced in mice by neonatal infection with lymphocyte choriomeningitis virus (LCM)	strain-related differences in susceptibility to chronic disease associated with ability to eliminate virus	39
LCM-induced disease in mice	susceptible strains produce low-affinity antibody and are poor at antigen elimination	40, 42, 43
Repeated antigen injections of rabbits and preimmunized rats	lesions in kidneys, lungs, heart, ovary and intestine	96, 97
Repeated protein injections into mice genetically selected to produce high- and low-affinity antibody	low-affinity mice have more severe antigen–antibody complex-mediated disease than do high-affinity mice	37, 54

4.5c). Longcope[24] showed in 1913 that repeated injection of small amounts of foreign serum protein into previously sensitized animals resulted in a chronic nephritis and, extending this observation and those of others[25, 128], Dixon and his colleagues[26] developed a model of chronic disease based on the postulate that the continued presence in the circulation of soluble complexes would result in a progressive, chronic disease. Rabbits were injected daily with varying amounts of antigen calculated to favour the production of soluble antigen–antibody complexes. The experiments showed a clear relationship between the presence of circulating complexes and the development of chronic glomerulonephritis. It was suggested that the relative amounts of antibody and antigen in the circulation were of critical importance in the development of the disease. Similar experiments employing fixed doses of antigen confirmed these observations[27]. Subsequent work by Christian and his colleagues[28] highlighted the importance of the quality of antibody in soluble complex formation. In these experiments, it was shown that only rabbits making non-

4.5d   Induction of disease by passive transfer of preformed complexes

Experimental procedure	Observations	Reference
Passive transfer of preformed complexes into rabbits	some evidence of glomerulonephritis and arteritis	17
Passive transfer of preformed complexes prepared with rabbit antibody into mice and rats	glomerulonephritis, arteritis and endocarditis induced	98
Passive transfer of preformed rabbit antibody–antigen complexes to mice	severe proliferative glomerulo-nephritis but deposition predominantly mesangial	30
Passive transfer of preformed rabbit antibody–antigen complexes to mice	strain-related differences in renal localization of complexes; inverse correlation with strain susceptibility to anaphylaxis	99
Passive transfer of preformed rabbit antibody–antigen complexes into mice	increased kidney localization with complexes prepared with reduced and alkylated antibodies	100
Passive transfer of preformed complexes with rabbit antibody of defined affinity to mice	complexes prepared with high-affinity antibody localized in mesangium, low-affinity complexes localized in glomerular basement membrane	59
Passive transfer of preformed complexes with rabbit antibody of defined avidity to mice	high-avidity complexes localized in the mesangium; low-avidity complexes gave rise to diffuse proliferative glomerulonephritis with subepithelial deposits	60
Passive transfer of preformed rabbit antibody–antigen complexes to mice after *in situ* formation of complexes in the glomerulus	increased renal deposition of complexes in mice with *in situ* complexes	101

precipitating antibody (of low avidity?) were susceptible to the development of glomerulonephritis, whereas those animals producing precipitating antibody eliminated the antigen efficiently and did not develop the disease. In addition, it has been shown that a decrease in the precipitating activity of antibody and production of low-avidity antibody occurred in rabbits developing membranous glomerulonephritis after prolonged antigen administration[29].

The passive induction of glomerulonephritis by large or repeated injections of preformed antigen–antibody complexes has been widely employed as a model for glomerulonephritis in rats and mice (Table 4.5d). However, there is some evidence that the disease produced in this way, usually with complexes prepared with heterologous antibodies, may be somewhat different to that produced after injection of antigen *in vivo*[30]. While it has proved comparatively easy to induce glomerular lesions by chronic antigen administration, particularly in rabbits, attempts to produce rheumatoid-like joint lesions by similar regimens have not been so successful. The occurrence of joint lesions during the induction of acute serum sickness in rabbits was briefly described by Hawn and Janeway[31] and rheumatoid-like joint lesions have been described by Coombs and his colleagues[32, 33] in a small proportion of rabbits receiving repeated injections of bovine serum or cows' milk proteins. However, the development of these lesions did not correlate with the development of kidney lesions[34]. Genetic factors appear to be important in the production of experimental joint lesions since stain differences in susceptibility have been shown following chronic antigen administration in rabbits[33], following articular injection of antigen in mice[35] and in susceptibility to adjuvant-induced anthritis in rats[36]. Attempts to induce joint lesions in rats and mice by chronic antigen administration and by persistent lactic dehydrogenase virus infection have so far been unsuccessful[37, 38].

THE ROLE OF ANTIBODY AFFINITY IN CHRONIC ANTIGEN–ANTIBODY COMPLEX DISEASE

A key development in the study of experimental antigen–antibody complex disease was the work on lymphocytic choriomeningitis (LCM) virus infection of mice[39]. This work extended the studies of antigen–antibody complex disease involving non-replicating protein antigens to include replicating antigens and showed that there were clear strain-related differences in susceptibility to chronic antigen–antibody complex disease in mice neonatally infected with the virus. Those strains which developed chronic disease (e.g. $B_{10}D_2$ new, SWR/J) were unable to clear the virus, whereas the strains not developing the disease (A/Jax, C_3H) cleared the virus efficiently. Convincing evidence for the presence of circulating complexes of virus and antibody and their renal localization was presented which showed this disease to be due to antigen–antibody complexes.

Soothill and Steward[40], in extending the work on mechanisms underlying chronic antigen–antibody complex disease, argued that on clinical and immunological grounds susceptibility to chronic disease should be viewed as a further example of immunodeficiency. Based on clinical observations that immunodeficiency is broadly antigen-non-specific, is likely to be under genetic control and that individuals can produce functionally poor antibodies[41] in addition to the animal work described above, Soothill and Steward proposed that antigen–antibody complex disease arises as a result of a genetically controlled low-affinity antibody response which fails to eliminate antigen, and favours the production and subsequent tissue localization of antigen-excess complexes. The complexes deposited in tissues may therefore contain either low-affinity antibody or, perhaps more likely, that small proportion of high-affinity antibody present in a low average affinity antibody population.

It was shown that those strains of mice susceptible to LCM-induced chronic disease ($B_{10}D_2$ new and SWR/J) produced lower affinity antibody to a variety of antigens than did mice not susceptible to chronic disease (C_3H and A/Jax)[40, 42]. In extending these observations, it was demonstrated that antibody of low affinity was much less efficient at antigen elimination than was antibody of higher affinity[43]. That antibody affinity is under genetic control has been convincingly demonstrated by breeding studies using both inbred mice[44, 45] and mice genetically selected for the production of either high- or low-affinity antibody to protein antigens injected in saline[46–48]. Those studies also provided evidence that antibody affinity was genetically controlled by mechanisms independent of those controlling antibody levels. It is possible that this control is expressed at the level of the macrophage[49, 50], the T-helper cell[40, 51] or the B cell[52]. However, irrespective of the level at which the genetic control is expressed, there is clearly an association between the genetically controlled production of low-affinity antibody to protein and hapten antigens and the susceptibility to chronic antigen–antibody complex disease induced by viral[39] and parasitic[53] infections. The availability of two genetically selected lines of mice, one producing high and the other low affinity to protein antigens, afforded an ideal opportunity to investigate the relationship of antibody affinity to the development of chronic antigen–antibody complex disease following repeated injection of protein antigen. In the first of a series of experiments[54], high- and low-affinity mice were injected intraperitoneally five times a week with human serum albumin (HSA) in saline. During the experiment, the doses of antigen were adjusted to maintain the animals in antigen excess so that doses received ranged from 0.25 mg/day at the start of the experiment to 2.0 mg/day for the last 2 weeks. The severity and pattern of disease induced in the two lines of mice was studied in terms of levels and size of circulating complexes of antibody and HSA, the effect on glomerular filtration rate, the number of deaths due to renal failure, intensity and pattern of localization of antigen–antibody complexes in the kidneys and the amount and affinity of antibody which could be eluted from glomeruli of injected animals. The results obtained are summarized in Table 4.6 and show that a greater renal localization of antigen–antibody complexes occurred in low- than in high-affinity mice, as evidenced by a greater intensity of fluorescence and three times more anti-HSA antibody eluted from the kidneys of low- than of high-affinity mice. In the low-affinity mice the complexes were mainly on the basement membrane, whereas in high-affinity mice they were predominantly mesangial. However, although more low-affinity mice showed decreased glomerular filtration and more low-affinity mice died, presumably of renal failure, the effect of the chronic injection of antigen on these two aspects was not significantly different between the two lines.

In a subsequent series of experiments[37], 100 high- and low-affinity line mice were injected repeatedly with fixed doses of protein antigen rather than with varying doses as described above. Groups of mice received either 0.25, 0.5, 1.0 or 1.5 mg BSA daily for 6 weeks and glomerular filtration rates were determined weekly. After 41–44 injections of BSA, the mice were killed and various

Table 4.6   Antigen–antibody complex disease in generation 10 low- and high-affinity mice following daily injection of varying doses of HSA

	High-affinity mice	Low-affinity mice
Circulating antigen–antibody complexes:		
level*	++	++
size	⩾19S	9–11S
Impairment of glomerular filtration†	↓	↓↓
Deaths due to renal failure	1/12	4/12
Complex deposition by immunofluorescence‡		
intensity	+	+++
localization	predominantly mesangium	predominantly basement membrane
Antibody eluted from glomeruli		
amount	+	+++
affinity	high	high
Circulating free antibody affinity	high	low

* Circulating complexes determined by globulin precipitation following injection of [^{125}I]HSA
† Glomerular filtration measured by clearance of [^{51}Cr]EDTA[102]
‡ Immunofluorescence with both FITC-labelled anti-mouse globulin and FITC-labelled anti-HSA antisera
  Data from reference 54

Table 4.7   Summary of the induction of antigen–antibody complex disease in high- and low-affinity mice by the repeated injection of a fixed dose of antigen (BSA)

	High-affinity mice	Low-affinity mice
Circulating antigen–antibody complexes*		
solid-phase C1q	±	+
solid-phase K	++	+++
solid-phase RF	−	++
Impairment of glomerular filtration†	−	↓↓↓
Complex deposition by immunofluorescence‡		
intensity anti-Ig	+	+++
anti-C3	+	+
anti-BSA	−	++
localization	mesangium	mesangium plus basement membrane
Knee joint lesions	−	−

* Methods of Devey et al.[55]
† Methods of Knight et al.[102]
‡ Using FITC-conjugated antisera
  Data from reference 37

parameters of antigen–antibody complex-mediated disease were measured (Table 4.7). Under these experimental conditions the two lines of mice differed significantly in their response to daily injections of albumin. Low-affinity mice had higher levels of circulating antigen–antibody complexes using three solid-phase radioimmunoassays—C1q, conglutinin and rheumatoid factor[55]—and a greater intensity of fluorescent deposits using FITC-labelled antibodies to mouse immunoglobulin and BSA than did high-affinity mice. Furthermore, at all dose levels of BSA, low-affinity mice had a greater impairment of glomerular filtration than did high-affinity mice.

The pattern of localization of antigen–antibody complexes in the two lines of mice was predominantly mesangial in the high-affinity mice, whereas in the low-affinity mice fluorescent deposits were seen both in the mesangium and on the basement membrane. Mice receiving the higher dose of antigen showed an early transient decrease in glomerular filtration rate probably analogous to the early acute glomerulonephritis described by previous workers[27]. However, at the time the animals were killed the greatest impairment of glomerular filtration rate was seen in animals receiving the lowest doses of BSA; these animals also had higher levels of circulating immune complexes and a greater intensity of fluorescence in kidney sections when stained with FITC-conjugated anti-BSA and anti-mouse C3 compared with mice receiving higher doses of antigen. A greater intensity of glomerular fluorescence with FITC-conjugated anti-mouse immunoglobulin was seen in the higher antigen dose groups. It may be noted that no mice died of apparent renal failure in this experiment. However, it has subsequently been shown in a similar experiment that 50% mortality occurred in low-affinity mice receiving daily injections of 0.25 mg HSA when these were continued for a longer period of time[56].

These results with genetically selected high- and low-affinity mice demonstrate that mice selected to produce a lower average affinity antibody response to protein antigens develop more severe chronic antigen–antibody complex disease than mice selected to produce higher affinity antibody. The low-affinity mice had:

(1) higher levels of circulating complexes;
(2) more intense deposits of antigen–antibody complexes and complement in the glomeruli;
(3) glomerular basement membrane disposition of complexes; and
(4) a more severe impairment of glomerular filtration.

In this context it is of interest that mesangial deposition of complexes in human lupus nephritis is associated with a better prognosis than proliferative and membranous glomerulonephritis[57], although it may be associated with impaired glomerular filtration[58].

Similar results to those above have been described after prolonged immunization of rabbits with ovalbumen where development of diffuse membranous glomerulonephritis was associated with the production of non-precipitating antibodies of low avidity and mesangioproliferative glomerulonephritis with precipitating antibodies of high avidity[29]. In passive acute nephritis in mice, differences were observed in the renal localization of passively transferred DNP protein–anti-DNP complexes composed of rabbit antibodies with differing affinities[59]. Complexes with high-affinity anti-DNP antibodies localized predominantly in the mesangial region whereas complexes with lower-affinity antibody localized on the basement membrane. In a similar model it has been shown that passively transferred complexes prepared with rabbit antibodies of high avidity prepared over a wide range of antigen excess localized in the mesangial areas of the mouse kidney, whereas complexes prepared with low-affinity antibodies gave rise to diffuse proliferative glomerulonephritis with subepithelial deposits[60].

Germuth and Rodriguez[4] have suggested that small soluble antigen–antibody complexes (Class I in their terminology) localize on the glomerular basement membrane to form subepithelial deposits whereas larger, less soluble complexes (Type II) localize in the subendothelial mesangial region. Thus the observations on chronic antigen–antibody complex disease in high- and low-affinity antibody-producing mice[37,54], in rabbits[29] and in the passive model of antigen–antibody complex disease[59,60] can be interpreted in the light of these suggestions. According to this view, the mesangial deposits seen with complexes composed of high-affinity antibody and in our high-affinity mice could arise as a result of the localization of larger (Class II) complexes involving higher-affinity antibody. Smaller, more stable complexes comprising predominantly low-affinity antibody in our low-affinity mice would localize on the basement membrane in a manner analogous to the Class I complexes of Germuth and Rodriguez. However, preliminary elution studies have demonstrated[54] (Table 4.6) that the antibody which could be recovered from the kidneys of both high- and low-affinity line mice was of high affinity. These results are not therefore in total accord with the hypothesis presented above, but the possibility does exist that low-affinity antibody actually deposited in the low-affinity mice kidneys was lost during the practically difficult isolation procedure. Alternatively, the antibody localized may have indeed been of high affinity deposited in an antigen-excess form—arising out of the failure of the low-affinity antibody to eliminate all the antigen.

The research from the authors' and other laboratories described in this section indicates that antibody affinity is an important factor in the production and subsequent localization of injurious antigen–antibody complexes. The genetically controlled production of low-affinity antibody is clearly associated with the development of chronic disease but the mechanisms involved are at present not clear. The results of experiments to determine the immunochemical characteristics of localized complexes will be of particular importance in defining the precise role played by antibody affinity in chronic antigen–antibody complex disease.

ANIMAL MODELS OF SYSTEMIC LUPUS ERYTHEMATOSUS

Two animal models of human systemic lupus have contributed significantly to the understanding of the pathogenesis of this disease—the New Zealand black/white F_1 hybrid mouse (NZB/W) and canine lupus. More recently, two genetically distinct strains of mice—MRL/l and the BXSB—have been described which develop an acute lupus-like disorder and these will no doubt contribute further to knowledge of the disease (see below).

Murine systemic lupus erythematosus

Studies of the NZB mouse and its hybrids as models of human systemic lupus have been extensively reviewed by several authors[61–65] and therefore only a brief discussion will be included here. The role of antigen–antibody complexes in the disease of these animals must be viewed in the context of the very numerous 'abnormalities' in immunological functions which have been described in them. Some of these abnormalities are listed in Table 4.8. There is some debate as to the importance of all these observations to the pathogenesis of the lupus syndrome but nevertheless it is clear that these mice do appear to have a genetically determined immunoregulatory defect which predisposes to viral infection, autoimmunity, antigen–antibody complex disease and malignancy.

Table 4.8 Immunological abnormalities described in New Zealand mice

Atrophy of thymus
Premature competence of T and B cells
Spontaneous polyclonal B-cell activation
B-cell hyperactivity
Antibodies to nuclear antigens and DNA
Deficiency of tolerance induction
T-cell abnormalities:
    deficiency of suppressor T cells
    deficiency of Thy 123$^+$ cells
    loss of θ^+ cells late in life
    loss of recirculating T cells
    abnormal T-cell cytotoxicity
Phagocytic cell defects

Immunoglobulin and complement components have been demonstrated by immunofluorescence in the glomeruli of NZB/W mice together with DNA and the envelope glycoprotein antigen, gp 70, of murine leukoviruses[66, 67]. Following the elution of diseased glomeruli, antibodies to DNA, nuclear antigens and viral antigens have been demonstrated in the eluates. These observations, together with the presence in the serum of antibodies to nuclear antigens (and DNA), circulating antigen–antibody complexes[68, 69] and complexes consisting of gp 70–anti-gp 70[70] indicate that the antigen–antibody complex disease of these mice involves responses to DNA (and other nuclear antigens) and to the viral antigen gp 70. Electron microscopy and immunofluorescence studies have also been presented which indicate that complexes may also be deposited in the choroid plexus of the brain of NZB/W mice[71]. The possible role of antibody affinity in the development of antigen–antibody complex disease in the New Zealand mice has been investigated. NZB, NZW and NZB/W mice produce low-affinity antibody to protein antigens injected in saline, at values similar to those mice prone to LCM-induced chronic disease[72] and NZB mice produce low avidity anti-red-cell antibodies[73]. However, unlike most other strains, the NZB and NZB/W mice show marked variations in affinity with age of immunization[74].

Furthermore, antibodies to ds DNA in the sera of NZB/W mice show similar age-related variations in avidity. In both male and female NZB/W mice the avidity of anti-DNA antibody in the serum increased up to the age of 20 weeks, and thereafter fell with increasing age. The variation was more marked in males but the avidity of anti-DNA in the female was always lower than that in males[75] and levels of antibody were always higher in the females. It therefore appears that the time of onset and severity of the murine lupus syndrome is associated with the presence of increasing levels of low-avidity anti-DNA antibody in the serum. It is of course possible that high-avidity antibody may have been removed from the serum *in vivo* as complexes deposited in the kidneys, leaving low-avidity antibody in the circulation. However, preliminary experiments have shown that the anti-DNA antibody which can be eluted from diseased NZB/W kidneys forms readily dissociable complexes with [¹²⁵I]DNA, i.e. low-avidity antibody (Steward, unpublished observations). This work suggests that low antibody affinity production may

Table 4.9   Summary of histological changes observed in murine lupus

Mouse strain	Sex	Histological observations			
		Kidneys	Heart	Blood vessels	Joints
NZB/W	♀	chronic glomerulo-nephritis (95%)	infarcts (15%)	no vasculitis	—
MRL/1	♀	acute or subacute nephritis (100%)	infarcts (33%)	acute polyarteritis (55%)	arthritis (16%)
MRL/1	♂	subacute glomerulo-nephritis (100%)	infarcts (13%)	acute polyarteritis (56%)	arthritis (22%)
BX5B	♂	acute or subacute glomerulo-nephritis (100%)	infarcts (20%)	no vasculitis	—

Figures in parentheses show percentages of affected animals
Data from reference 69

play some part in the development of chronic antigen–antibody complex disease in these mice.

Recently, two strains of mice from the Jackson Laboratories have been described which develop murine lupus—the BXSB, a recombinant inbred strain derived from a cross between a C57B1/6 female and an SB/Le male, and the MRL/1 strain whose genome is derived mainly (75%) from strain LG/J but also 13% from AKR, 12% from C3H and 0.3% from C57B1/6. Mice of both BXSB and MRL/1 strains develop a more acute disease than the NZB/W mice[69] and, in addition to renal and vascular system involvement, the MRL/1 mice develop arthritis in the rear legs and feet associated with the presence of IgM antiglobulin in the serum. Other changes resulting from the deposition of antigen–antibody complexes include polyarthritis and myocardial infarcts (see Table 4.9). The arthritis developed by 20% of the MRL/1 mice was reported to be very reminiscent of rheumatoid arthritis with destruction of articular cartilage, synovial proliferation, pannus formation and occasional joint effusions.

Canine lupus

Lewis et al.[76] have described a spontaneous multisystem disease in outbred dogs which was characterized by autoimmune haemolytic anaemia, thrombocytopenia, proteinuria, nephritis, arthritis and lymphadenopathy. Laboratory findings include LE cells, positive direct antiglobulin tests to rheumatoid factor, antibodies to ds DNA and RNA and DNA–histone complexes. The disease primarily affects young female dogs and often terminates in renal failure. Following extensive breeding experiments, no evidence for a genetic basis for the disease was obtained[77]. Subsequently, experiments involving the transfer into newborn dogs of cell-free filtrates prepared from spleens of dogs with the disease demonstrated that the injected dogs developed serological abnormalities which characterize SLE–antinuclear antibodies, antibodies to ds DNA and positive LE cell tests[78]. Furthermore, serological abnormalities could similarly be transferred to mice, together with the subsequent development of lymphomas. These results were interpreted as suggesting the presence of a virus in canine lupus which is capable of inducing some of the serological abnormalities characterizing SLE in dogs and mice and may also be capable of activating a latent murine leukaemia virus. Although antigen–antibody complexes are likely to play a role in canine lupus, no formal evidence of their involvement in the disease has been presented.

VIRUS-ASSOCIATED ANTIGEN–ANTIBODY COMPLEX DISEASE IN ANIMALS

In addition to the valuable information obtained from experiments with non-replicating antigens, our understanding of chronic antigen–antibody complex disease has been significantly extended by the study of disease induced by replicating antigens such as viruses. Circulating complexes of virus (or viral antigen) and antibody frequently occur in viral infections in mice, mink, horses, pigs and dogs and it is likely that such complexes are the immuno-pathogenetic agents which induce glomerulonephritis and vasculitis in these animals with a pathology which is very similar to that seen in much human disease. The evidence in favour of this conclusion is that virus, host antibody to the virus (or viral antigen) and complement can be shown to be deposited in a granular form in the glomeruli and in blood vessels, and that circulating complexes of virus and antibody can be detected in infected animals. The literature on virus-associated antigen–antibody complex diseases in animals is extensive (see reference 71 for review) but the relevant data are summarized in Table 4.10.

Table 4.10   Animal models of virus-associated antigen–antibody complex disease

Virus	Animal species	Circulating complexes	Vasculitis	Nephritis
Lymphocytic choriomeningitis	mice	yes	yes	yes
Lactic dehydrogenase	mice	yes	no	yes
Oncornaviruses:				
Moloney leukaemia	mice	yes	no	yes
Murine sarcoma	mice	yes		yes
Gross leukaemia	mice	yes		yes
Friend leukaemia	mice			yes
Rauscher leukaemia	mice			yes
Polyoma	mice		yes	yes
Coxsackie B4	mice			yes
ECHO 9	mice			yes
Hog cholera	pigs		yes	yes
Aleutian disease	mink	yes	yes	yes
Infectious anaemia	horses	yes	yes	yes

Data modified from reference 71

CONCLUSIONS

The experimental study of the role of antigen–antibody complexes in disease during the last 70 or so years has resulted in a formidable amount of published information and several theories to explain 'immune complex disease'. However, what is clear from the studies so far is that many factors are involved in the formation, persistence in the circulation and subsequent tissue localization of antigen–antibody complexes.

A number of these factors are tabulated in Table 4.11, from which it will be seen that some are likely to be of greater general significance than others in antigen–antibody complex disease. The evidence available at present suggests that the existence of circulating complexes in disease does not necessarily

Table 4.11 Factors involved in the formation, clearance, and tissue deposition of antigen–antibody complexes

Factor	Comment	Reference
Amount of antibody	chronic antigen administration in rabbits: high response—no disease intermediate response—chronic disease low response—no disease	26, 27
Quality and affinity of antibody	chronic antigen administration in rabbits: non-precipitating antibody response—chronic disease precipitating antibody response—no disease	28, 29
	chronic antigen–antibody complex disease of mice in association with the production of low-affinity antibody	37, 40, 54
	nephritis in acute and chronic serum sickness in rabbits associated with low-affinity antibody production	29, 103
Immunoglobulin class and subclass of antibody	binding to macrophage and neutrophilic granulocyte receptors is most marked with IgG1 and IgG3 in man	104, 105
	antinuclear antibody deposited in glomeruli of NZB/W mice predominantly IgG2a	66
	onset of antigen–antibody complex disease of NZB/W mice associated with a 'switch' from IgM to IgG anti-ds DNA response	106, 107
Valence of antigen	polyvalence of antigen required for lattice formation and antigen–antibody complex elimination; failure of host to 'recognize' antigenic determinants could result in production and persistence of small antigen–antibody complexes	108, 109
Antibody–antigen ratio of complexes	complexes of slight to moderate antigen excess persist in the circulation	110
	complexes $> Ag_2Ab_2$ rapidly cleared	111–113
	complexes $< Ag_2Ab_2$ persist, i.e. Ag_1Ab_2–Ag_2Ab_1	
Size of complexes	complexes $> 19S$ rapidly cleared	109, 114
	complexes with reduced and alkylated antibodies persist irrespective of size	115
	complexes must exceed 19S to be trapped in vessel walls (guinea-pig) in conditions of increased vascular permeability	114
Vascular permeability	increased vascular permeability results in increased deposition of antigen–antibody complexes	116, 117
	This deposition inhibited by antihistamine treatment	118

Table 4.11   Factors involved in the formation, clearance, and tissue deposition of antigen–antibody complexes—*continued*

Factor	Comment	Reference
Complement	activation of complement and binding of complement components to complexes attracts phagocytic cells but in experimental rabbits not involved in the clearance of complexes requirements for complement fixation parallel those for rapid RES clearance of complexes	111
Complement	complement is involved in tissue damage following deposition of complexes, but not always	26, 119
Reticuloendothelial function	pathogenic antigen–antibody complexes may persist because of:	
	(a) genetic functional deficiency of RES	49, 50
	(b) functional deficiency of RES arising from effect of drugs	120, 121
	(c) functional deficiency of RES arising from malnutrition	122
	(d) functional deficiency of RES arising from 'RES fatigue'	123
	(e) differences in density and affinities of receptor sites for IgG on macrophages	124
Antiglobulins— (rheumatoid factor (anti-Fc) or anti-antibody)	antiglobulin response may enhance clearance of antigen–antibody complexes by: (a) increasing size of soluble complexes (b) increasing lattice structure of soluble complexes (c) rendering non-complement fixing complexes able to fix complement	18
Immunoconglutinin	may react with complement in complexes to enhance their clearance	125
Hydrodynamic factors	hypertension intensifies lesions of acute serum sickness	126
	turbulence, high blood flow and high intracapillary pressure favour antigen–antibody complex deposition	
Antigen localization	DNA localized on GBM prior to subsequent formation of complexes *in situ*; *in situ* localization of aggregated BSA and *in situ* complex formation enhances subsequent localization of passively transferred complexes	127
		101

imply that such complexes are actually involved in the disease process. The possibility exists that the complexes detected in the circulation are in fact those remaining after the phlogistic complexes have been deposited in the tissues. This highlights the point that we just do not know what is the significance of circulating complexes, nor do we know the precise nature of the complexes actually involved in tissue-damaging reactions. Recently, experimental approaches have been developed for the isolation both of circulating and tissue-localized antigen–antibody complexes in diseases of experimental animals and of man. By such approaches it is likely that the characteristics of the antibody involved in phlogistic complexes (in terms of antibody affinity, immunoglobulin class, complement-fixing ability, etc.) and the nature of the antigenic structures concerned will be determined.

To conclude on a rather speculative note, if the association of low-affinity antibody production with susceptibility to chronic disease is confirmed by further *in vivo* experimentation and by the immunochemical approaches described above, then serious consideration should be given to possible immunotherapy aimed at enhancing antibody affinity as a means of treating chronic antigen–antibody complex disease.

Acknowledgments

Work in the authors' laboratory cited in this article was supported by the Medical Research Council, the Wellcome Trust and the Arthritis and Rheumatism Council.

References

1. Weigle, W. O. (1961). Fate and biological action of antigen:antibody complexes. *Adv. Immunol.*, **1**, 283
2. Unanue, E. R. and Dixon, F. J. (1967). Experimental glomerulonephritis. Immunological events and pathogenetic mechanisms. *Adv. Immunol.*, **6**, 1
3. Cochrane, C. G. and Koffler, D. (1973). Immune complexes disease in experimental animals and man. *Adv. Immunol.*, **16**, 185
4. Germuth, F. G. and Rodriguez, E. (1973). *Immunopathology of the Renal Glomerulus.* (Boston: Little, Brown and Co.)
5. Zvaifler, N. J. (1973). The immunopathology of joint inflammation in rheumatoid arthritis. *Adv. Immunol.*, **16**, 265
6. Erhardt, C. C., Mumford, P. and Maini, R. N. (1979). The association of cryoglobulinaemia with modules, vasculitis and fibrosing alveolitis in rheumatoid arthritis and their relationship to serum C1q binding activity and rheumatoid factor. *Clin. Exp. Immunol.*, **38**, 405
7. Pauling, L., Pressman, D. and Grossberg, A. L. (1944). Serological properties of simple substances. VII. Quantitative theory of inhibition by haptens of precipitation of heterogeneous antisera with antigens and comparison with experimental results for polyhaptenic simple substances and for azoproteins. *J. Am. Chem. Soc.*, **66**, 784
8. Sips, R. (1948). On the structure of a catalyst surface. *J. Chem. Phys.*, **16**, 490
9. Steensgaard, J., Steward, M. W. and Frich, T. (1980). The significance of antibody affinity in antigen:antibody reactions demonstrated by computer simulation. *Mol. Immunol.*, **17**,689
10. Lambert, P. H., Dixon, F. J., Zubler, R. H., Agnello, V., Cambiaso, C., Casali, P., Clarke, J., Cowdery, J. S., McDuffie, F. C., Hay, F. C., MacLennan, I. C. M., Masson, P., Müller-Eberhardt, H. J., Penttinen, K., Smith, M., Tappeiner, G., Theofilopoulos, A. N. and Verroust, P. (1979). A WHO collaborative study for the evaluation of eighteen methods for detecting immune complexes in serum. *J. Clin. Lab. Immunol.*, **1**, 1
11. Almeida, J. and Waterson, A. P. (1969). Immune complexes in hepatitis. *Lancet*, **2**, 983

12. Pagnelli, R., Levinsky, R. J., Brostoff, J. and Wraith, D. G. (1979). Immune complexes containing food proteins in normal and atopic subjects after oral challenge and effect of sodium cromoglycate on antigen absorption. *Lancet*, 1, 1270

13. Heidelberger, M. (1939). Quantitative absolute methods in the study of antigen:antibody reactions. *Bacteriol. Rev.*, 3, 49

14. Marrack, J. R. (1938). *The Chemistry of Antigens and Antibodies*. (London: HMSO)

15. Steensgaard, J. and Frich, J. R. (1979). A theoretical approach to precipitation reactions. Insight from computer simulation. *Immunology*, 36, 279

16. Jacobsen, C. and Steensgaard, J. (1979). Evidence of a two stage nature of precipitation reactions. *Molec. Immunol.*, 16, 571

17. Germuth, F. G. and McKinnon, G. E. (1957). Studies on the biological properties of antigen:antibody complexes. I: Anaphylactic shock induced by soluble antigen:antibody complexes in unsensitized normal guinea-pigs. *Bull. J. Hopkins Hosp.*, 101, 13

18. Tesar, J. T. and Schmid, F. R. (1970). Conversion of soluble immune complexes into complement fixing aggregates by IgM-rheumatoid factor. *J. Immunol.*, 105, 1206

19. Christian, C. L. (1969). Immune complex disease. *N. Engl. J. Med.*, 280, 878

20. Arthus, M. (1903). Injection répétés de sérum de cheval chez le lapin. *C. R. Soc. Biol.*. 55, 817

21. Arthus, M. and Breton, M. (1903). Lésions cutanées produit par les injections de sérum de cheval chez le lapin anaphylactisé par et pour ce sérum. *C.R. Soc. Biol.*, 55, 1478

22. von Pirquet, C. E. (1911). Allergy. *Arch. Intern. Med.*, 7, 259

23. Longcope, W. T. and Rackemann, F. M. (1918). The relation of circulating antibodies to serum disease. *J. Exp. Med.*, 27, 341

24. Longcope, W. T. (1913). The production of experimental nephritis by repeated proteid intoxication. *J. Exp. Med.*, 18, 678

25. Rich, A. R. and Gregory, J. E. (1943). The experimental demonstration that periarteritis nodosa is a manifestation of hypersensitivity. *Bull. J. Hopkins Hosp.*, 72, 65

26. Dixon, F. J., Feldman, J. D. and Vazquez, J. J. (1961). Experimental glomerulonephritis. The pathogenesis of a laboratory model resembling the spectrum of human glomerulonephritis. *J. Exp. Med.*, 113, 899

27. Germuth, F. G., Senterfit, L. B. and Pollack, A. D. (1967). Immune complex disease. I. Experimental acute and chronic glomerulonephritis. *Johns Hopkins Med. J.*, 120, 225

28. Pincus, T., Haberkern, R. and Christian, C. L. (1968). Experimental chronic glomerulonephritis. *J. Exp. Med.*, 127, 819

29. Kuriyama, T. (1973). Chronic glomerulonephritis induced by prolonged immunization in the rabbit. *Lab. Invest.*, 28, 224

30. Okumura, K., Kondo, Y. and Tada, T. (1971). Studies on passive serum sickness. I. The glomerular fine structure of serum sickness nephritis induced by preformed antigen: antibody complexes in the mouse. *Lab. Invest.*, 24, 383

31. Hawn, C. V. Z. and Janeway, C. A. (1947). Histological and serological sequences in experimental hypersensitivity. *J. Exp. Med.*, 85, 571

32. Poole, A. R. and Coombs, R. R. A. (1977). Rheumatoid-like joint lesions in rabbits injected intravenously with bovine serum. *Int. Arch. Allergy Appl. Immunol.*, 54, 97

33. Oldham, G. and Coombs, R. R. A. (1980). Early rheumatoid-like joint lesions in rabbits injected with foreign serum or milk proteins. III: Influence of concomitant IgE-like antibodies and of the breed of rabbit. *Int. Arch. Allergy Appl. Immunol.*, 61, 81

34. Poole, A. R., Oldham, G. and Coombs, R. R. A. (1978). Early rheumatoid-like lesions in rabbits injected with foreign serum: relationship to localization of immune complexes in the lining tissues of joints and cellular content of synovial fluid. *Int. Arch. Allergy Appl. Immunol.*, 57, 135

35. Brackertz, D., Mitchell, G. F. and Mackay, I. R. (1977). Antigen-induced arthritis in mice. I: Induction of arthritis in various strains of mice. *Arth. Rheum.*, 20, 841

36. Swingle, K. F., Jaques, L. W. and Kvam, D. C. (1969). Differences in the severity of adjuvant arthritis in four strains of rats. *Proc. Soc. Exp. Biol. Med.*, **132**, 608

37. Devey, M. E. and Steward, M. W. (1980). The induction of chronic antigen:antibody complex disease in selectively bred mice producing either high or low affinity antibody to protein antigens. *Immunology*, **41**, 303

38. Oldham, G., Poole, A. R., Brownson, J. M., Mahy, B. W. J. and Coombs, R. R. A. (1980). Experiments in mice and rats on the induction of joint lesions following injections of serum and in chronic virus infection. *Int. Arch. Allergy Appl. Immunol.*, **62**, 213

39. Oldstone, M. B. A. and Dixon, F. J. (1969). Pathogenesis of chronic disease associated with persistent lymphocytic choriomeningitis viral infection. I. Relationship of antibody production to disease in neonatally infected mice. *J. Exp. Med.*, **129**, 583

40. Soothill, J. F. and Steward, M. W. (1971). The immunopathological significance of the heterogenicity of antibody affinity. *Clin. Exp. Immunol.*, **9**, 193

41. Blecher, T. E., Soothill, J. F., Voyce, M. A. and Walker, W. H. C. (1968). Antibody deficiency syndrome: a case with normal immunoglobulin levels. *Clin. Exp. Immunol.*, **3,** 47

42. Petty, R. E., Steward, M. W. and Soothill, J. F. (1972). The heterogenicity of antibody affinity in inbred mice and its possible immunopathologic significance. *Clin. Exp. Immunol.*, **12**, 231

43. Alpers, J. H., Steward, M. W. and Soothill, J. F. (1972). Differences in immune elimination in inbred mice. The role of low affinity antibody. *Clin. Exp. Immunol.*, **12**, 121

44. Steward, M. W. and Petty, R. E. (1976). Evidence for the genetic control of antibody affinity from breeding studies with inbred mouse strains producing high and low affinity antibody. *Immunology*, **30**, 789

45. Kim, Y. T. and Siskind, G. W. (1978). Studies on the control of antibody synthesis. XII: Genetic influences on antibody affinity. *Immunology*, **34**, 669

46. Katz, F. E. and Steward, M. W. (1975). The genetic control of antibody affinity in mice. *Immunology*, **29**, 543

47. Katz, F. E. and Steward, M. W. (1976). Studies on the genetic control of antibody affinity: the independent control of antibody levels and affinity in Biozzi mice. *J. Immunol.*, **117**, 477

48. Steward, M. W., Reinhardt, M. C. and Staines, N. A. (1979). The genetic control of antibody affinity. Evidence from breeding studies with mice selectively bred for either high or low affinity antibody production. *Immunology*, **37**, 697

49. Passwell, J. H., Steward, M. W. and Soothill, J. F. (1974). Intermouse strain differences in macrophage function and its relationship to antibody responses. *Clin. Exp. Immunol.*, **17**, 159

50. Morgan, A. G. and Soothill, J. F. (1975). Relationship between macrophage clearance of PVP and affinity of anti-protein antibody response in inbred mouse strains. *Nature (London)*, **254**, 711

51. Gershon, R. K. and Paul, W. E. (1971). Effect of thymus-derived lymphocytes on amount and affinity of anti-hapten antibodies. *J. Immunol.*, **106**, 872

52. Steward, M. W., Gaze, S. E. and Petty, R. E. (1974). Low affinity antibody production in mice—a form of immunological tolerance? *Eur. J. Immunol.*, **4**, 751

53. Soothill, J. F., Smith, M. D. and Morgan, A. G. (1975). Immunodeficiency and the allergic effects of parasitic infection. In Taylor, A. E. R. and Müller, R. (eds.) *Pathogenic Processes in Parasitic Infections* (British Society for Parasitology, Symposia). (Oxford: Blackwell Scientific Publications)

54. Steward, M. W. (1979). Chronic immune complex disease in mice: the role of antibody affinity. *Clin. Exp. Immunol.*, **38**, 414

55. Devey, M. E., Taylor, J. and Steward, M. W. (1980). Measurement of antigen:antibody complexes in mouse sera by conglutinin, C1q and rheumatoid factor solid phase binding assays. *J. Immunol. Meth.*, **34**, 191

56. Reinhardt, M. C., Devey, M. E., Collins, M., Gregory, B. and Steward, M. W. (1981). The effect of protein deficiency on the development of chronic antigen–antibody complex disease in mice. *Clin. Exp. Immunol.* (in press)

57. Baldwin, D. S., Gluck, M. C., Lowenstein, J. and Gallo, G. R. (1978). Lupus nephritis. Clinical course as related to morphological forms and their transitions. *Am. J. Med.*, **62**, 12

58. Appel, G. B., Silva, F. G., Pirani, C. L., Meltzer, J. I. and Eshes, D. (1978). Renal involvement in systemic lupus erythematosus. *Medicine*, **57**, 371

59. Koyama, A., Niwa, Y., Shigematsu, H., Taniguchi, M. and Tada, T. (1978). Studies of passive serum sickness. II : Factors determining localization of antigen : antibody complexes in the murine renal glomerulus. *Lab. Invest.*, **38**, 253

60. Germuth, F. G., Rodriguez, E., Lorelle, C. A., Trump, E. I., Milano, L. and Wise, O'L. (1979). Passive immune complex glomerulonephritis in mice: models for various lesions found in human disease. I : High avidity complexes and mesangio proliferative glomerulonephritis. II : Low avidity complexes and diffuse proliferative glomerulonephritis with subepithelial deposits. *Lab. Invest.*, **41**, 360

61. Howie, J. B. and Helyer, B. J. (1968). The immunology and pathology of NZB mice. *Adv. Immunol.*, **9**, 215

62. East, J. (1970). Immunopathology and neoplasms in New Zealand Black (NZB) and SJL/J mice. *Prog. Exp. Tumour Res.*, **13**, 84

63. Talal, N. and Steinberg, A. D. (1974). The pathogenesis of autoimmunity in New Zealand Black mice. *Curr. Top. Microbiol. Immunol.*, **64**, 79

64. Talal, N. (1975). Animal models for systemic lupus erythematosus. *Clin. Rheum. Dis.*, **1**, 485

65. Dixon, F. J. (1979). The pathogenesis of murine systemic lupus erythematosus. *Am. J. Pathol.*, **97**, 10

66. Lambert, P. H. and Dixon, F. J. (1968). Pathogenesis of the glomerulonephritis of NZB/W mice. *J. Exp. Med.*, **127**, 507

67. Yoskiki, T., Mellors, R. C., Strand, M. and August, J. T. (1974). The viral envelope glycoprotein of murine leukemia virus and the pathogenesis of immune complex glomerulonephritis of New Zealand mice. *J. Exp. Med.*, **140**, 1011

68. Steward, M. W. and Powis, P. A. (1977). Antibody affinity and immune complex disease. In Feltkamp, T. E. W. (ed.) *Non-articular Forms of Rheumatoid Arthritis*, p. 23. (Leiden: Netherlands League against Rheumatism, Stafleu's Scientific Publishers)

69. Andrews, B. S., Eisenberg, R. A., Theofilopoulous, A. N., Izui, S., Wilson, C. B., McConahey, P. J., Murphy, E. D., Roths, J. B. and Dixon, F. J. (1978). Spontaneous murine lupus-like syndromes: clinical and immunopathological manifestation in several strains. *J. Exp. Med.*, **148**, 1198

70. Izui, S., McConahey, P. J., Theofilopoulous, A. N. and Dixon, F. J. (1979). Association of circulating retroviral gp70–antigp70 immune complexes with murine systemic lupus erythematosus. *J. Exp. Med.*, **149**, 1099

71. Oldstone, M. B. A. (1975). Virus neutralization and virus-induced immune complex disease. *Prog. Med. Virol.*, **19**, 84

72. Petty, R. E. and Steward, M. W. (1972). Relative affinity of antiprotein antibodies in New Zealand mice. *Clin. Exp. Immunol.*, **12**, 343

73. Elkerbout, E. A. S. and Hijmans, W. (1974). Relative avidity of antibodies towards sheep red blood cells in New Zealand Black mice. *Immunology*, **26**, 901

74. Petty, R. E. and Steward, M. W. (1977). Relationship of antibody affinity to onset of immune complex disease in New Zealand mice. *Ann. Rheum. Dis.*, **36**, 39

75. Steward, M. W., Katz, F. E. and West, N. J. (1975). The role of low affinity antibody in immune complex disease. The quantity of anti-DNA antibodies in NZB/W/F1 mice. *Clin. Exp. Immunol.*, **21**, 121

76. Lewis, R. M., Schwartz, R. S. and Henry, W. B. (1965). Canine systemic lupus erythematosus. *Blood*, **25**, 143

77. Lewis, R. M. and Schwartz, R. S. (1971). Canine systemic lupus erythematosus: genetic analysis of an established breeding colony. *J. Exp. Med.*, **134**, 417

78. Lewis, R. M., Andre-Schwartz, J., Harris, G. S., Hirsch, M. S., Black, P. H. and Schwartz, R. S. (1973). Canine systemic lupus erythematosus: transmission of serologic abnormalities by cell-free filtrates. *J. Clin. Invest.*, **52**, 1893

79. Friedmann, U. (1909). Weitere Untersuchungen über den Mechanismus der Anaphylaxie. *Z. Immunitaetsforsch.*, **2**, 591

80. Friedeberger, E. (1909). Kritik der Theorien über die Anaphylaxie. *Z. Immunitaetsforsch.*, **2**, 208

81. Opie, E. L. (1924). Inflammatory reaction of the immune animal to antigen (Arthus phenomenon) and its relation to antibodies. *J. Immunol.*, **9**, 231

82. Kulka, A. M. (1942). Studies on antibody:antigen mixtures. 1. Effect on normal living excised tissue. *J. Immunol.*, **43**, 273

83. Humphrey, J. H. and Jaques, R. (1955). The release of histamine and 5-hydroxy-triptamine (serotonin) from platelets by antigen:antibody reactions *in vitro. J. Physiol.*, **128**, 9

84. Cochrane, C. G. and Weigle, W. O. (1958). The cutaneous reaction to soluble antigen: antibody complexes. A comparison with the Arthus phenomenon. *J. Exp. Med.*, **108**, 591

85. Lepow, I. H., Wurz, L., Ratnoff, O. D. and Pillemer, L. (1954). Studies on the mechanism of inactivation of human complement by plasma and by antigen:antibody aggregates. I. The requirement for a factor resembling C1 and the role of Ca^{+++}. *J. Immunol.*, **73**, 146

86. Mackenzie, G. M. and Leake, W. H. (1921). Relation of antibody and antigen to serum disease susceptibility. *J. Exp. Med.*, **33**, 601

87. More, R. H. and Waugh, D. (1949). Diffuse glomerulonephritis produced in rabbits by massive injections of bovine serum gamma globulin. *J. Exp. Med.*, **89**, 541

88. Talmage, D. W., Dixon, F. J., Bukantz, S. C. and Dammin, G. J. (1951). Antigen elimination from the blood as an early manifestation of the immune response. *J. Immunol.*, **67**, 243

89. Schwab, L., Moll, F. C., Hall, T., Brean, H., Kirk, M., Hawn, C. V. Z. and Janeway, C. A. (1950). Experimental hypersensitivity in the rabbit. Effect of inhibition of antibody formation by X-radiation and nitrogen mustards on the histologic and serologic sequences and on the behaviour of serum complement, following single large injections of foreign proteins. *J. Exp. Med.*, **91**, 505

90. Dixon, F. J., Vazquez, J. J., Weigle, W. O. and Cochrane, C. G. (1958). Pathogenesis of serum sickness. *Arch. Pathol.*, **65**, 18

91. Lukens, F. D. W. and Longcope, W. T. (1931). Experimental acute glomerulonephritis. *J. Exp. Med.*, **53**, 511

92. McLeod, N. and Finney, G. G. (1932). Acute experimental glomerulitis following injection of *Streptococcus viridans* into the renal artery. *Bull. J. Hopkins Hosp.*, **51**, 380

93. Bell, E. T., Clawson, B. J. and Hartzell, T. B. (1925). Experimental glomerulonephritis. *Am. J. Pathol.*, **1**, 247

94. Wood, C. and White, R. G. (1955). Experimental glomerulo-nephritis produced in mice by subcutaneous injection of heat killed *Proteus mirabilis*. *Br. J. Exp. Pathol.*, **37**, 49

95. McLean, C. R., Fitzgerald, J. D. L., Younghusband, O. Z. and Hamilton, J. D. (1951). Diffuse glomerulonephritis induced in rabbits by small intravenous injections of horse serum. *AMA Arch. Pathol.*, **51**, 1

96. Brentjens, J. R., O'Connell, D. W., Pawlowski, I. B., Hsu, K. C. and Andres, G. A. (1974). Experimental immune complex disease of the lung. The pathogenesis of a laboratory model resembling certain human interstitial lung diseases. *J. Exp. Med.*, **140**, 105

97. Arisz, L., Noble, B., Milgrom, M., Brentjens, J. R. and Andres, G. A. (1979). Experimental chronic serum sickness in rats: a model of immune complex glomerulonephritis and systemic immune complex deposition. *Int. Arch. Allergy Appl. Immunol.*, **60**, 80

98. McClusky, R. T. and Benacerraf, B. (1959). Localization of colloidal substances in vascular endothelium. A mechanism of tissue damage. II: Experimental serum sickness with acute glomerulonephritis induced passively in mice by antigen:antibody complexes in antigen excess. *Am. J. Pathol.*, **35**, 275

99. Ford, P. M. (1975). Passive serum sickness in the mouse: effect of interstrain differences on glomerular deposition of immune complexes. *Br. J. Exp. Pathol.*, **56**, 199

100. Haakenstad, A. O., Striker, G. E. and Mannik, M. (1976). The glomerular deposition of soluble immune complexes prepared with reduced and alkylated antibodies and intact antibodies in mice. *Lab. Invest.*, **35**, 293

101. Ford, P. M. and Kosatka, I. (1980). The effect of *in situ* formation of antigen:antibody complexes in the glomerulus on subsequent glomerular localization of passively administered immune complexes. *Immunology*, **39**

102. Knight, J. G., Adams, D. D. and Purves, H. D. (1977). The genetic contribution of the NZB mouse to the renal disease of the NZB × NZW hybrid. *Clin. Exp. Immunol.*, **28**, 352

103. Dreesman, G. R. and Germuth, F. G. (1972). Immune complex disease. IV: The nature of the circulating complexes associated with glomerulonephritis in the acute BSA-rabbit system. *J. Hopkins Med. J.*, **130**, 335

104. Abramson, N., Gelfand, E. W., Jandz, J. H. and Rosen, F. S. (1970). The interaction between human monocytes and red cells: specificity for IgG subclasses and IgG fragments. *J. Exp. Med.*, **132**, 1207

105. Messner, R. P. and Jelinek, J. (1970). Receptors for human γG globulin on human neutrophils. *J. Clin. Invest.*, **49**, 2165

106. Steward, M. W. and Hay, F. C. (1976). Changes in immunoglobulin class and subclass of anti-DNA antibodies with increasing age in NZB/W F₁ hybrid mice. *Clin. Exp. Immunol.*, **26**, 363

107. Papoian, R., Pillarisetty, R. and Talal, N. (1977). Immunological regulation of spontaneous antibodies to DNA and RNA. II: Sequential switch from IgM to IgG in NZB/NZW F₁ mice. *Immunology*, **32**, 75

108. Christian, C. L. (1970). Character of non-precipitating antibodies. *Immunology*, **18**, 457

109. Lightfoot, R. W., Drusin, R. E. and Christian, C. L. (1970). Properties of soluble immune complexes. *J. Immunol.*, **105**, 1493

110. Weigle, W. O. (1958). Elimination of antigen:antibody complexes from sera of rabbits. *J. Immunol.*, **81**, 204

111. Mannik, M., Arend, W. P., Hall, A. P. and Gilliland, B. C. (1971). Studies on antigen: antibody complexes. I. Elimination of soluble complexes from rabbit circulation. *J. Exp. Med.*, **133**, 713

112. Mannik, M. and Arend, W. P. (1971). Fate of preformed immune complexes in rabbits and rhesus monkeys. *J. Exp. Med.*, **134**, 195

113. Arend, W. P. and Mannik, M. (1971). Studies on antigen:antibody complexes. II: Quantification of tissue uptake of soluble complexes in normal and complement-depleted rabbits. *J. Immunol.*, **107**, 63

114. Cochrane, C. G. and Hawkins, D. (1968). Studies on circulating immune complexes. III: Factors governing the ability of circulating complexes to localize in blood vessels. *J. Exp. Med.*, **127**, 137

115. Haakenstad, A. O. and Mannik, M. (1976). The disappearance kinetics of soluble immune complexes prepared with reduced and alkylated antibodies and with intact antibodies in mice. *Lab. Invest.*, **35**, 283

116. Benacerraf, B., Sebestyen, M. and Cooper, N. S. (1959). The clearance of antigen:antibody complexes from the blood by the reticulo-endothelial system. *J. Immunol.*, **82**, 131

117. Cochrane, C. G. (1971). Mechanism involved in the deposition of immune complexes in tissues. *J. Exp. Med.*, **134**, 755

118. Kniker, W. T. and Cochrane, C. G. (1968). The localization of circulating immune complexes in experimental serum sickness. *J. Exp. Med.*, **127**, 119

119. Allison, A. C. and Houba, V. (1976). Immunopathology due to complexes of antigen and antibody (type III reactions) in parasitic infections. In Cohen, S. and Sadum, E. (eds.) *Immunology of Parasitic Infections*, p. 436. (Oxford: Blackwell Scientific Publications)

120. Morgan, A. G. and Steward, M. W. (1976). Macrophage clearance function and immune complex disease in New Zealand Black/White hybrid mice. *Clin. Exp. Immunol.*, **26**, 133

121. Haakenstad, A. O., Case, J. B. and Mannik, M. (1975). Effect of cortisone on the disappearance kinetics and tissue localization of soluble immune complexes. *J. Immunol.*, **114**, 1153

122. Passwell, J. M., Steward, M. W. and Soothill, J. F. (1974). The effects of protein malnutrition on macrophage function and the amount and affinity of antibody response. *Clin. Exp. Immunol.*, **17**, 491

123. Haakenstad, A. O. and Mannik, M. (1974). Saturation of the reticuloendothelial system with soluble immune complexes. *J. Immunol.*, **112**, 1939

124. Arend, W. P. and Mannik, M. (1973). The macrophage receptor for IgG: number and affinity of binding sites. *J. Immunol.*, **110**, 1455

125. Lachmann, P. J. (1967). Conglutinin and immunoconglutinins. *Adv. Immunol.*, **6**, 479

126. Fisher, E. R. and Bark, J. (1961). Effect of hypertension on vascular and other lesions of serum sickness. *Am. J. Pathol.*, **39**, 665

127. Izui, S., Lambert, P. H. and Miescher, P. A. (1976). *In vitro* demonstration of a particular affinity of glomerular basement membrane and collagen for DNA. *J. Exp. Med.*, **144**, 428

128. Germuth, F. G. (1953). A comparative histologic and immunologic study in rabbits of induced hypersensitivity of the serum sickness type. *J. Exp. Med.*, **97**, 257

5
Complement

K. WHALEY and A. EL-GHOBAREY

INTRODUCTION

The human complement system consists of a complex series of at least 18 plasma proteins (Table 5.1). These proteins have now been isolated in pure form and their molecular interactions are now reasonably well understood. As a result the complement system can be divided into four groups of proteins on the basis of their known actions. Two groups are involved in the generation of enzymes which cleave C3 and C5, the classical and alternative pathway proteins. The third (C3), fifth (C5), sixth (C6), eighth (C8) and ninth (C9) components form the terminal sequence, and one group of proteins serves to modulate complement activation. We propose to discuss in turn the interactions of the proteins in each of these groups, describe the biological activities of their cleavage products, and finally review our knowledge of the contributions complement activation and complement deficiency play in the pathogenesis of systemic lupus erythematosus (SLE) and rheumatoid arthritis (RA).

THE CLASSICAL PATHWAY

Immune complexes containing antibody of the IgM class or the IgG1, IgG2 or IgG3 subclasses can activate the classical pathway. The activation process involves the interaction of the precursor C1 macromolecule with the Cγ2 domain of IgG[1] or Cμ4 of IgM[2], with the acquisition of proteolytic activity. C1 consists of three distinct proteins held together by calcium. C1q is the recognition subunit of C1, and interacts with immune complexes. Following this interaction it undergoes a conformational change which leads to activation of C1r. C1r is a precursor enzyme which is activated following the complexing of C1q with immune complexes. C$\overline{1r}$, a serine esterase, activates

93

Table 5.1 Physicochemical characteristics of complement proteins

Proteins	Serum concentrations (μg/ml)	Molecular weight	Polypeptide chains	Cleavage products	Electrophoretic mobility
Classical pathway					
C1q	250	400 000	18 (6 × 3)	—	γ2
C1r	100	190 000	1	1 heavy chain 1 light chain	β1
C1s	80	85 000	1	1 heavy chain 1 light chain	α2
C4	430	204 000	3	C4a, C4b C4c, C4d	β1
C2	30	117 000	1	C2a, C2b	β2
Alternative pathway					
Factor B	150	93 000	1	Ba, Bb	β2
Factor D	2	25 000	1	—	α
Properdin	30	220 000	4	—	γ2
Terminal sequence					
C3	1300	190 000	2	C3a, C3b, C3c, C3d, C3e	β1
C5	75	185 000	2	C5a, C5b, other peptides	β1
C6	60	128 000	1	—	β2
C7	60	121 000	1	—	β2
C8	80	153 000	3	—	γ1
C9	50	79 000	1	—	α
Control proteins					
C1 inhibitor	180	105 000* 90 000	1	—	α2
C4-binding protein	?	540–590 000	8	—	β
C3b inactivator	50	100 000	2	—	β2
β1H globulin	300	150 000	1	—	β
S protein	?	88 000	2	—	α
Anaphylotoxin inactivator	?	300 000	8	—	α

*It appears that there are two forms of this protein in human serum

C1s by a limited proteolytic cleavage to form $\overline{C1s}$, which carries the enzymatic site of the C1 macromolecule. $\overline{C1s}$ cleaves its two natural substrates, the α chain of C4 to form C4a and C4b, and C2 to form C2a and C2b. In the presence of magnesium ions C4b and C2a bind to form $\overline{C4b2a}$ ($\overline{C42}$), the classical pathway C3 convertase (Figure 5.1) (see reference 3 for review).

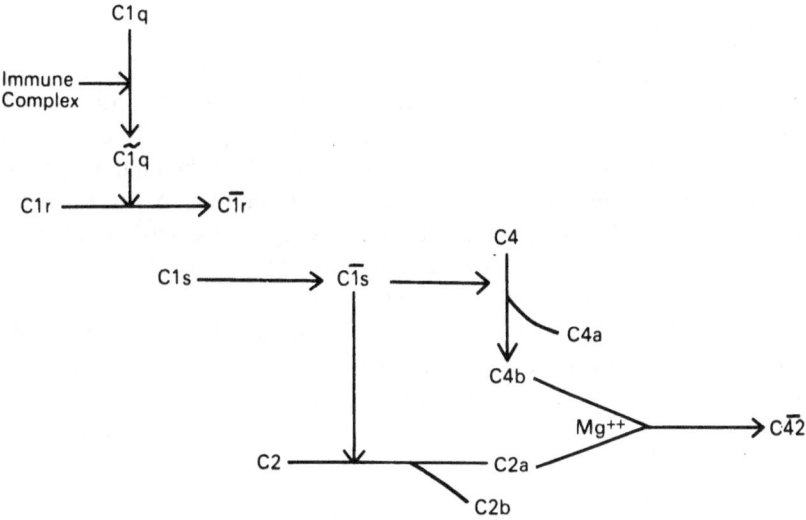

Figure 5.1 Steps involved in activation of the classical pathway. The constituent proteins are denoted by numerical symbols. A bar over a symbol (e.g. $\overline{C1r}$) shows that the component is in its active form. The ˜ over a symbol shows that it has undergone a conformational change

THE ALTERNATIVE PATHWAY

The proteins involved in the formation of the C3 convertase are C3b, the major cleavage product of C3, factor B (B) and $\overline{D}$ and properdin (P). The reaction sequence is as follows: C3b, in the presence of magnesium ions, binds with factor B, to form a low-efficiency C3 cleaving enzyme ($\overline{C3bB}$). Factor $\overline{D}$, a serine esterase, cleaves the B in C3b$\tilde{B}$ to form $\overline{C3bBb}$, the unstable alternative pathway C3 convertase[4,5]. Properdin, by binding to C3b, stabilizes $\overline{C3bBb}$ by slowing the rate at which Bb decays from the complex[6]. The properdin-stabilized alternative pathway C3 convertase is designated $\overline{C3bBbP}$. One of the important components of the alternative pathway C3 convertase is C3b, itself a cleavage product of C3. Thus a positive feedback loop has been established, which clearly requires careful regulation. This control is mediated by two plasma proteins C3b inactivator (C3bINA) and β1H-globulin. As there are two such control proteins two questions are raised:

(1) Why does recruitment of the alternative pathway positive feedback loops occur in the presence of these control proteins?

(2) How do substances which activate the alternative pathway circumvent these controls?

In order to answer these two questions it is first necessary to explain the actions of these control proteins (see below).

Terminal events

Cleavage of C3 by either the classical or alternative pathway C3 convertases results in the formation of C3a and C3b. C3b lying in close apposition to the C3 convertases alters their specificities, and they acquire C5 convertase activity[7-9]. C5 convertases cleave C5 into C5a and C5b; the final enzymatic step in the complement cascade. Following formation of C5b, one molecule each of C6 and C7 bind to it in sequence. Once the $\overline{C5b67}$ complex is assembled, C8 is incorporated, its binding requiring the presence of C5b, C6 and C7. Three molecules of C9 can bind to each C8 molecule to complete the formation of the C5b–9 membrane attack complex[10]. This complex, by its integration into cell membranes, causes lysis. A slow rate of lysis follows the insertion of C5b–8[11] but the inclusion of C9 greatly accelerates this process.

MODULATION OF COMPLEMENT ACTIVATION

It is probable that the complement system is undergoing continual low-grade turnover, and it therefore is not surprising that there are integral control processes which can be subdivided into three groups, on the basis of their different mechanisms. The early stages of complement activation, the generation of C3 and C5 convertases, is highly inefficient. Cleavage of C4, C3 and C5 generates the molecules C4b, C3b and C5b having transient binding sites, being active for less than 100 ms[12]. The natural decay of certain components offers a further level of control. C2a decays from $\overline{C42}$ and $\overline{C423b}$[13]. Bb decays from $\overline{C3bBb}$ and $\overline{C3bBbP}$[6] and C5b decays from cell membranes[14]. Regeneration of these enzymes occurs if the native molecules are reintroduced and the components required for their activation are present. The presence of plasma proteins which modulate the activities of certain complement components provides the third level of control.

$\overline{C1}$ inhibitor

This glycoprotein inhibits a number of serine esterase enzymes by binding on or near their active sites. These include $\overline{C1s}$, $\overline{C1r}$, plasmin, plasminogen activator, Hageman factor and its active fragments, kallikrein and PF/dil (permeability factor of dilution). Deficiency of this protein results in the clinical picture of hereditary angio-oedema[15] in which the uncontrolled activation of C$\overline{1}$ increases C4, C2[16] and C3 turnover[17] with the generation of C2-kinin, a polypeptide released by the action of plasmin on C2[18].

C4 binding protein (C4-bp)

This is the most recently described regulatory protein of the complement system[19]. It stoichiometrically binds to C4b, and is required for the complete enzymatic catalysis of C4b to C4c and C4d by C3b inactivator[20]. In this respect the actions of C4-bp are the same as those of the 10S globulin of Shirishai and Stroud[21], which probably indicates that they are identical molecules. C4-bp accelerates the decay of C$\overline{42}$[22].

C3b inactivator (C3bINA)

C3bINA, initially called conglutinogen activating factor (KAF)[23], is an enzyme which acts on C3b and requires a cofactor, β1H globulin (see below), for its activity. The α chain of C3B is cleaved, the resultant molecule C3bi being unable to form the classical pathway C5 convertase[24] and the alternative pathway C3 and C5 convertases[7, 25]. Immune adherence, the binding of C3b-coated particles with C3b receptors, is also inhibited[26]. The complete degradation of C3b to C3c and C3d requires the presence of β1H-globulin (see below) and other proteases[27].

Hereditary deficiency of C3bINA[28, 29] or immunochemical removal of C3bINA from serum[30] results in uncontrolled alternative pathway turnover. This occurs because C3b, formed during the normal low-grade turnover of the complement system, is not degraded and so interacts with factors B and $\overline{D}$ and properdin to form C$\overline{3bBbP}$ and thereby amplify C3 cleavage.

β1H-globulin

This plasma protein stoichiometrically binds to C3b[31–34] and by this property plays an important role in the control of the alternative pathway at three levels. By its binding to C3b it inhibits the C5 convertase activity of EAC$\overline{4235}$[31] and the formation of C$\overline{3bBb}$ and C$\overline{3bBbP}$[31]. Thus the end results of these actions are similar to the effects of C3bINA. However, once C$\overline{3bBbP}$ has been formed, the site of C3bINA enzymatic attack on C3b is concealed and C3bINA control is circumvented[32]. β1H, by contrast, restores control by displacing Bb from C$\overline{3bBbP}$, thereby re-rendering C3b susceptible to the actions of C3bINA[32, 35]. The third action of β1H is to potentiate the rate and extent of inactivation of C3b by C3bINA[32]. Not only is the inactivation of C3b potentiated, but the further degradation of fluid-phase C3b by C3bINA requires β1H. For the formation of C3c and C3d, a further proteolytic cleavage is required[27]. Plasmin probably mediates this final step.

Hereditary deficiency of β1H presents in a similar way to C3bINA deficiency (Thompson, R. A., personal communication). The immunochemical depletion of β1H from serum results in uncontrolled turnover of the alternative pathway, which can be abrogated by adding pure β1H but not C3bINA[36].

S protein

The C5b–9 membrane attack complex is capable of being integrated into cell membranes, resulting in lysis. In free solution the nine isolated components C3, B, P, $\overline{\text{D}}$, C5, C6, C7, C8 and C9 at their serum concentrations are capable of forming the C5b–9 complex[37] and lysing Gram-negative bacteria even in the presence of C3bINA and β1H in their correct serum concentrations[38]. The 'S' protein was identified as an extra constituent of the C5b–9 complex purified from serum[39]. It is now appreciated that this protein competes for the labile binding site on C5b–7 to restrict its incorporation with cell membranes. Very low-density serum lipoproteins acting in identical fashion also control the insertion of C5b–7 into cell membranes[40, 41].

'Activation' of the alternative pathway

There are two observations which help in understanding the mechanisms of turnover of the alternative pathway (Figure 5.2).

(1) Purified C3*, factors B and D and properdin in 'free solution' form a low-efficiency C3-converting enzyme. When C3b is formed as a result of C3 cleavage by this enzyme, $\overline{\text{C3bBbP}}$, a higher efficiency enzyme, is formed[43].

(2) Hereditary deficiency of C3bINA[28, 29] or its immunochemical removal from serum[30] results in uncontrolled activation of the alternative pathway. These observations show that C3b must be being formed continuously, and the presence of C3bINA controls its activity, to limit the alternative pathway 'tickover'.

Therefore in the absence of control proteins unrestricted formation of $\overline{\text{C3bBbP}}$ occurs. Applying this conclusion a number of workers have shown that in pathological states turnover of the alternative pathway occurs under conditions in which the influence of C3bINA and/or β1H is circumvented. When cobra venom factor (CoVF) is introduced into serum, alternative pathway activation occurs. It is now known that CoVF is cobra C3b which is resistant to mammalian C3bINA[44] and β1H[45].

Nephritic factor (NeF), found in the sera of some patients with mesangiocapillary glomerulonephritis, is associated with intense activation of the

---

*C3 is now known to contain an active carbamyl group, probably a thio-ester, in the α chain at the point of cleavage by C3 convertases. This group can react with water to form a C3b-like C3 molecule, which can interact with B to form a C3 convertase[42].

alternative pathway. NeF has been shown to be an oligoclonal immuno-globulin which has activity for C3bBb[46-48]. The antigen with which it reacts is presumably present at the junction of the two constituent proteins, and by binding them together it reduces the rate of decay of the convertase[49] and prevents the accelerated decay dissociation of β1H[35].

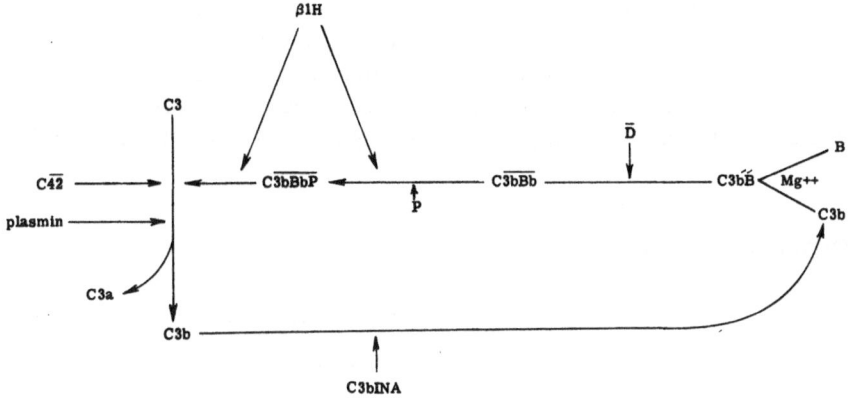

Figure 5.2 Steps involved in the activation of the alternative pathway. The constituent proteins are denoted by alphabetic symbols. A bar over a symbol (C3bBb) shows that it is in its active form. The ′ over a symbol shows that it has undergone a conformational change

When complex polysaccharides on the surface of yeasts such as zymosan, Gram-negative bacteria, or rabbit erythrocytes, are introduced into serum there is obvious alternative pathway activation. The explanation for this phenomenon has recently been elucidated by Fearon and Austen[50-53]. These authors have shown that during the normal low-grade fluid-phase turnover of C3 some C3b binds to the surface of these particles and in some way their surfaces offer a microenvironment which is protected from the activities of the control proteins. The observation that these particles were relatively deficient in sialic acid, whereas sheep erythrocyte membranes were relatively rich in sialic acid, offered an interesting line of approach to this problem[54]. Neur-aminidase treatment of sheep erythrocytes resulted in their acquiring the ability to turnover of the alternative pathway[33, 52]. Furthermore using inbred strains of mice, the ability of mouse erythrocytes to 'activate' the alternative pathway was shown to be inherited in a Mendelian fashion. Erythrocytes with membranes with high sialic acid content produced little turnover and those with low sialic acid content produced high turnover. In studies of the F_1 and F_2 hybrid progeny of matings between strains of mice having high and low erythrocyte sialic acid content, and their back-crosses with the parent strains, these characteristics could not be segregated[55] suggesting that both are geneti-cally controlled at a single autosomal locus.

The association constant for the binding of β1H with C3b is decreased on surfaces having a low sialic acid content, thereby favouring the formation of $C\overline{3bBb}$[56].

The observation that increasing magnesium ion concentration of serum causes alternative pathway turnover occurs because the association constant of B for C3b is increased, thereby circumventing the actions of $\beta1H$[56].

These experiments have now led us to the concept that agents which activate the alternative pathway are not really activating agents; rather, they permit amplification of the pre-existing low-grade turnover of the system. When alternative pathway turnover is seen in immune-complex disease such as SLE and RA, it probably occurs because increased classical pathway activity produces C3b at a rate exceeding the inactivating capacity of C3bINA and $\beta1H$.

BIOLOGICAL ACTIVITIES

Table 5.2   Biological activities generated during complement activation

Activity	Mediators
Cytolysis	C5b–9
Reactive lysis	$C\overline{567}$ + C8 and C9
Vasopermeability	C-kinin C3a C5a
Chemotaxis	C5a, Ba (? $C\overline{567}$)
Mobilization of PMN from bone marrow	C3e
Macrophage spreading	Bb
Lysosomal enzyme secretion	? C3b
Opsonization	C3b, C4b
Phagocytosis	C3b, C4b
Intracellular killing of bacteria	C3b
Solubilization of immune complexes	C3b
Antibody production	? C3

Cytolysis

This activity first drew attention to the existence of the complement system, as it was noted that a heat-labile serum factor was required in addition to antibody for the lysis of bacteria. Lysis of many cell types including erythrocytes; nucleated cells, such as Kreb's ascites cells, rat peritoneal mast cells and Chinese hamster lung cells; bacteria; and subcellular particles such as platelets, mycoplasmae and viruses occurs (see reference 57 for review).

The observations that complement can lyse pure lipid liposomes[58] suggests that proteolysis is unlikely to be the cause of the lytic event. Furthermore phospholipase activity has not been detected[58–60]. The most probable explanation for cytolysis is that the C5b–9 complex is inserted into the cell membrane to form a hydrophilic channel which permits the passage of water and electrolytes, eventually leading to osmotic lysis[61].

Electron-microscopic examination of cell membranes which have been lysed by complement reveal characteristic 'holes', about 10 nm in diameter with a 2.5 nm electron-lucent ring[62]. These lesions do not appear prior to the action of the components C5–C9[63, 64]. Dourmashkin[65] has studied the electron-microscopic appearances of developing complement lesion, and shown that at the C5b–7 stage 'folacious' particles projecting from the cell membrane were formed. Following the addition of C8 these particles enlarged and developed a variable number of arms. Not until the C5b–9 stage was reached, however, did the lesions appear as the typical hollow cylinders projecting from the cell membrane and partly penetrating it. The C5b–9 complex isolated from the membranes of lysed cells has the same appearance as the complement lesion in membranes, and is capable of being reincorporated into artificial lipid vesicles[66]. It is therefore fairly safe to assume that the C5b–9 complex is inserted into the cell membrane, and becomes the 'complement lesion'. The integration of the C5b–9 complex explains the release of membrane lipid[60, 67], intercalar particle aggregation[68], rearrangement of membrane lipids[67] and non-osmotic membrane-swelling[69], yet the exact mechanism by which lysis is produced is not clear. The centre of the cylinder takes up the silicotungsten stain, and therefore could represent a transmembrane channel. However, the C5b–9 cylinder has never been shown to penetrate the full thickness of lipid vesicles[66, 70], although it has been shown to increase ion permeability of lipid bilayers[71].

It is possible that the transmembrane channel does not pass through the centre of the C5b–9 complex, but rather that the lipophilic C5b–9 complex grossly distorts the lipid bilayers, forming a channel immediately adjacent to the complex. Once the C5b–9 complex has been assembled on cell membranes there are apparently three steps required for the lysis to occur. The first step is temperature-dependent, and is associated with the insertion of the complex into the cell membrane. Prior to this step the complex is trypsin-sensitive, whereas afterwards it is trypsin-resistant. Following the insertion of the complex into the membrane two further steps can be distinguished, one of which is blocked by a variety of metal salts and the other blocked by high-molarity EDTA[72, 73]. Only when these three steps have been completed are the cell contents released.

Anaphylotoxins and chemotaxis

Cleavage of C3 or C5 by their respective convertases yields C3a and C5a respectively*. Both C3a and C5a possess anaphylotoxic activity, the latter

---

*It has recently been suggested that C4a has weak anaphyylotoxic activity.

being approximately ten times more potent than the former[74]. As anaphylotoxins they react with receptors on mast cells and basophils with subsequent degranulation. These granules contain vasoactive amines such as histamine and their release is associated with increased vascular permeability. Anaphylotoxins also cause smooth muscle contraction. C5a but not C3a is chemotactic for polymorphs and macrophages[75] even after its anaphylotoxic activity has been removed by anaphylotoxin inactivator.

The trimolecular complex $\overline{C5b67}$ has been thought to possess chemotactic properties[76] but this is now considered unlikely. The *in vitro* assembly of the alternative pathway convertase $\overline{C3bBb}$ is associated with the generation of chemotactic activity[77] probably because the Ba fragment is released. Ba, but not Bb or native B, is chemotactic for polymorphonuclear leukocytes[78]. The isolated Bb fragment interacts with macrophage cell membranes, increasing the ruffling of the membrane and causing cytoplasmic spreading[79].

Modulation of immune-complex-mediated effects

Immune complexes interact with complement proteins, and as a result the complexes undergo changes which can completely alter their biological activities.

The recognition and gross removal of complexes from the circulation by the cells of the mononuclear phagocytes system appears to be a complement-independent phenomenon[80]. If complexes are injected intravenously into normal mice, some bind to the cellular constituents of the blood and some stay in the plasma. Within a short period of time the complexes are released from the cells and circulate in the plasma from which they are removed[81]. This complex-releasing activity (CRA), which may play a role in protecting the body from the injurious effects of immune complexes, requires an intact alternative pathway[82]. Solubilization of immune precipitates occurs as a consequence of complement activation. This process requires an intact alternative pathway but proceeds more efficiently in the presence of an intact classical pathway[83–85]. The mechanism of solubilization is not enzymatic, but is a consequence of the intercalation of C3b, and perhaps C4b into the antigen–antibody lattice[84, 85]. As a result of the intercalation of C3b the harmful effects of immune complexes may be abrogated.

The presence of C3b or C4b on immune complexes permits this interaction with receptors on the surface of certain cells such as erythrocytes, mononuclear phagocytes, polymorphonuclear leukocytes and certain classes of lymphocytes. This interaction was termed immune adherence by Nelson[86]. The biological consequences of this phenomenon vary depending upon the cell type involved; for instance phagocytic cells show enhanced phagocytosis[87, 88].

An important recent observation is that following the binding of C3b to the C3b receptor, the intracellular killing of organisms is enhanced[89]. The role of

C3b receptors on lymphocytes is controversial; perhaps they are important in the production of antibody. It has been suggested that complement together with antigen provides a second signal for the production of antibody[90] but this concept is probably incorrect, especially as a T-lymphocyte-independent antibody response can be obtained[91, 92] in the absence of C3. There are studies reporting that T-lymphocyte-dependent antibody responses require C3[91] probably because C3b could bring together macrophages and the two subsets of lymphocytes required for this response. In contrast, normal antibody responses occurred in a patient with a genetically determined complete deficiency of C3[93]. The formation of B memory cells is impaired in decomplemented rabbits[94] perhaps also because C3 is required for the transport of aggregated IgG and immune complexes into the germinal centres[95].

Rabbit, but not human, platelets have C3b receptors, and C3b-coated complexes cause selective release of granule content or total lysis of the platelet, depending upon the size of the complex[96]. Human platelets, by means of Fc receptors, bind complexes in the absence of complement. When zymosan is incubated with human plasma, it acquires the ability to stimulate secretion by human platelets. This reaction requires an intact alternative pathway and fibrinogen, but not the classical pathway components[97].

Micro-organisms and complement

Opsonization

The attachment of bacteria to macrophages is facilitated by their being coated with C3b and/or C4b. C3b can coat Gram-negative bacteria by the alternative pathway as described earlier. In immune individuals opsonization may be achieved by IgG antibody, C4b, C3b or all three.

Antiviral activity of complement

Measles-virus infected cells coated with antibody will lyse in the presence of human serum; a reaction requiring an intact alternative pathway[98]. The efficiency of the neutralization pathway[98]. The efficiency of the neutralization of certain type viruses by antibody is enhanced by C1, C4 and C2[99]. RNA tumour viruses possess a C1q receptor, which binds C1q, thereby activating C1. Virolysis occurs in human but not guinea-pig serum[100]. The efficiency of antibody-dependent cytotoxicity of virus-infected cells by leukocytes is increased by adding complement[101].

Complement in SLE

Classical pathway activation

Evidence for classical pathway activation in SLE comes from the detection of circulating immune complexes[102, 103], reduced serum levels of the classical pathway components C1, C4 and C2[104], the glomerular deposition of immune complexes and classical pathway components[105, 106] and the hypercatabolism of C4[17].

In the routine laboratory abnormalities of the classical pathway are more frequently observed than abnormalities of the alternative pathway: generally speaking the levels of immune complexes rise during exacerbations and levels of complement proteins drop. When one compares values measured on serum samples taken serially over a long period of time (Figure 5.3) it becomes

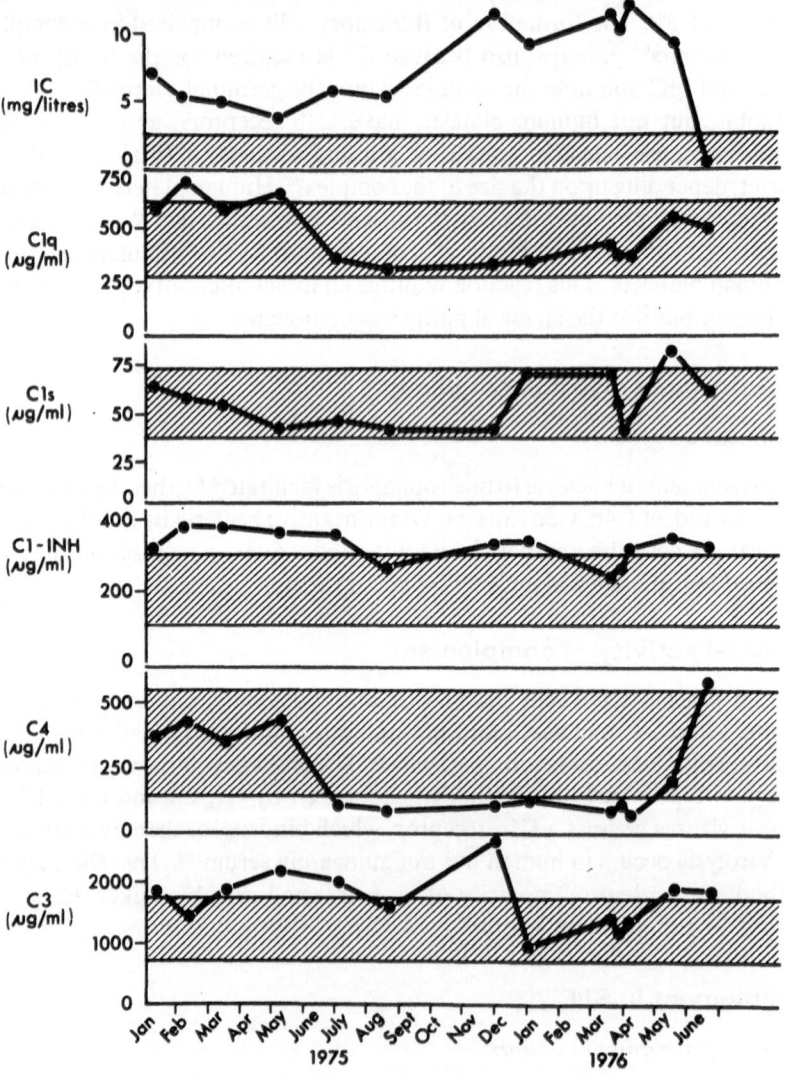

Figure 5.3 Serial measurements of the serum concentrations of C3, C4, CĪ-INH, C1s, C1q and immune complexes in a patient with SLE (shaded areas represent normal ranges)

obvious that the measurements which correlate best with disease activity are immune complexes and C4, with the former providing a somewhat more sensitive index than the latter. The concentrations of the C1 subcomponents change with disease activity but rarely fall into the subnormal range, and C3 may be normal in patients who have severe disease and pronounced comp-

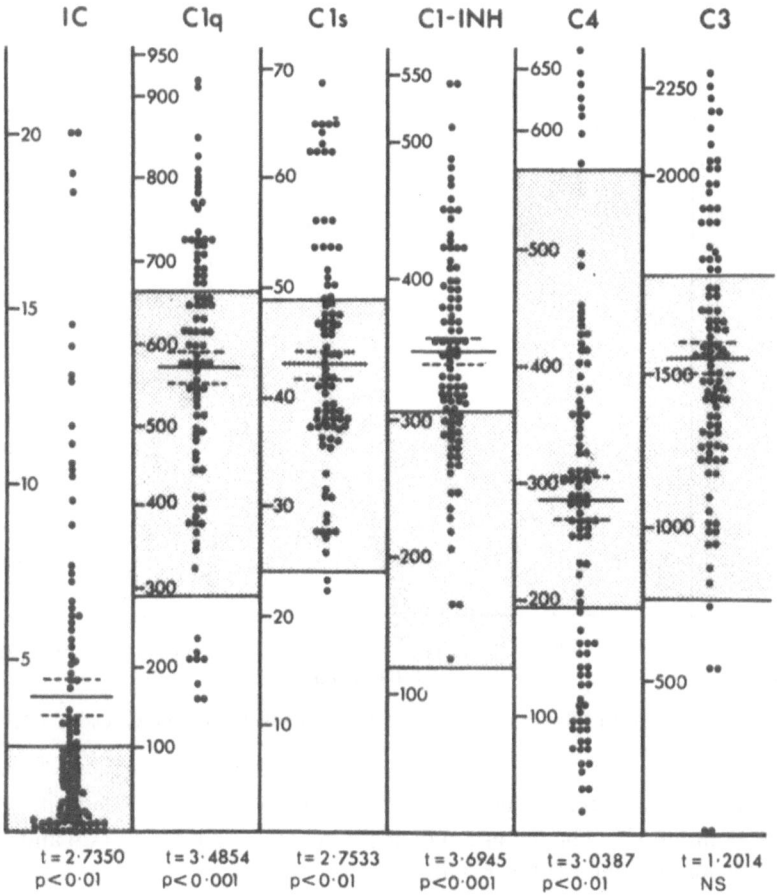

Figure 5.4 Serum concentrations of immune complexes and classical pathway components and CĪ-INH in SLE (——mean ± ----- SEM; shaded areas represent normal ranges)

lement activation. These conclusions are confirmed when one measures levels of these components in patients with severe SLE, and one plots them against the normal range: levels of immune complexes are frequently raised and C4 concentrations are most frequently reduced (Figure 5.4).

Serum concentrations of the regulatory protein CĪ inhibitor are usually elevated (Figure 5.4) but there are data which suggest that it is hyper-catabolized:

(1) Concentrations dip when C4 levels are at their lowest (Figure 5.3).
(2) Occasionally, subnormal levels are seen in SLE (in the absence of heredi-
    tary deficiency of the protein).
(3) Levels of immune complexes correlate inversely with C$\bar{1}$-inhibitor levels
    (Figure 5.5), suggesting that when high levels of immune complexes are
    activating C1, increased consumption of C$\bar{1}$ inhibitor occurs.

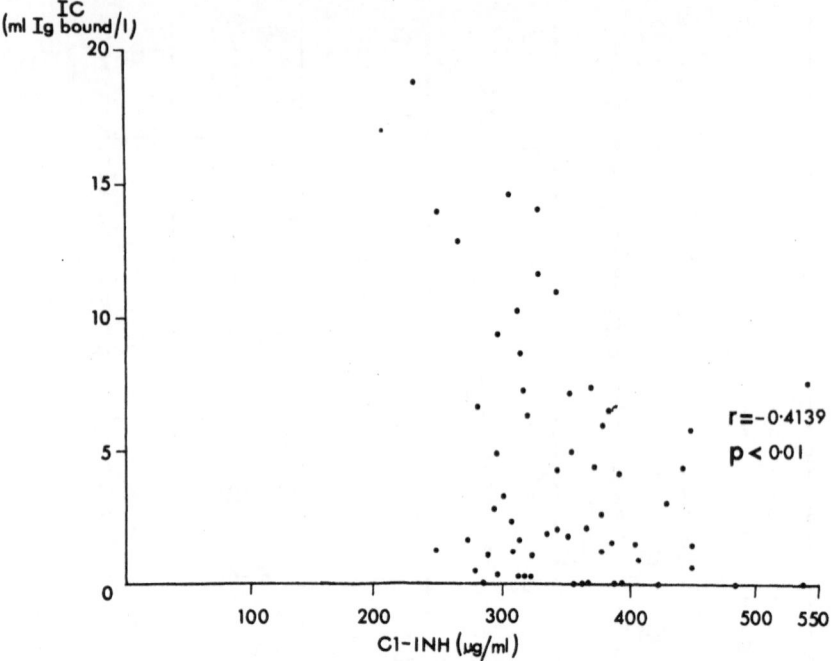

Figure 5.5 Correlation between serum concentrations of immune complexes and C$\bar{1}$-INH in
SLE

(4) Immunofluorescence studies of renal biopsies in SLE show deposition of
    C$\bar{1}$ inhibitor[107]. The pattern of deposition of C$\bar{1}$ inhibitor and C4 and C1s
    are closely similar (Figure 5.6).

Thus in SLE there is evidence that increased catabolism of C$\bar{1}$ inhibitor occurs
and suggests that perhaps this protein is playing a regulatory role in this
disease.

Alternative pathway activation

Although complement activation in SLE is primarily by the classical pathway,
significant alternative pathway activation occurs, as shown by reduced serum
levels of factor B and properdin[108, 109], the presence of factor B cleavage
products[110], glomerular localization of factor B and properdin[104, 106] and the
increased catabolism of factor B[17, 111] and properdin[112].

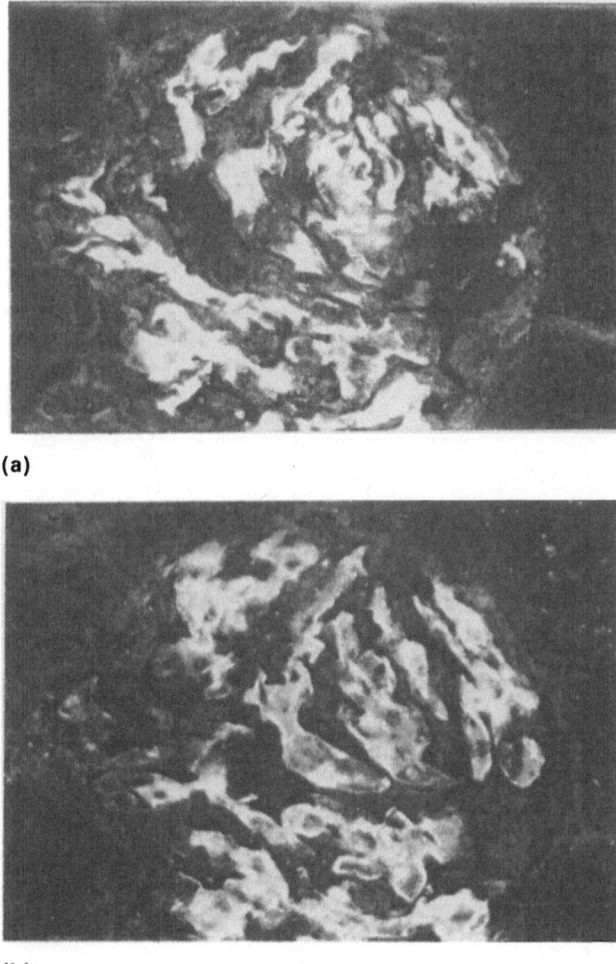

(a)

(b)

Figure 5.6 Immunofluorescence localization of (a) C1s, and (b) C̄1-INH in serial sections of a renal biopsy taken from a patient with SLE (magnification × 750)

Although the mean serum levels of factor B and properdin are frequently reduced in patients who have severe disease with nephritis[109], non-renal cases of SLE rarely have low levels of either, despite much reduced C4 levels. Despite the normal levels of the alternative pathway proteins, however, increased turnover of factor B can be shown by the presence of increased levels of its cleavage product Ba (Figure 5.7). Similarly, increased C3 turnover in SLE is shown by elevated levels of the cleavage product, C3d, despite normal concentrations of C3 (Figure 5.7). The increased turnover of the alternative pathway in SLE is probably secondary to the intense activation of the classical pathway. It was suggested[113] that nephritic factor-like substances were present

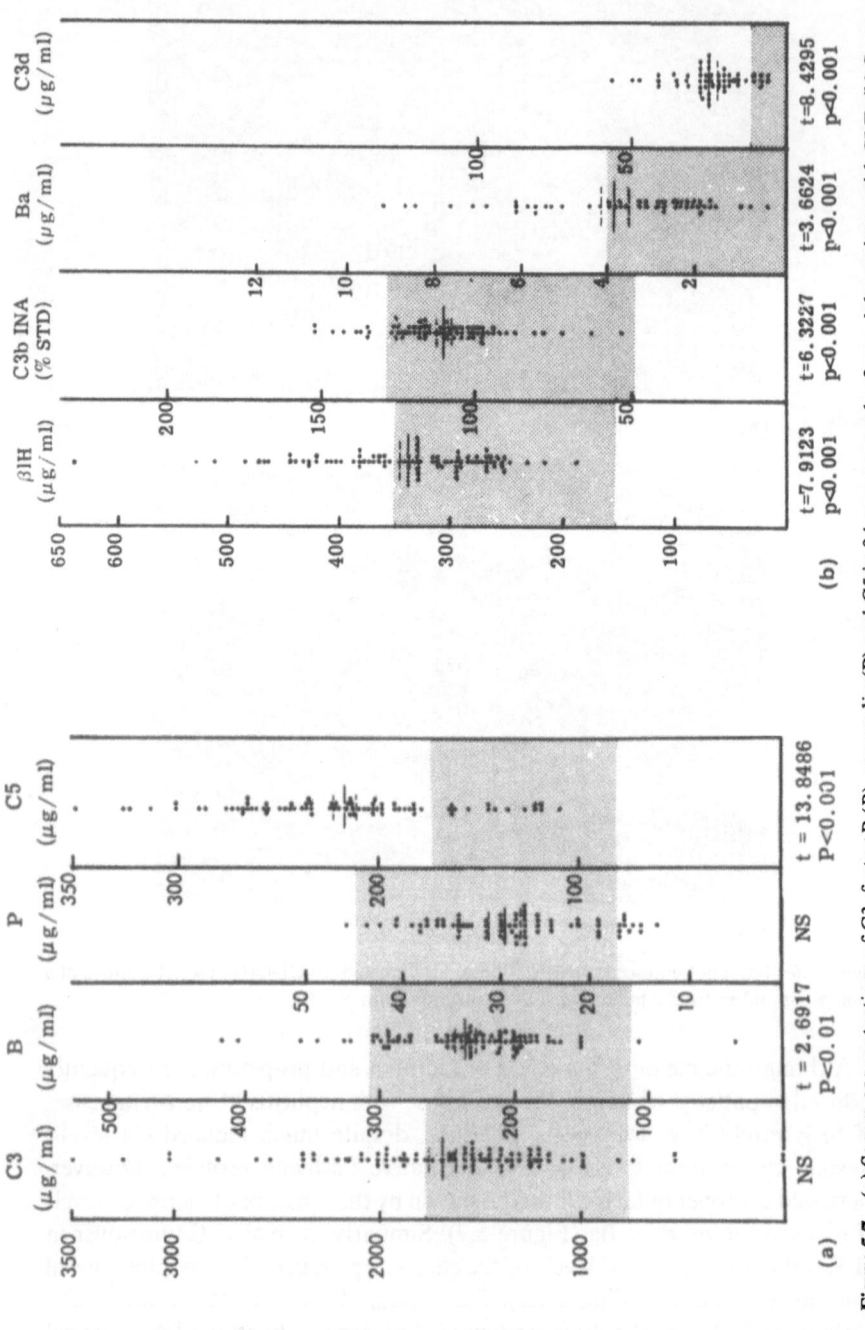

Figure 5.7 (a) Serum concentrations of C3, factor B (B), properdin (P) and C5 in 94 serum samples from eight patients with SLE. (b) Serum concentrations of β1H, C3bINA and plasma concentrations of Ba and C3d in SLE. Shaded areas represent the normal ranges

in SLE sera, causing direct activation of the alternative pathway, but this finding has not been confirmed[109]. In fact, serum levels of immune complexes show negative correlations with the levels of the alternative pathway proteins B and P (Figure 5.8), indicating that the extent of classical pathway activation dictates the rate of turnover of the alternative pathway. If, as seems likely, the increased alternative pathway turnover seen in SLE is secondary to the generation of C3b, by the classical pathway, then the serum concentrations of the control proteins C3b inactivator and β1H ought to be of central importance in controlling the extent of turnover. Our early studies[25, 109] showed that reduced serum concentrations of C3bINA and β1H occurred during exacerbations of SLE, especially when C3 levels were reduced. The reductions in levels of β1H were more pronounced than those of C3bINA. When we examined the correlations between the serum concentrations of C3bINA or β1H and the serum concentrations of C4, C3, B and P we found that concentrations of C3bINA correlated only with B levels, whereas β1H levels correlated well with concentrations of C3, B and P. From these observations it was concluded that low levels of the control proteins permitted increased turnover of the alternative pathway thereby increasing C3, B and P utilization. Thus low levels of the proteins were associated with low levels of C3, B and P, and high concentrations of the control proteins, which would reduce alternative pathway turnover, were associated with high levels of C3, B and P. These correlations could also arise if the synthetic rates of these proteins were controlled by common stimuli. In more recent studies, we have examined the relationships between the concentrations of C3bINA and β1H and the concentrations of the cleavage products Ba and C3d (Figure 5.7). If the rate of turnover of B can be expressed as Ba/B (concentration of cleavage product/ concentration of total factor B), and if C3bINA and/or β1H concentrations are critical in controlling the rate of turnover of the alternative pathway, then high levels of C3bINA and/or β1H should be associated with reduced alternative pathway turnover (i.e. Ba/B low). Conversely, low levels of the control proteins should be associated with increased turnover (Ba/B high). Thus, if our previous conclusion was correct, then the serum concentrations of C3bINA and/or β1H should show a negative correlation with Ba/B. However, we found no correlations between either protein and Ba/B, which would lead to the conclusion that the absolute levels of the control proteins are not important in controlling the extent of alternative pathway turnover in SLE. We have recently confirmed this finding by measuring serum C3bINA and β1H levels in 15 patients undergoing factor B metabolic studies. We found that the serum concentrations of these two proteins were totally unrelated to either the catabolic or synthetic rates of this protein, or to the intravascular/ extravascular distribution of the protein (Whaley and Arroyave, unpublished observations).

Despite the fact that our conclusions argue that the absolute levels of these control proteins do not dictate the extent of alternative turnover in SLE, there

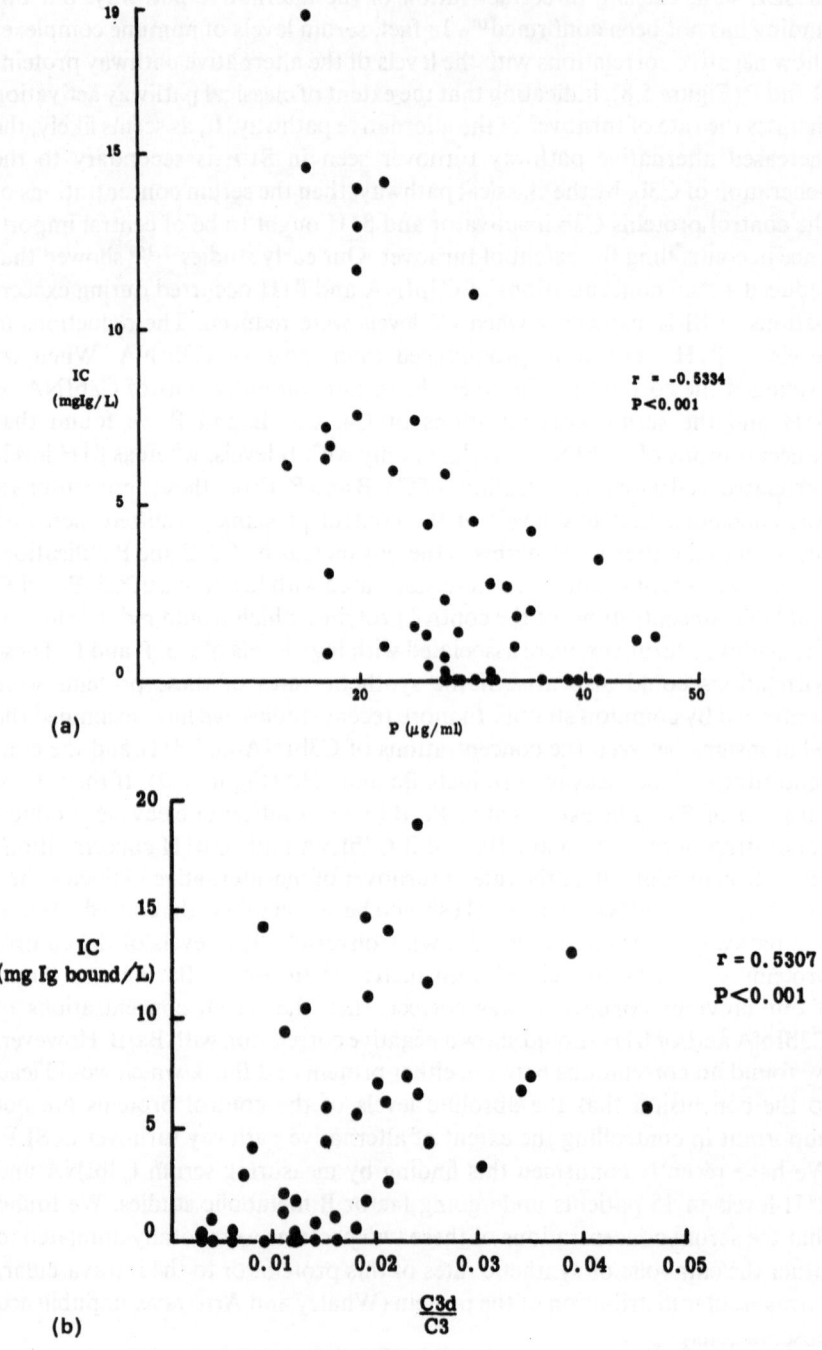

Figure 5.8   Relationship between serum concentrations of (a) immune complexes and properdin, and (b) immune complexes and C3d/C3 in SLE

is considerable evidence for increased utilization of β1H in this disease. Whenever C3 is detected in the glomeruli of renal biopsies from these patients, β1H is always present[107] and their distribution patterns are identical. Likewise β1H may be found with C3 in skin biopsy samples from these patients[114].

Table 5.3   Factor B metabolism and serum C3bINA and β1H concentrations in SLE

Patient	F.C.R (%/h)	E : P ratio	β1H (μg/ml)	C3bINA (% std.)
1	1.36	0.83	252	81
2	1.69	1.28	302	143
3	1.95	1.22	372	143
4	1.77	1.10	286	84
5	2.19	0.79	230	88
6	2.72	0.44	272	109
7	2.20	0.66	157	103
8	1.51	0.95	272	110
9	2.16	0.58	213	95
10	1.78	0.91	288	95
11	1.85	0.75	221	68
12	2.59	0.53	291	118
13	2.42	0.93	252	146
14	2.04	1.05	198	96
15	2.82	0.93	252	130

The evidence supporting hypercatabolism of C3bINA in SLE is less conclusive. Occasionally this enzyme may be detected in the glomeruli during immunofluorescence examination[107], but its pattern of distribution is focal and segmental, which is difficult to explain. The infrequent detection of C3bINA in SLE renal biopsies is almost certainly due to the weak binding of C3bINA to C3b and it is impossible to detect consumption of the protein during complement activation *in vitro*[115].

Complement activation in rheumatoid arthritis

In contrast to SLE, in which complement activation is seen in the blood, in RA serum complement levels are usually elevated except in patients with vasculitis[116]. However, when the synovial fluid is examined, evidence of complement activation is obvious. High concentrations of immune complexes[103,117], reduced concentrations of C1 and its subcomponents C4 and C2[118,119] and the presence of C4 cleavage products[120] all show that classical pathway activation occurs in synovial fluid. Although C$\bar{1}$-INH levels are occasionally reduced in RA synovial fluid, the mean levels do not differ from those found in DJD. There are reduced concentrations of B and P[121,122] and the presence of factor B cleavage products[123-125]. As we have been unable to detect nephritic factor-like substances in RA synovial fluid, it is probable that activation of the alternative pathway in RA results from C3 turnover by the classical pathway convertase. Although the serum concentrations of C3bINA and β1H are high in RA, their synovial fluid concentrations are sometimes extremely low, but their mean levels do not differ from those found in DJD. As in SLE, both in RA serum and synovial fluid the concentrations of C3bINA and β1H correlate well with levels of C3, B and P[25, 126] but again no correlation could be found between the concentrations of C3bINA or β1H and Ba/B. This observation re-emphasizes the probability that concentrations of these two control proteins do not play a major role in dictating the rate of turnover of the alternative pathway in RA. Krick and his colleagues[127] came to a similar conclusion when they found that catabolic rates of B in RA patients were unrelated to the serum concentrations of C3bINA or β1H.

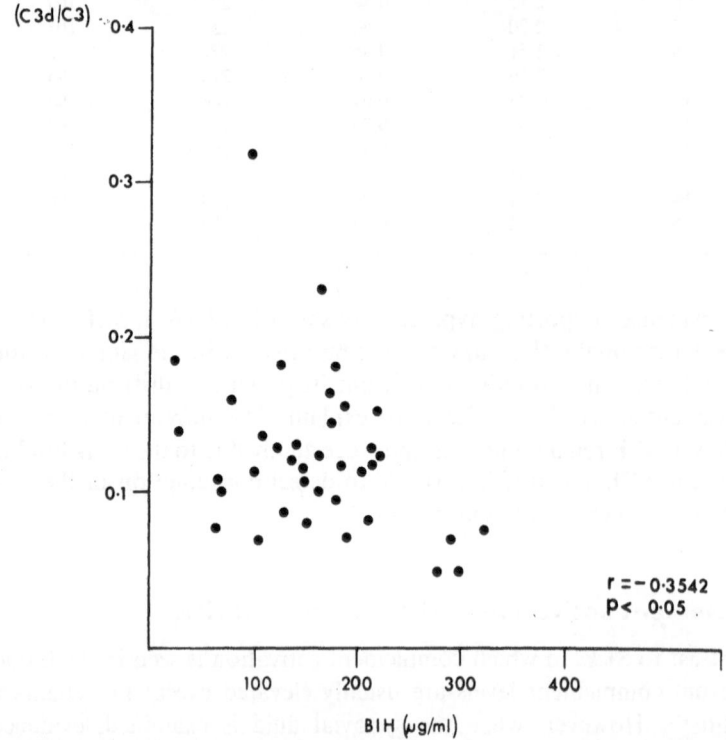

Figure 5.9   Negative correlation between synovial fluid β1H concentrations and C3 turnover (represented as C3d/C3)

We have found a negative correlation between synovial fluid β1H concentrations and C3d/C3 (Figure 5.9). This correlation probably reflects the increased consumption of β1H with accelerated C3 turnover. Thus in both RA and SLE there is little evidence to suggest that the absolute concentrations of the control proteins of the alternative pathway play a significant role in regulating turnover of the alternative pathway. This conclusion is unexpected as absolute deficiency of C3bINA[28, 29] and immunochemical depletion of either C3bINA[30] or β1H[36] results in uncontrolled alternative pathway turnover. However, to reduce turnover of the alternative pathway to its normal level in these depleted sera, one requires to add only between 25 and 50% of their original concentrations. Thus under normal conditions there is a great deal of 'spare' control protein available, which may account for the lack of correlation between B turnover and control protein concentration. Furthermore, measurement of the specific functional activities of $\overline{\text{CI}}$-INH, C3bINA and β1H in normals, SLE and rheumatoid arthritic patients showed that the activity of these control proteins was proportional to their immunochemical concentrations in all three groups. It is also possible that B turnover may be produced by tissue proteases rather than the more specific mechanisms involved in complement activation. Such a mechanism has been proposed by Goldstein and Weissmann[128].

Complement deficiency and connective tissue disease

As a result of the development of techniques for measuring individual components, genetically determined deficiencies of ten complement proteins and two regulatory proteins, $\overline{\text{CI}}$-INH and C3bINA, have been described. Recently there has been a spate of case reports describing genetically determined

Table 5.4 Reported complement component deficiencies and associated connective tissue diseases

Component	Associated diseases	MHC linkage
C1r	Glomerulonephritis; SLE	No
C1s	SLE	
C4	SLE	Yes
C2	SLE; discoid LE; anaphylactoid purpura; Still's; dermatomyositis; 'synovitis'; Hodgkin's	Yes
C3	Severe recurrent infections	No
C5	SLE, recurrent infections	No
C6	Gonococcaemia	Yes
C7	Raynaud's sclerodactyly	No
C8	Gonococcaemia	Yes (1/3)
$\overline{\text{CI}}$-INH	Hereditary angio-oedema; SLE	No
C3bINA	Severe recurrent infections	

Data from reference 135

deficiencies of the complement system in association with glomerulonephritis or connective tissue diseases, usually an SLE-like syndrome, although anaphylactoid purpura, dermatomyositis, Raynaud's syndrome with sclerodactylly discoid LE, and synovitis of the hip have been recorded (Table 5.4). None of the reported cases of C3, C6 or C3bINA deficiency have had associated connective tissue disease. The important association of complement deficiency and connective tissue disease has been re-emphasized by the finding of heterozygous C2 deficiency in 12 families with Still's disease[129].

The association of complement deficiency with connective tissue disease in which complement activation is reputed to play a pathogenetic role is curious; one would have expected complement deficiency to exert a protective effect. Three possible explanations can be proposed. Firstly, C1, C4 and C2 increase the efficiency of neutralization of certain viruses[99] and oncornaviruses activate the classical pathway in the absence of antibody, with resultant virolysis[100], Clearly, therefore, complement deficiency could permit certain viruses to replicate, and perhaps produce disease. Against this argument is the observation that only a few viruses show enhanced neutralization and that patients with complement deficiency do not show an undue frequency of viral infections.

A second mechanism whereby complement deficiency could lead to disease would be by failure of opsonization of immune complexes. Thus complexes may circulate and fail to be removed by normal host defence mechanisms and be deposited in the tissues with consequent inflammation.

The third explanation, and perhaps the most likely, stems from the findings that the genes controlling C2, C4 and factor B polymorphism, and C2, C4 and possibly C8 deficiency are located on the sixth chromosome in the region of the major histocompatibility complex. In mice and guinea-pigs, genes controlling immune responses (Ir genes) have been demonstrated in, or near, the major histocompatibility loci. It is likely that Ir genes in the human are similarly situated. Thus complement deficiencies may be linked to Ir genes, and the latter, rather than the complement deficiency, predispose to the increased frequency of certain rheumatoid diseases.

There are also an increasing number of reports of complement proteins in certain lymphocyte membranes. C4 inhibits the mixed lymphocyte reaction in the human[124]. Perlmann et al.[125] have shown the C8 in lymphocyte membranes is required for cytotoxic reactions. Factor B is present in certain lymphocyte membranes and can form a C3 convertase with cobra venom factor[126], and Budzco et al.[127] have shown that certain malignant lymphoma cell lines carry a preformed alternative pathway C3 convertase. Thus the complement system may not only be a plasma protein system, but also a system of membrane proteins, perhaps involved in cell co-operation. This proposal is supported by the observations of Dierich and Landen[128] who were able to form bridges between cells bearing different complement components which interact with each other.

Acknowledgment

This work was supported by grants HERT 532 and 564 from the Scottish Hospital Endowment Research Trust.

References

1. Kehoe, J. M. and Fougereau, M. (1969). Immunoglobulin peptide with complement fixing activity. *Nature (London)*, **224**, 1212

2. Hurst, M. M., Volanakis, J. E., Stroud, R. M. and Bennett, J. C. (1975). Cī fixation and classical complement pathway activation by a fragment of the Cµ4 domain of IgM. *J. Exp. Med.*, **142**, 1322

3. Porter, R. R. (1977). Structure and activation of the early components of complement. *Fed. Proc.*, **36**, 2191

4. Fearon, D. T., Austen, K. F. and Ruddy, S. (1973). Formation of a hemolytically active cellular intermediate by the interaction between properdin factors B and D and the activated third component of complement. *J. Exp. Med.*, **138**, 1305

5. Fearon, D. T., Austen, K. F. and Ruddy, S. (1973). Properdin factor D: characterization of its active site and isolation of the precursor form. *J. Exp. Med.*, **139**, 355

6. Fearon, D. T. and Austen, K. F. (1975). Properdin: binding to C3b and stabilization of the C3b-dependent C3 convertase. *J. Exp. Med.*, **142**, 856

7. Daha, M. R., Fearon, D. T. and Austen, K. F. (1976). C3 requirements for formation of alternative pathway C5 convertase. *J. Immunol.*, **117**, 630

8. Medicus, R. G., Gotze, O. and Müller-Eberhard, H. J. (1976). Alternative pathway of complement: recruitment of precursor properdin by the labile C3/C5 convertase and the potentiation of the pathway. *J. Exp. Med.*, **144**, 1076

9. Vogt, W., Schmidt, G., Von Buttlar, B. and Dieminger, L. (1978). A new function of the activated third component of complement: binding to C5, an essential step for C5 activation. *Immunology*, **34**, 29

10. Kolb, W. B., Haxby, J. A., Arroyave, C. M. and Müller-Eberhard, H. J. (1972). Molecular analysis of the membrane attack mechanism of complement. *J. Exp. Med.*, **135**, 549

11. Stolfi, R. L. (1968). Immune lytic transformation: a state of reversible damage generated as a result of the reaction of the eighth component in the guinea-pig complement system. *J. Immunol.*, **100**, 46

12. Müller-Eberhard, H. J. (1975). Complement. *Ann. Rev. Biochem.*, **44**, 697

13. Borsos, T., Rapp, H. J. and Mayer, M. M. (1961). Studies on the second component of complement. II. The nature of the decay of EAC'1 42. *J. Immunol.*, **87**, 326

14. Cooper, N. R. and Müller-Eberhard, H. J. (1970). The reaction mechanism of human C5 in immune hemolysis. *J. Exp. Med.*, **132**, 775

15. Donaldson, V. H. and Evans, R. R. (1963). A biochemical abnormality in hereditary angioneurotic oedema. Absence of serum inhibitor of C1-esterase. *Am. J. Med.*, **35**, 37

16. Ruddy, S. and Austen, K. F. (1967). A stoichiometric assay for the fourth component of complement in whole human serum using EAC'1a^{SP} and functionally pure human second component. *J. Immunol.*, **99**, 1162

17. Ruddy, S., Carpenter, C. B., Chin, K. W., Knostman, J. N., Soter, N. A., Gotze, O., Müller-Eberhard, H. J. and Austen, K. F. (1975). Human complement metabolism: an analysis of 144 studies. *Medicine*, **54**, 165

18. Donaldson, V. H., Rosen, F. S. and Bing, D. H. (1977). Role of the second component of complement (C2) and plasmin in kinin release in hereditary angioneurotic edema (H.A.N.E.) plasma. *Trans. Assoc. Am. Phys.*, **90**, 174

19. Scharfstein, J., Ferreira, A., Gigli, I. and Nussenzweig, V. (1978). Human C4-binding protein. I. Isolation and characterization. *J. Exp. Med.*, **148**, 207

20. Fujita, T., Gigli, I. and Nussenzweig, V. (1978). Human C4-binding protein. II. Role in proteolysis of C4b by C3b-inactivator. *J. Exp. Med.*, **148**, 1044

21. Shirishai, S. and Stroud, R. M. (1975). Cleavage products of C4b produced by enzymes in human serum. *Immunochemistry*, **12**, 935

22. Gigli, I., *et al.* (1979). *Proc. Natl. Acad. Sci. USA*, **76**, 6596

23. Lachmann, P. J. and Müller-Eberhard, H. J. (1968). The demonstration in human serum of conglutinogen-activating factor and its effects on the third component of complement. *J. Immunol.*, **100**, 691

24. Ruddy, S. and Austen, K. F. (1969). C3 inactivator of man. I. Hemolytic measurement by the inactivation of cell-bound C3. *J. Immunol.*, **102**, 533

25. Whaley, K., Schur, P. H. and Ruddy, S. (1976). C3b inactivator in the rheumatic diseases. Measurement by radial immunodiffusion by inhibition of formation of properdin pathway C3 convertase. *J. Clin. Invest.*, **57**, 1554

26. Tamura, N. and Nelson, R. A. (1967). Three naturally-occurring inhibitors of components of complement in guinea-pig or rabbit serum. *J. Immunol.*, **99**, 582

27. Pangburn, M. K., Schreiber, R. D. and Müller-Eberhard, H. J. (1977). Human complement C3b inactivator: isolation, characterization, and demonstration of an absolute requirement for the serum protein β1H for cleavage of C3b and C4b in solution. *J. Exp. Med.*, **146**, 257

28. Abramson, N., Alper, C. A., Lachmann, P. J., Rosen, F. S. and Jondl, J. H. (1971). Deficiency of C3 inactivator in man. *J. Immunol.*, **107**, 19

29. Thompson, R. A. and Lachmann, P. J. (1977). A second case of human C3b inhibitor (KAF) deficiency. *Clin. Exp. Immunol.*, **27**, 23

30. Nicol, P. A. E. and Lachmann, P. J. (1973). The alternate pathway of complement activation. The role of C3 and its inactivator (KAF). *Immunology*, **24**, 259

31. Whaley, K. and Ruddy, S. (1976). Modulation of C3b hemolytic activity by a plasma protein distinct from C3b inactivator. *Science*, **193**, 1011

32. Whaley, K. and Ruddy, S. (1976). Modulation of the alternative pathway by β1H globulin. *J. Exp. Med.*, **144**, 1147

33. Pangburn, M. K. and Müller-Eberhard, H. J. (1978). Complement C3 convertase: cell restriction of β1H control and generation of restriction on neuraminidase-treated cells. *Proc. Natl. Acad. Sci. USA*, **75**, 241

34. Conrad, D. H., Carlo, J. R. and Ruddy, S. (1978). Interaction of β1H globulin with cell-bound C3b: quantitative analysis of binding and influence of alternative pathway components on binding. *J. Exp. Med.*, **147**, 1792

35. Weiler, J. M., Daha, M. R., Austen, K. F. and Fearon, D. T. (1976). Control of the amplification convertase of complement by the plasma protein β1H. *Proc. Natl. Acad. Sci. USA*, **73**, 3268

36. Whaley, K. and Thompson, R. A. (1978). Requirements for β1H globulin and C3b inactivator in the control of the alternative complement pathway in human serum. *Immunology*, **35**, 1045

37. Schreiber, R. D. and Müller-Eberhard, H. J. (1978). Assembly of the cytolytic alternative pathway of complement from 11 isolated plasma proteins. *J. Exp. Med.*, **148**, 1722

38. Schreiber, R. D., Morrison, D. C., Podack, E. R. and Müller-Eberhard, H. J. (1979). Bactericidal activity of the alternative complement pathway generated from 11 isolated plasma proteins. *J. Exp. Med.*, **149**, 870

39. Podack, E. R., Kolb, W. P. and Müller-Eberhard, H. J. (1977). The SC5b–7 complex: formation, isolation, properties and submit composition. *J. Immunol.*, **119**, 2024

40. Lint, T. F., Behrands, C. L. and Gewurz, H. (1977). Serum lipoproteins and C567-INH activity. *J. Immunol.*, **119**, 883

41. Podack, E. R., Kolb, W. P. and Müller-Eberhard, H. J. (1978). The C5b–6 complex: formation, isolation and inhibition of its activity by lipoprotein and the S-protein of serum. *J. Immunol.*, **120**, 1841

42. Pangburn. M. K. and Müller-Eberhard, H. J. (1980). *J. Exp. Med.*, **152**, 1115

43. Fearon, D. T. and Austen, K. F. (1976). Properdin: initiation of alternative complement pathway. *Proc. Natl. Acad. Sci. USA*. **72**. 3220

44. Alper. C. A. and Balavitch. D. (1976). Cobra venom factor: evidence for its being altered cobra C3 (the third component of complement). *Science*. **191**. 1275

45. Nagaki, K., Iida, K., Okubo, M. and Inai, S. (1978). Reaction mechanisms of β1H globulin. *Int. Arch. Allergy Appl. Immunol.*, **57**, 221

46. Daha, M. R., Austen, K. F. and Fearon, D. T. (1978). Heterogeneity, polypeptide chain composition and antigenic reactivity of C3 nephritic factor. *J. Immunol.*, **120**, 1389

47. Davis, A. E., Ziegler, J. B., Gelfond, E. W., Rosen, F. S. and Alper, C. A. (1977). Heterogeneity of nephritic factor and its identification as an immunoglobulin. *Proc. Natl. Acad. Sci. USA*, **71**, 3980

48. Scott, D. M., Amos, N., Sissons, J. G. P., Lachmann, P. J. and Peters, D. K. (1978). The immunoglobulin nature of nephritic factor (NeF). *Clin. Exp. Immunol.*, **32**, 12

49. Daha, M. R., Fearon, D. T. and Austen, K. F. (1976). C3 nephritic factor (C3NeF): stabilization of fluid phase and cell-bound alternative pathway convertase. *J. Immunol.*, **116**, 1

50. Fearon, D. T. and Austen, K. F. (1977). Activation of the alternative complement pathway due to resistance of zymosan-bound amplification convertase to endogenous regulatory mechanisms. *Proc. Natl. Acad. Sci. USA*, **74**, 1683

51. Fearon, D. T. and Austen, K. F. (1977). Activation of the alternative complement pathway with rabbit erythrocytes by circumvention of the regulatory action of endogenous control proteins. *J. Exp. Med.*, **146**, 22

52. Fearon, D. T. (1978). Activation of the alternative complement pathway by *E. coli*: resistance of bound C3b to inactivation by C3bINA and β1H. *J. Immunol.*, **120**, 1772 (abstr.)

53. Fearon, D. T. (1978). Regulation by membrane sialic acid of β1H-dependent decay-dissociation of the amplification C3 convertase of the alternative complement pathway. *Proc. Natl. Acad. Sci. USA*, **75**, 1971

54. Aminoff, D., Bell, W. C., Fulton, I. and Ingebrigtsen, N. (1976). Effect of sialidase on the viability of erythrocytes in the circulation. *Am. J. Hematol.*, **1**, 419

55. Nyedegger, U., Fearon, D. T. and Austen, K. F. (1979). 'Regulation by an autosomal locus of the inverse relationship between membrane sialic acid content and the capacity of mouse erythrocytes to activate the human alternative complement pathway.' Presented at the Fourth European Complement Workshop

56. Kazatchkine, M. D., Fearon, D. T. and Austen, K. F. (1979). Human alternative complement pathway membrane associated sialic acid regulates the competition between B and β1H for cell-bound C3b. *J. Immunol.*, **122**, 75

57. Barkas, T. (1978). Biological activities of complement. *Biochem. Soc. Trans.*, **6**, 798

58. Inoue, K. and Kinsky, S. C. (1970). Fate of phospholipids in liposomal model membranes damaged by antibody and complement. *Biochemistry*, **9**, 4767

59. Lachmann, P. J., Bowyer, D. E., Nicol, P., Dawson, P., Dawson, R. M. C. and Munn, E. A. (1973). Studies on the terminal stages of complement lysis. *Immunology*, **24**, 135

60. Kinoshita, T., Inoue, K., Okada, M. and Akiyama, Y. (1977). Release of phospholipids from liposomal model membrane damaged by antibody and complement. *J. Immunol.*, **119**, 73

61. Mayer, M. M. (1972). Mechanism of cytolysis by complement. *Proc. Natl. Acad. Sci. USA*, **69**, 2954

62. Borsos, T., Dourmashkin, R. R. and Humphrey, J. H. (1964). Lesions in erythrocyte membrane caused by immune haemolysis. *Nature (London)*, **202**, 251

63. Humphrey, J. H. and Dourmashkin, R. R. (1969). The lesions in cell membranes caused by complement. *Adv. Immunol.*, **11**, 75

64. Packman, C. H., Rosenfeld, S. I., Weed, R. I. and Leddy, J. P. (1976). Complement-induced ultrastructural membrane lesions: requirements for terminal components. *J. Immunol.*, **117**, 1883

65. Dourmashkin, R. R. (1978). The structural events associated with the attachment of complement components to cell membranes in reactive lysis. *Immunology*, **35**, 205

66. Bhakdi, S. and Tranum-Jensen, J. (1978). Molecular nature of the complement lesion. *Proc. Natl. Acad. Sci. USA*, **75**, 5655

67. Giavedoni, E. B. and Dalmasso, A. P. (1976). The induction by complement of a change in KCNS dissociable membrane lipids. *J. Immunol.*, **116**, 65

68. Bhakdi, S., Speth, V., Knufermann, H., Wallach, D. F. H. and Fischer, H. (1974). Complement-induced changes in the coarse structure of sheep erythrocyte membranes: a study by freeze-etch electron microscopy. *Biochim. Biophys. Acta*, **356**, 300

69. Valet, G. and Opferkuch, W. (1975). Mechanism of complement-induced cell lysis. Demonstration of a three-step mechanism of EAC1-8 lysis by C9, and a non-osmotic swelling of erythrocytes. *J. Immunol.*, **115**, 1028

70. Iles, G. H., Seeman, P., Naylor, D. and Cinader, B. (1973). Membrane lesions in immune lysis. Surface rings, globule aggregates and transient openings. *J. Cell Biol.*, **56**, 528

71. Michaels, D. W., Abramovitz, A. S., Hammer, C. H. and Mayer, M. M. (1976). Increased ion permeability of planar lipid bilayer membranes after treatment with C56–9 cytolytic attack mechanism of complement. *Proc. Natl. Acad. Sci. USA*, **73**, 2852

72. Frank, M. M., Rapp, H. J. and Borsos, T. (1965). Studies on the terminal steps of immune hemolysis. II. Resolution of the E* transformation reaction into multiple steps. *J. Immunol.*, **94**, 295

73. Boyle, M. D. P., Langone, J. J. and Borsos, T. (1979). Studies on the terminal stages of immune hemolysis. IV. Effect of metal salts. *J. Immunol.*, **122**, 1209

74. Johnson, A. R., Hughli, T. E. and Müller-Eberhard, H. J. (1975). Release of histamine from rat mast cells by the complement peptides C3a and C5a. *Immunology*, **28**, 1067

75. Fernandez, H. N., Henson, P. M., Otani, A. and Hugli, T. E. (1978). Chemotactic response to human C3a and C5a anaphylotoxins. I. Evaluation of C3a and C5a leukotaxis *in vitro* and under simulated *in vivo* conditions. *J. Immunol.*, **120**, 109

76. Ward, P. A., Cochrane, C. G. and Müller-Eberhard, H. J. (1966). Further studies on the chemotactic factor of complement and its formation *in vivo*. *Immunology*, **11**, 141

77. Ruddy, S., Austen, K. F. and Goetzl, E. J. (1975). Chemotactic activity derived from interaction of factors D̄ and B of the properdin pathway with cobra venom factor or C3b. *J. Clin. Invest.*, **55**, 587

78. Hadding, U., Hamuro, J. and Bitter-Suermann, D. (1978). Biological activities of the purified Ba fragment derived from guinea-pig factor B of the alternative pathway. *J. Immunol.*, **120**, 1776 (abstr.)

79. Götze, O., Bianco, C. and Cohn, Z. A. (1979). The induction of macrophage spreading by factor B of the properdin system. *J. Exp. Med.*, **149**, 373

80. Arend, W. P. and Mannik, M. (1971). Studies on antigen–antibody complexes: II. Quantification of tissue uptake of soluble complexes in normal and complement-depleted rabbits. *J. Immunol.*, **107**, 63

81. Miller, G. W., Steinberg, A. D., Green, I. and Nussenzweig, V. (1975). Complement-dependent alterations in the handling of immune complexes by NZB/W mice. *J. Immunol.*, **114**, 1166

82. Miller, G. W., Saluk, P. H. and Nussenzweig, V. (1973). Complement-dependent release of immune complexes from the lymphocyte membrane. *J. Exp. Med.*, **138**, 495

83. Czop, J. and Nussenzweig, V. (1976). Studies on the mechanism of solubilization of immune precipitates by serum. *J. Exp. Med.*, **143**, 615

84. Takahashi, M., Tack, B. F. and Nussenzweig, V. (1977). Requirements for the solubilization of immune aggregates by complement. Assembly of a factor B-dependent C3 convertase on the immune complexes. *J. Exp. Med.*, **145**, 86

85. Takahashi, M., Takahashi, S., Brade, V. and Nussenzweig, V. (1978). Requirements for the solubilization of immune aggregates by complement. The role of the classical pathway. *J. Clin. Invest.*, **61**, 349

86. Nelson, R. A. (1953). The immune adherence phenomenon. An immunologically specific reaction between micro-organisms and erythrocytes leading to enhanced phagocytosis. *Science*, **118**, 733

87. Gigli, I. and Nelson, R. A., Jr (1968). Complement dependent immune phagocytosis. I. Requirements for C'1, C'4, C'2, C'3. *Exp. Cell Res.*, **51**, 45

88. Wellek, B., Hahn, H. H. and Opferküch, W. (1975). Evidence for macrophage C3d-receptor active in phagocytosis. *J. Immunol.*, **114**, 1643

89. Leigh, P. C. J., Van den Barselaar, M. Th., Van Zwet, T. L., Daha, M. R. and Van Furth, R. (1979). Requirement of extracellular complement and immunoglobulin for intracellular killing of micro-organisms by human monocytes. *J. Clin. Invest.*, **63**, 772

90. Dukor, P., Schumann, G., Gisler, R. H., Dierich, M., Konig, W., Hadding, U. and Bitter-Suerman, D. (1974). Complement-dependent B-cell activation by cobra venom factor and other mitogens. *J. Exp. Med.*, **139**, 337

91. Pepys, M. A. (1974). Role of complement in induction of antibody production *in vivo*. Effect of cobra venom factor and other C3 reactive agents on thymus-dependent and thymus-independent antibody responses. *J. Exp. Med.*, **140**, 126

92. Pryzma, J. and Humphrey, J. H. (1975). Prolonged C3 depletion by cobra venom factor in thymus-deprived mice and its implication for the role of C3 as an essential second signal for B-cell triggering. *Immunology*, **28**, 569

93. Alper, C. A., Colten, H. R., Gear, J. S. S., Robson, A. R. and Rosen, F. S. (1976). Homozygous C3 deficiency: The role of C3 in antibody production, CTs-induced vaso-permeability, and cobra venom-induced passive hemolysis. *J. Clin. Invest.*, **57**, 222

94. Klaus, G. G. B. and Humphrey, J. H. (1977). The generation of memory cells. I. The role of C3 in the generation of B memory cells. *Immunology*, **33**, 31

95. Papamichail, M., Guttierez, C., Embling, P., Johnson, P., Holborow, E. J. and Pepys, M. G. (1975). Complement dependence of localization of aggregated IgG in germinal centres. *Scand. J. Immunol.*, **4**, 343

96. Henson, P. M. and Cochrane, C. G. (1969). Immunological induction of increased vascular permeability. II. Two mechanisms of histamine release from rabbit platelets involving complement. *J. Exp. Med.*, **129**, 167

97. Zucker, M. B., Grant, R. A., Alper, C. A., Goodkofsky, I. and Lepow, I. H. (1974). Requirements for complement components and fibrinogen in zymosan-induced release reaction of human platelets. *J. Immunol.*, **113**, 1744

98. Perrin, L., Joseph, B. S., Cooper, N. R. and Oldstone, M. B. A. (1976). Mechanism of injury of virus-infected cells by antiviral antibody and complement: participation of IgG, F(ab')$_2$, and the alternative complement pathway. *J. Exp. Med.*, **143**, 1027

99. Daniels, C. A., Borsos, T., Rapp, H. J., Snyderman, R. and Notkins, A. L. (1970). Neutralization of sensitized virus by purified components of complement. *Proc. Natl. Acad. Sci. USA*, **65**, 528

100. Welsh, R. M., Cooper, N. R., Jensen, F. C. and Oldstone, M. B. A. (1975). Human serum lysis RNA tumor viruses. *Nature (London)*, **257**, 612

101. Rouse, B. T., Grewal, A. S. and Babiuk, L. A. (1977). Complement enhances antiviral antibody-dependent cell cytotoxicity. *Nature (London)*, **266**, 456

102. Nydegger, U. E., Lambert, P. E., Gerber, H. and Meischer, P. A. (1974). Circulating immune complexes in the serum in systemic lupus erythematosus and in carriers of hepatitis B antigen. Quantitation by binding to radiolabelled Clq. *J. Clin. Invest.*, **54**, 297

103. Scullion, M., Balint, G. and Whaley, K. (1979). Evaluation of the Clq solid-phase binding assay for immune complexes. A clinical and laboratory study. *J. Clin. Lab. Immunol.*, **2**, 15

104. Schur, P. H. (1975). Complement in lupus. In Rothfield, N. F. (ed.) *Clinics in Rheumatic Diseases, Systemic Lupus Erythematosus*. Vol. I, pp. 519–543. (London: W. B. Saunders Co. Ltd.)

105. Koffler, D., Agnello, V., Carr, R. I. and Kunkel, H. G. (1969). Variable patterns of immunoglobulin and complement deposition in the kidneys of patients with systemic lupus erythematosus. *Am. J. Pathol.*, **56**, 305

106. Verroust, P. J., Wilson, C. B., Cooper, N. R., Edgington, T. S. and Dixon, F. J. (1975). Glomerular complement components in human glomerulonephritis. *J. Clin. Invest.*, **53**, 77

107. Moseley, H. L. and Whaley, K. (1979). Evidence for the glomerular modulation of complement activation. *J. Clin. Lab. Immunol.*, **2**, 9

108. Gwyn-Williams, D., Peters, D. K., Fallows, J., Petrie, A., Kourilsky, O., Morel-Maroger, L. and Cameron, J. S. (1974). Studies of serum complement in the hypocomplementaemic nephritides. *Clin. Exp. Immunol.*, **18**, 391

109. Whaley, K., Schur, P. H. and Ruddy, S. (1979). Relative importance of C3b inactivator and β1H globulin in the modulation of the properdin amplification loop in systemic lupus erythematosus. *Clin. Exp. Immunol.*, **36**, 408

110. Perrin, L. H., Lambert, P. H. and Meischer, P. A. (1975). Complement breakdown products in plasma from patients with systemic lupus erythematosus and patients with membranoproliferative or other glomerulonephritids. *J. Clin. Invest.*, **56**, 165

111. Charlesworth, J. A., Gwyn-Williams, D., Sherington, E., Lachmann, P. and Peters, D. K. (1974). Metabolic studies of the third component of complement and the glycerine-rich beta-glycoprotein in patients with hypocomplementemia. *J. Clin. Invest.*, **53**, 1578

112. Ziegler, J. B., Rosen, F. S., Alper, C. A., Grupe, W. and Lepow, I. H. (1975). Metabolism of properdin in normal subjects and patients with renal disease. *J. Clin. Invest.* **56**, 761

113. Arroyave, C. M., Wilson, M. R. and Tan, E. M. (1976). Serum factors activating the alternative complement pathway in autoimmune disease: description of two different factors from patients with systemic lupus erythematosus. *J. Immunol.*, **116**, 821

114. Carlo, J. R., Rothfield, N. F. and Ruddy, S. (1979). Demonstration of β1H globulin together with C3 in the dermal–epidermal junction of patients with systemic lupus erythematosus. *Arth. Rheum.*, **22**, 13

115. Whaley, K., Ward, D. J. and Ruddy, S. (1978). Modulation of the properdin amplification loop in membranoproliferative and other forms of glomerulonephritis. *Clin. Exp. Immunol.*, **35**, 101

116. Franco, A. E. and Schur, P. H. (1971). Hypocomplementemia in rheumatoid arthritis. *Arth. Rheum.*, **14**, 231

117. Winchester, R. J., Agnello, V. and Kunkel, H. G. (1970). Gammaglobulin complexes in synovial fluids of patients with rheumatoid arthritis: partial characterization and relationship to lowered complement levels. *Clin. Exp. Immunol.*, **6**, 689

118. Fostiropoulos, G., Austen, K. F. and Bloch, K. J. (1965). Total hemolytic complement (CH^{50}) and second component of complement (C2^{hu}) activity in serum and synovial fluid. *Arth. Rheum.*, **8**, 219

119. Ruddy, S. and Austen, K. F. (1970). The complement system in rheumatoid synovitis: I. An analysis of complement component activities in rheumatoid synovial fluids. *Arth. Rheum.*, **13**, 713

120. Perrin, L. H., Shiraishi, S., Stroud, R. M. and Lambert, P. H. (1975). Detection and quantitation in plasma and synovial fluid of a fragment of human C4 with mobility generated during the activation of the complement system. *J. Immunol.*, **115**, 32

121. Ruddy, S., Fearon, D. T. and Austen, K. F. (1975). Depressed synovial fluid levels of properdin and properdin factor B in patients with rheumatoid arthritis. *Arth. Rheum.*, **18**, 289

122. Whaley, K. (1978). Modulation of complement activation: a pharmacotherapeutic goal. In Dumonde, D. C. and Jasani, M. K. (eds.) *The Recognition of Anti-Rheumatic Drugs*, pp. 55–68. (Lancaster: MTP Press)

123. Zvaifler, N. J. (1974). Rheumatoid arthritis: an extravascular immune complex disease. *Arth. Rheum.*, **17**, 297

124. Lambert, P. H., Nydegger, U. E., Perrin, L. H., McCormick, J., Fehr, K. and Meischer, P. A. (1975). Complement activation in seropositive and seronegative rheumatoid arthritis.

^{125}I C1q binding capacity and complement breakdown products in serum and synovial fluid. *J. Rheumatol.*, **6**, 52

125. El-Ghobarey, A. and Whaley, K. (1979). Alternative pathway complement activation in rheumatoid arthritis. *J. Rheumatol.*, **7**, 453

126. Whaley, K., Widener, H. and Ruddy, S. (1977). Modulation of the alternative pathway amplification loop in rheumatic disease. In Opferkuch, K., Rother, K. and Schultz, D. R. (eds.) *Clinical Aspects of the Complement System* (International Symposium, Bochum), pp. 999–111. (Stuttgart: Thième)

127. Krick, E. H., de Heers, D. H., Kaplan, R. A., Arroyave, C. M. and Vaughan, J. H. (1978). Metabolism of factor B of serum complement in rheumatoid arthritis. *Clin. Exp. Immunol.*, **34**, 1

128. Goldstein, I. M. and Weismann, G. (1974). Generation of C5-derived lysosomal enzyme-releasing activity (C5a) by lysates of leukocyte lysosomes. *J. Immunol.*, **113**, 1583

129. Glass, D., Raum, D., Gibson, D., Stillman, J. and Schur, P. H. (1976). Inherited deficiency of the second component of complement. Rheumatic disease associations. *J. Clin. Invest.*, **58**, 853

130. Ferrone, S., Pellegrino, M. A. and Cooper, N. R. (1976). Expression of C4 on human lymphoid cells and possible role in immune phenomena. *Science*, **193**, 109

131. Perlmann, P., Perlmann, H. and Lachmann, P. J. (1974). Lymphocyte-associated complement: role of C8 in certain cell-mediated lytic reactions. *Scand. J. Immunol.*, **3**, 77

132. Hobart, M. J. and Lachmann, P. J. (1976). Allotypes of complement components in man. *Transplant Rev.*, **32**, 26

133. Budzco, D. B., Lachmann, P. J. and McConnell, I. (1976). Activation of the alternative complement pathway by lymphoblastoid cell lines derived from patients with Burkitt's lymphoma and infectious mononucleosis. *Cell Immunol.*, **22**, 98

134. Dierich, M. P. and Landen, B. (1977). Complement bridges between cells. Analysis of a possible cell–cell interaction mechanism. *J. Exp. Med.*, **146**, 1484

135. Ruddy, S. (1977). Complement, rheumatic diseases and the major histocompatibility complex. *Clin. Rheum. Dis.*, **3**, 215

6
Immunogenetics and Rheumatology

D. F. ROBERTS and J. WENTZEL

In the last decade there has been a remarkable development in knowledge of immunogenetics as applied to man. Genetic factors have been shown to be implicated at a number of points in both the humoral and cellular immune responses. In the humoral response, following the definition of the molecular structure of the immunoglobulins, the number of genes controlling the regions of their several chains has been indicated, and also how they act[1]. The marker allotypes, the *Gm, Inv* and *Am* groups, have been shown to be due to single amino acid substitutions which are point mutations in the sequences coding for the chains of immunoglobulin[2]. Besides these qualitative differences, some genetic influence on the level of the immunoglobulins in apparently healthy individuals has been demonstrated[3], and though many deficiencies are non-genetic the inherited bases of several, especially of IgA and IgM, have been established[4-8]. In the complement system, similarly, there are polymorphisms—different alleles at the same locus producing slightly different substances—in each of the components of complement except C5, and again there are genes responsible for a deficiency of specific components[9-13]. The existence of genetically controlled circulating antibodies has long been known.

At the cellular level, blood-group antigens on the red cells were the earliest to be discovered[14]. Lymphocytes have provided particularly vigorous development, notably in the exploration of the human chromosome major histocompatibility region[15, 16], the identification of a large number of alleles at the loci controlling the HLA-A and HLA-B antigens, and rather smaller numbers at the HLA-C and D loci. The differentiation of B and T cells by rosetting and immunofluorescence has led to the identification of B cell types and T cell types, again under genetic control, and indeed another major polymorphic system of cell surface antigens (reminiscent of mouse Ia antigens) has been established in man.

These developments have had a profound effect on rheumatology. It was perhaps prophetic that discovery of the *Gm* groups originated in a study of rheumatoid factor in the blood of patients with rheumatoid arthritis[17].

SOME GENETIC CONSIDERATIONS

Antibodies are immunoglobulin molecules each composed of four polypeptide chains, two light chains (each about 200 amino acids) and two heavy chains (each about 400 amino acids), the chains being joined by disulphide bonds[18]. The amino acid sequences of the chains show great variety at the *N*-terminal end of the polypeptide, the variable region, as opposed to the invariable remainder, the constant region. The variable regions of adjacent light and heavy chains give a configuration to that part of the molecule which combines with the antigen. Each variable region of an immunoglobulin polypeptide chain has three hypervariable regions, considerably increasing its specificity.

Controlling these structures are the genes. There appear to be three linkage groups, probably on separate chromosomes, two for the light chains (one each for kappa and lambda) and one for heavy chains. Each such linkage group contains sets of genes for the variable region (the *V* genes), closely linked to the genes for the constant regions (the *C* genes). In man there appear to be at least 10 genes or gene sets for the C-region and four for the V-region of the heavy chains, two for the constant and five for the variable region of the lambda light chains, and only one for the constant and three for the variable region of the kappa light chains.

At a specific point in these gene sets are located the genes determining the allotypes. The *Gm* (standing for *g*enetic *m*arker or *gam*maglobulin) system comprises some 24 factors, each inherited according to simple Mendelian laws, and these are characteristic of the IgG heavy chains only, most being located in the Fc fragment but *Gm 3*, *4* and *17* in the Fd fragment. The *Inv* factors (standing for *in*hibitor *v*), with only three factors, are found in the light chains of the kappa type only.

A major area of genetic as well as clinical interest is the association between susceptibility to different diseases and genes of the major histocompatibility system in man. At about the middle of the short arm on chromosome no. 6, in what is known as the major histocompatibility region, there are several closely linked loci. Antigens controlled by several of these loci are serologically detectable, and are notable for their great polymorphism. At the HLA-A locus there appear to be available some 20 different alleles, of which about a dozen are routinely tested for in most laboratories working with the histocompatibility system. At the HLA-B locus there appear to be about 25 to 30 alleles available, and most laboratories test for about 15 of these. At the C locus there are some eight alleles, of which five are routinely tested for. These antigens are usually identified on lymphocytes by microcytotoxicity testing, but they also exist in many other tissues. Alleles at the fourth locus (the HLA-D locus) have not usually been sought serologically, being lymphocyte-defined by mixed lymphocyte culture. Lymphocytes from different individuals when mixed together stimulate proliferation, by an amount depending upon the number of gene differences at this locus in the two individuals. There would be virtually no stimulation when the two individuals are identical at this locus, but pronounced stimulation where there are one or two gene differences between them. Inhibition of DNA synthesis of one participant's cells, rendering them incapable of responding but not affecting their stimulating capacity, allows the response of one population of cells at a time to be studied. Once homozygotes at this locus are identified, then their cells can be incorporated in the reaction with an unknown individual, and so the particular genes present in the latter can be determined. There also appears to be a minor locus contributing to this reaction.

These histocompatibility loci are very close together on the chromosome; crossing over between the A and B loci occurs on only 0.8% and between the B and D loci on 1% of occasions. A curious feature about the genes present in the major histocompatibility region is that there is linkage disequilibrium, that is to say a tendency for some combinations of genes that are linked together to occur much more frequently than expected by chance in the population. For example, the combinations HLA-1 and B8, A3-B7, and A2-B12 occur much more often than would be expected from the frequency of the particular alleles. Similar disequilibrium has been observed to include the C and D loci. The fact that these loci have been identified does not preclude the possibility that there may be other genes within the same region, some of which may have similar functions to the HLA genes.

Related to the major histocompatibility region is one locus governing the serologically detected B-cell alloantigens, that determining the Ly-Li system which is close to that for HLA-D. However, there appear to be several loci involved, one of which governing the Ly-Co system is outside the HLA region. The Li gene products are sufficiently well-defined to allow their attribution to a distinct DR locus (= D related), with at least seven alleles designated DR W1 to DR W7; it is indeed likely that the DRW specifities are essentially those of the D locus but detected by a different technique.

Other genes are thought to occur in this region, though evidence for them is still only circumstantial. It has been postulated that genetic factors other than those already mentioned are responsible for eliciting a delayed hypersensitivity reaction during transplantation. These HDR genes are believed to map within the major histocompatibility region, since they segregate with the HLA haplotype in family studies, and to be closer to the A and B loci than to the D. In animals, immune response (*Ir*) genes exist, as has been shown by studies of the inheritance of the immune response to artificially made antigens. Such genes are transmitted as dominants, and are linked to the genes controlling the major histocompatibility antigens. The *Ir* gene product is thought to be a receptor for antigens on the T lymphocytes. The existence of *Ir* genes in man remains to be demonstrated, but if the animal analogy holds they can be expected to lie in or close to the major histocompatibility region; indeed the strong HLA associations with disease have been interpreted as indicating their occurrence.

Certainly within this region occur several of the genes affecting the complement system, the series of proteins present in the serum and which complement the action of antibodies in the defence against invasive proteins. The complement system is a complex system of factors activated by antibody–antigen interactions, forming a triggered protein cascade; that is to say, the activation of one component by a trigger activates a further component, which in turn activates another further down the cascade. Each component is under separate genetic control. The genetics of the system is known through the occurrence of specific factor deficiencies, partial deficiencies, and the occurrence of genetically distinct variant forms of each component except C5. Genes controlling the C2, C4, C8 and the proactivator of the C3 component of complement are known to be located in the major histocompatibility region.

IMMUNOGENETIC INVOLVEMENT IN RHEUMATOLOGY

So much attention has been given to the association of the HLA system with various rheumatological disorders that it is easy to overlook their other immunogenetic correlations. There is evidence that both the production of circulating antibody and the establishment of cell-mediated or delayed hypersensitivity reactions may be disturbed in rheumatoid arthritis (RA). The rheumatoid factor (RF) is an antibody found in the serum of many rheumatoid arthritis patients. This is generally considered to be an autoantibody or constellation of autoantibodies and reacts with the patient's own γ-globulin, although in some patients it reacts with IgG which possesses *Gm* groups different from the patient's own. RF may react with IgG of human, guinea-pig or rabbit origin and occasionally all these reactions may be detected in the same patient's serum[19].

RF is usually IgM, is produced by plasma cells of lymph nodes and in the synovium, and may circulate in complexes with seven IgG molecules or dissociated into 7S and 19S fragments. However, some rheumatoid sera show complexes of intermediate size (9–17S) composed entirely of IgG molecules; these are particularly relevant in rheumatoid synovitis, and it seems that IgG antiglobulins also occur in some seronegative rheumatic conditions such as ankylosing spondylitis, psoriatic arthropathy and Still's disease. It has been suggested that intermediate complexes of 11–15S formed by an IgG rheumatoid factor and seven IgG molecules may be implicated in the pathogenesis of vasculitis and of pulmonary fibritis, and RF itself is known to be capable of becoming attached to the walls of small blood vessels[19].

The appearance of RF is thought more likely to be a consequence than a cause of rheumatoid arthritis. Not all patients with RA have circulating RF, while it may be detected in normal subjects and in patients with some viral, bacterial and parasitic infections, and indeed most subjects with IgM RF antiglobulin activity in their serum do not have rheumatoid arthritis; hence the ability to synthesize RF, presumably genetically controlled, is not restricted to RA patients alone. However, RA is more severe and its extra-articular complications are more frequent in the presence of high-titre RF. IgM RF activates the classical complement pathway through its own sites of complement attachment and the ability of rheumatoid RF to fix complement is particularly important in rheumatoid synovitis. In view of the genetic involvement in the structure of these molecules and their affinities, the genetic relevance of these considerations is that only those individuals capable of producing them are susceptible to the trigger to do so, so that there is a genetic predisposition to these disorders; the question is how important that predisposition is in each of the various disorders. A similar argument applies to the other antibody types that occur: the antinuclear antibodies characteristic of SLE that are found in established rheumatoid patients with vasculitis; the granulocyte-specific RNA of Felty's syndrome.

Abnormalities in the cell-mediated immune response have also been described in RA. The response to dinitrochlorobenzene is reduced in sero-positive RA although the tuberculin reaction is normal. There is an increase in the ratio of RNA to DNA in lymphocytes, suggesting increased protein synthesis, while lymphocyte transformation *in vitro* with mitogens such as phytohaemagglutinin gives abnormal results. The one-way mixed lymphocyte culture technique shows a marked reduction in the response of rheumatoid cells to other rheumatoid cells but a normal response to control cells and a normal ability to stimulate control cells[20, 21]. Similar impairment has been noted in cells from ankylosing spondylitis and psoriatic arthritis patients[22].

Rheumatic fever is a connective tissue disease which affects young people and is caused by an abnormal reaction to infection with β-haemolytic streptococcus. Tests for rheumatoid factor are negative. It has been suggested that repeated infection may lead to sensitization by the cross-reacting antigen in the streptococcal membrane and hence to an auto-immune type of disease process[69]. An antibody that binds to heart tissue is present in and is virtually unique to the serum of rheumatic fever patients[23]. A genetic factor was suggested as long ago as 1889, when Cheadle noted a familial aggregation. Early studies[24–26] suggested that susceptibility to rheumatic fever is based on a single autosomal gene, recessive in effect. This seems unlikely, for the inheritance of rheumatic fever does not follow a Mendelian pattern[27, 28], while a study of rheumatic fever patients and their monozygotic and dizygotic twins[29] showed that if single genetic factors operate they have only limited penetrance.

It is much more likely in this as in most rheumatological disorders (other than those where the joint involvement is secondary to some other simply inherited process, for example in alkaptonuria) that the aetiology is multifactorial and any genetic component polygenic (Figure 6.1). Liability to develop the disease is regarded as being under the control of a system of many genes situated at a number of loci interacting with each other. Some genes promote liability to this disease, their alleles the reverse, just as some genes promote tall stature and their alleles short. Liability of an individual to develop the disease depends on the loading of genes promoting it that he

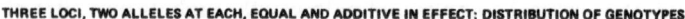

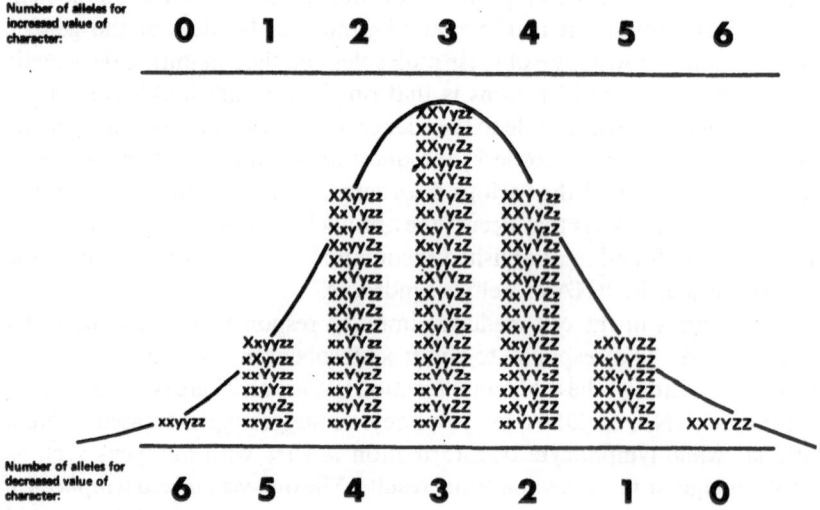

Figure 6.1 A simplified model of polygenic inheritance of a disorder. Here three loci are shown, at each of which the upper-case letter represents a gene making for increased liability and a lower-case letter for decreased liability. With all gene frequencies equal, the different combinations produce a histogram approaching a normal Gaussian curve, with which the fit would improve the greater the number of loci considered. The position of an individual in the distribution does not depend on whether he has a particular gene, but on the loadings that he has of the genes making for increased liability. Individuals of the same liability can therefore be genetically heterogeneous

possesses. Were it possible to plot the number of individuals of a given liability in the population, a Gaussian distribution curve would be produced, just as in the case of stature. Towards one end of the distribution in a given environment there occurs a threshold. Individuals who possess the appropriate loading of genes for susceptibility fall beyond this threshold and develop the disease. On this model first-degree relatives of patients have a higher risk of developing the disorder than do random members of the population, second-degree relatives a risk not quite so elevated but still above that for a random person

(Figure 6.2); these risks are considerably lower than those for simple Mendelian disorders. But just as stature can be influenced by differences in nutrition during growth, and improvement of nutrition for the whole population would shift the distribution curve so that fewer individuals fall beyond the threshold for small stature (Figure 6.3), so also environment may affect the position of an individual relative to the threshold for a rheumatological disorder. All the factors suggested as triggers for the condition, trauma, and stress would affect the position of the individual relative to the threshold. Thus on this model it is not the presence or absence of a particular gene that determines the development of the disorder, it is the loading of the relevant polygenes that determines the position of the individual relative to the threshold of clinical manifestation. Whether or not he transgresses it depends upon his exposure to the necessary environmental trigger. The relative importance of genetic factors in such disorders is assessed by the heritability—the proportion of the total variance in liability to develop the condition that is attributable to inheritance—expressed usually as a percentage.

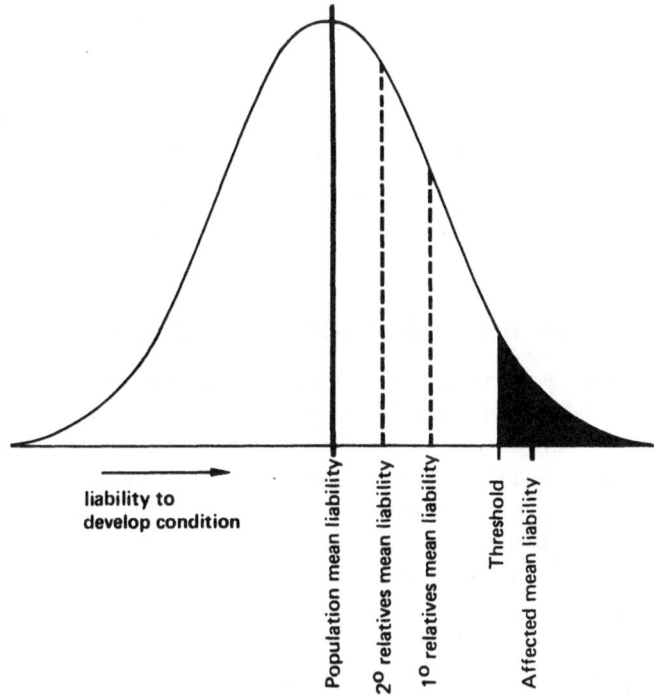

Figure 6.2 Since first-degree relatives have 50% of their genes in common, the first-degree relatives of patients have a mean liability halfway between that of the patients and the population as a whole. The second-degree relatives have one-quarter of their genes in common with the patients, so their mean liability falls three-quarters of the distance between the patient mean and the population mean and fewer of them transgress the threshold. The positions of the means and distributions give relatives of patients an increased incidence of the disorder

Such considerations show how widely ranging are the possibilities of immunogenetic influence in the rheumatological disorders. Most immuno-genetic investigation has, however, concentrated on the HLA associations.

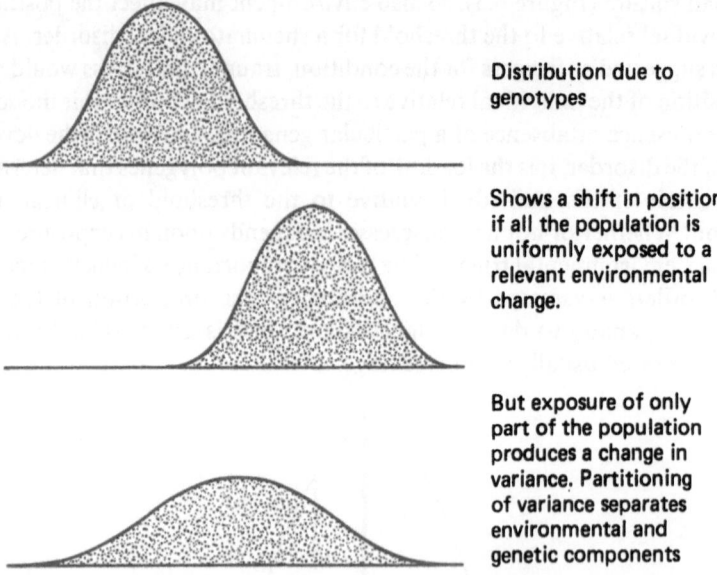

Distribution due to genotypes

Shows a shift in position if all the population is uniformly exposed to a relevant environmental change.

But exposure of only part of the population produces a change in variance. Partitioning of variance separates environmental and genetic components

Figure 6.3 Estimation of the genetic component in liability is achieved by analysis of variance from family data

HLA TYPES AND RHEUMATOLOGICAL DISEASE

The first report by Brewerton of a major association of HLA B27 with ankylosing spondylitis prompted many similar enquiries into this and other arthropathies[30]. Ankylosing spondylitis with its strong male predominance and familial incidence is an erosive arthropathy, starting usually with low-back pain and progressing throughout the spine and to the peripheral joints. Several hundred patients have now been investigated in over a dozen different studies, and there is no doubt at all about the closeness of the HLA associ-ation. Whereas B27 is present in about 8% of the population in Britain, it occurs in approximately 90% of patients. An individual born with HLA B27 would be some 87 times as likely to develop ankylosing spondylitis as some-body without that antigen[31]—that is to say, the relative risk is said to be 87. This association provides one marker of genetic predisposition as a primary basis for the disease. In practical terms it also provides a useful diagnostic tool in that it may help to assign to the correct category a patient presenting with symptoms which may or may not be those of ankylosing spondylitis, and so initiate treatment rather earlier than would otherwise be possible. Yet despite the closeness of the association, it is not absolute. It seems that only about 20% of HLA B27 positive subjects develop the disorder, as the number of individuals in the population who develop the disorder is lower than those with the HLA B27 antigen. Not only is the genetic predisposition necessary, but so is the trigger—whatever that may be—for the development of the disorder. Hence it is not yet possible to employ the B27 antigen in families to identify those at risk of developing ankylosing spondylitis with a view to preventive treatment. Figure 6.4 shows representative families.

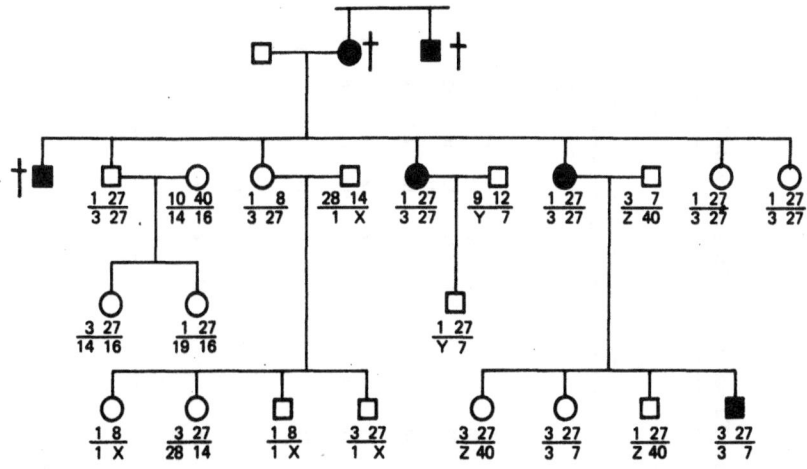

X, Y, Z unidentified HLA specificities

ANKYLOSING SPONDYLITIS

Figure 6.4a A family in which transmission of ankylosing spondylitis appears to parallel that of HLA-B27; only a proportion of those with B27 show the disorder

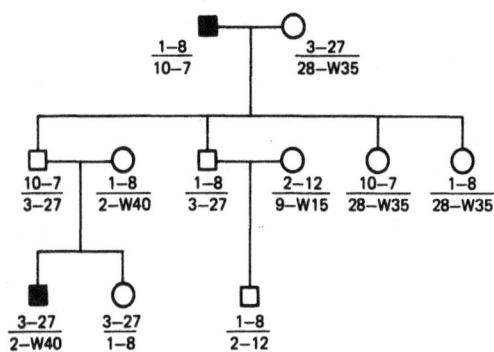

Figure 6.4b A family in which ankylosing spondylitis does not appear to be transmitted with the B27 gene

Table 6.1　Phenotype frequencies (%) of some selected HLA antigens in European RA patients and controls.

Ref.	No. of patients	No. of controls	A2		A3		A9		B5		B7		B13		B15		B27		B40		Cw3		Dw4		DRw4	
			Pat.	Cont.	Pat.	Cont.	Pat.	Cont.	Pat.	Cont.	Pat.	Cont.	Pat.	Cont.	Pat.	Cont.	Pat.	Cont.	Pat.	Cont.	Pat.	Cont.	Pat.	Cont.	Pat.	Cont.
43	122	384	18	30	11	20	25	29	21	18	7	13	7	8	21	10	14	3	21	9			69	13		24
82	28	456													4	4	9	14			18	7			61	
83	11	89																								
48	27	250	59	50			6	17			30	29			19	9	22	10	6	10						
84	45	686	67	55			27	10			11	29			18	26	49	13	9	14						
32	46	1200	51	48			20	22			17	23			11	11	13	10	13	9	20	16				
45	78																91									
85	104	102	62	54	28	26	12	27	13	8	23	14	3	7	13	23	10	6	14	10						
86	62	114	64	58			18	15			39															
87	54	398	54	50			15	19			0	3			4	4	4	5	6	4						
88	125	300	50	47	26	25	24	19	12	13	17	21	10	13	14	8	16	13	10	8						
89	39	51					11	20			24	21			19	10	19	9	13	16	33*	17	36	13		
90	38	700	63	50			56	25	50	33										0						
37	32																									
40	95	200																							77	34
46	70	120	66	45	34	48	7	20	11	11	18	20	9	3	27	18	36	16	14	18						
91	50	300	44	47			18	22			14	19					14	9	16	7						
41	119	906	49	48			20	22			13	25			11	8	8	8								
34	54	68																					54	16		
47	47	1967	60	54	17	27	17	23	13	11	15	27	2	4	19	18†	13	9	17	18	40	35†	54	44‡	70	28

*n = 30, †n = 1291, ‡n = 36, §n = 157

The related disorder of Reiter's syndrome shows a similar association with the B27 antigen. The resemblance is not perceptible in the acute stage of the full syndrome, which includes involvement of the skin, joints and mucous membranes, and only later may it resemble ankylosing spondylitis. In the several studies, the numbers of patients that have been investigated run into several hundred, and about 75% of them have the B27 antigen, representing a relative risk[31] of 37. Another related disorder, acute anterior uveitis, in which an appreciable proportion of patients shows ankylosing spondylitis, Reiter's disease, or sacro-iliitis, though mostly to a mild degree, shows the same B27 association. Several studies indicate that from 35 to 70% of patients carry the antigen, representing a relative risk[31] of 11. Besides this high relative risk for the condition in patients with this particular allele, the association has shown the existence of a common element in the aetiology, which has helped understanding of all three disorders.

Table 6.2   HLA antigen frequencies in RA—combined results from Table 6.1

Antigens	Patients		Controls		χ^2	p	Relative risk
	%	n	%	n			
A2	55.0	815	49.6	7499	8.20	<0.005	1.11
A3	24.9	358	26.5	2945	0.37	n.s.	
A9	19.8	847	20.4	7499	1.62	n.s.	
B5	15.0	406	12.2	2945	2.36	n.s.	
B7	17.7	815	22.5	7385	9.82	<0.005	
B13	8.6	374	5.5	2945	4.95	<0.05	1.56
B15	12.5	865	12.9	7669	0.07	n.s.	
B27	23.1	882	9.1	7664	169.2	≪0.001	2.54
B40	14.3	768	12.8	6607	1.30	n.s.	
Cw3	30.9	123	25.5	2542	1.49	n.s.	
Dw4	57.0	251	14.4	660	168.6	≪0.001	3.96
DRw4	68.3	271	27.5	652	131.8	≪0.001	2.48

Rheumatoid arthritis

Positive associations have been claimed in Europeans and European-derived populations between rheumatoid arthritis and HLA antigens A2, A9, A10[32]; B5, B13, B27, B40; Cw1[32], Cw3, Dw4, DRw3[33]; and DRw4[34]. Negative associations have been claimed with A3[35], A9, B7 and DRw2[33]. Increased frequencies of the HLA haplotypes A2–B27 in Europeans and A9–B5 in Iranians have also been alleged[36, 37]. Table 6.1 shows the results obtained by various workers for some selected HLA specificities, while Table 6.2 combines these results to give overall frequencies of antigens in patients and controls. The associations between RA and Dw4, DRw4 and B27 are highly significant, while the positive association with A2 and negative association with B7 are also significant, though at a much lower level.

HLA-Dw4 and DRw4 are believed by many to be the same antigen specificity (or equivalent antigen specificities) detected by different techniques. RA patients who have both DRw4 and rheumatoid factor are more likely to get a severe form of the disease[38] while healthy women[39] with rheumatoid factor do not have a higher incidence of Dw4 than the general population. Thus having both Dw4 (or DRw4) and RF in rheumatoid arthritis seems to indicate poor prognosis. DRw3 is also stated to be increased in severely affected patients with a high-titre RF[40].

HLA-B15, B40 and Cw1 are all found in linkage disequilibrium with Dw4, and reports of their increased frequency in RA can be explained on this basis. The raised incidence of B13 sometimes reported may be due to cross-reactions with B40.

The associations of B27 with ankylosing spondylitis is well established[30, 41] and it has been suggested that the excess of B27 in RA may be due to what is actually ankylosing spondylitis being misdiagnosed as RA. Julkunen, in a longterm study of AS patients[42], found the disease to begin as a joint disease in 38% of patients and in only 49% as a spondylitis and thus a degree of misdiagnosis is likely. The 7th International Histocompatibility Workshop, in an attempt to avoid this complication, excluded from its study of RA all patients with sacroiliitis or a family history of AS[43]. Nevertheless, a slight excess of B27 (16%) in patients compared with controls (8%) was found which is significant at the $p = 0.05$ level.

Table 6.3   Frequency of HLA-B27 in RA patients and controls

Reference	RA patients		Controls
	RF+	RF−	
45		91% (71/78)	
46	27% (11/41)	48% (14/29)	16% (19/120)
47	13% (6/47)*		9% (169/1967)
combined	19% (17/88)	79% (85/107)	9% (188/2087)

RF+ compared with controls, $\chi^2 = 9.34$, $p < 0.005$
RF− compared with controls, $\chi^2 = 418.3$, $p \ll 0.001$
RF+ compared with RF− $\chi^2 = 67.6$, $p < 0.001$
* 37/47 RA patients are RF+

HLA-B27 is more common in seronegative than seropositive RA[44–47]; the combined results (Table 6.3) show the incidence of B27 to be significantly higher ($p < 0.001$) in seronegative patients compared either to seropositive patients or to controls. However, the incidence of B27 in seropositive patients remains significantly higher (19%) than in controls (9%) ($p < 0.005$). This may represent either a genuine increase of B27 or a residue of yet-undiagnosed AS cases. The finding[48] that the increase of B27 in RA patients was significant compared with controls but not compared with the patients' first-degree relatives may be important here.

Table 6.4 Phenotype frequencies of some selected HLA antigens in European Still's disease patients and controls

Ref.	No. of patients	No. of controls	A2 Pat.	A2 Cont.	B7 Pat.	B7 Cont.	B15 Pat.	B15 Cont.	B27 Pat.	B27 Cont.	B40 Pat.	B40 Cont.	Cw1 Pat.	Cw1 Cont.	Dw3 Pat.	Dw3 Cont.	Dw4 Pat.	Dw4 Cont.	DRw4 Pat.	DRw4 Cont.
55	34	314	61	48	20	25	15	10	29	9										
54	46	1205							26	8	13	14			46	12				
60	63								32	8										
57	62	450	63	50	13	22	8	13	31	9	6	10								
92	47	326					49	26	17	14	13	15								
56	46								39											
93	26	267	65	47	19	26	11	10	42	6	19	12								
58	112	1863	66	50			20	9	26	8										
34	30–112	65–71	67	48	21	30	4	8	29	9	17	10								
94	24												13	5			11	16	7	30
53	35	1000	64	49	3	19	23	11	58	7	6	12								

Antigen

Keats and Barnes[45] suggest that the features of rheumatoid arthritis may be determined by closely linked immune response (*Ir*) genes (relating to spondylitis, sacroiliitis, peripheral small joint disease and oligoarthritis) either as separate entities or in various combinations, so that RA results from the expression of specific *Ir* genes within the major histocompatibility region. HLA-27 may be a marker for an aberrant immune response to some antigen(s), this aberration leading to arthritis. The observation[49, 50] that, of the patients with a *Yersinia* infection, those with B27 are more likely to contract arthritis strongly supports this idea. It has been suggested[51] that in patients not possessing B27 a dissociation may have occurred between the *Ir* and HLA genes.

Very little research has been reported on non-European RA patients. Toyoda *et al.*[52] found that in Japan, where RA is virtually absent from the population, B27 was not increased, but Bw22 occurred twice as frequently (48%) in RA patients as in controls. Nakagawa *et al.* (quoted in HLA and Disease Registry Report[31]) found no significant deviations.

Still's disease

Still's disease is a polyarthritis of children occurring usually between the ages of 1 and 3 in females and 2 and 16 in males. In the latter, it often appears to be triggered by the onset of puberty. Rheumatoid factor is not generally detectable. There appears to be little general agreement among rheumatologists as to what distinguishes 'Still's disease' from 'juvenile chronic polyarthritis' or 'juvenile rheumatoid arthritis'. For the present discussion, following the

Table 6.5   HLA antigen frequencies in Still's disease—combined results from Table 6.4

Antigens	Patients		Controls		χ^2	p	Relative risk
	%	n	%	n			
A2	64.3	305	48.9	5210	25.2	<0.001	1.31
B7	14.5	193	22.4	2922	6.14	<0.02	
B15	19.6	352	11.2	5111	22.0	<0.001	1.75
B27	31.1	495	8.1	5425	262.5	≪0.001	3.84
B40	13.2	326	12.6	4844	0.06	n.s.	
Dw3	46	35	12	69	13.4	<0.001	3.83
Dw4	11	112	16	65	1.27	n.s.	
DRw4	7	30	30	71	5.06	<0.05	

system of Veys *et al.*[53], the term 'juvenile chronic polyarthritis' (JCP) will be used to refer to the more common seronegative arthritis of children, 'juvenile rheumatoid arthritis' (JRA) to a seropositive arthritis with a disease pattern more closely resembling that of adult rheumatoid arthritis, and 'Still's disease' to the whole group.

HLA deviations reported in Still's disease are similar to those found in adult RA; increase in HLA-A2, B15 and B27 and a decrease in B7 (Table 6.4). Gershwin et al.[54] report a statistically significant increase in Dw3 (Table 6.5) while the decrease in DRw4 reported by Stastny[34] requires further investigation.

As with adult RA the increase of B27 in Still's disease can be largely attributed to overt or undiagnosed ankylosing spondylitis. About half the Still's disease patients with B27 had overt AS or a pauciarticular arthritis consistent with early AS[53, 55–58] while long-term studies show that over a period of around 15 years about 8% of patients develop AS[56, 59]. However, not all patients with B27 develop AS[56] and many workers believe that the excess of B27 'far exceeds the possible future outcome in ankylosing spondylitis'[60].

Besides spondylitis, B27 appears to be associated with sacroiliitis in Still's disease. Veys et al.[53] found B27 in 19 out of 20 (95%) seronegative patients with sacroiliitis but in only 11% of patients without sacroiliitis, while Gibson et al.[61] found the incidence of B27 to be only 15% in 123 patients without sacroiliitis or spondylitis.

The few reports on juvenile chronic polyarthritis show antigen frequencies very similar to those found for Still's disease[56, 62]. This is hardly surprising as the majority of Still's disease patients are probably JCP. In juvenile rheumatoid arthritis, by contrast, B27 appears not to be raised. Veys et al.[53] found no B27 in six JRA patients, while Edmonds et al.[56] found no B27 in 11 such patients.

Mitsui et al.[63] found no significant variation in the frequencies of Japanese patients with 'juvenile rheumatoid arthritis', but an excess of A9 and B40 ($p < 0.001$). However, it is not clear from this paper what proportion of the patients were JCP and what JRA.

Rheumatic fever and rheumatic heart disease

Joysey et al.[64] found an increased incidence of HLA-B15 in rheumatic heart disease patients. Leirisalo et al.[50] found an increased incidence of Bw35 in rheumatic fever patients, and of B18 in those patients who had had carditis. Ward et al.[65] found significantly more A29 and Aw30/Aw31 in heart disease patients with a history of rheumatic fever compared with those without such history but not compared with normal controls. Other studies of mixed groups of rheumatic fever/rheumatic heart disease patients have suggested higher frequencies of B17[66] and lower of A3[35] and A28[66].

Table 6.6 shows the data obtained by various workers for some HLA-A and B locus specificities. Combining the data (Table 6.7) suggests that overall there is a slight excess of B15 and B27 in all patients with slightly raised frequencies of B17 and Bw35 in rheumatic fever patients and of A2 in rheumatic heart disease patients. None of these increases, however, is dramatic. A reduced frequency of B5 postulated by Leirisalo[50], on the basis of the finding by

Table 6.6   HLA phenotype frequencies of some selected HLA antigens in European rheumatic fever and/or rheumatic heart disease patients and controls

			Antigen																								
			A2		A3		A9		A28		B5		B7		B13		B15		B17		B18		B27		Bw35		B40	
Ref.	No. of patients	No. of controls	Pat.	Cont.	Pat.	Cont.	Pat.	Cont.	Pat.	Cont.	Pat.	Cont.	Pat.	Cont.	Pat.	Cont.	Pat.	Cont.	Pat.	Cont.	Pat.	Cont.	Pat.	Cont.	Pat.	Cont.	Pat.	Cont.
66	50*	514	62	53	14	27	20	19	0	2	12	12	26	31	8	4			22	6			4	7	6	9	16	16
35	76*	177	51	46	15	28	25	22	5	5	16	9	18	26	8	4	4	3					11	6	21	22	7	12
50	109†	326	59	55	46	42	17	18	12	12	10	13	28	29	6	8	25	26	5	4	9	5	14	14	37	19	11	15
65	75†	1000	45	47	31	30	17	17	4	6	10	10	33	27	5	4	7	15	9	10	8	8	14	8	11	14	7	13
64	94‡	1507	64	52	25	25	13	18	9	5	11	9	21	27	8	8	17	6	10	8	3	4	10	8	18	11	12	13
50	86‡	326	65	55	37	42	17	18	11	12	8	13	14	29	8	8	27	26	3	4	8	5	17	14	23	19	28	15
65	133‡	1000	54	47	32	30	20	17	4	6	8	10	32	27	5	4	10	15	5	10	9	8	11	8	11	14	11	13

* Mixed rheumatic fever and rheumatic heart disease, † rheumatic fever, ‡ rheumatic heart disease

Table 6.7   HLA antigen frequencies in RF/RHD—combined results from Table 6.6

Antigen	Controls %	RF/RHD patients			RF patients			RHD patients			All patients		
		%	χ^2	p	%	χ^2	p	%	χ^2	p	%	χ^2	p
A2	50.5	55.6	1.05	n.s.	53.3	0.42	n.s.	60.1	10.12	<0.005	57.1	9.06	<0.05
A3	28.4	14.3	11.32	<0.001	39.7	10.31	<0.005	31.3	1.07	n.s.	30.3	0.90	n.s.
A9	18.3	23.0	1.50	n.s.	17.4	0.05	n.s.	16.9	0.28	n.s.	18.3	0	n.s.
A28	5.2	2.4	1.47	n.s.	7.6	1.46	n.s.	7.3	2.56	n.s.	6.4	1.20	n.s.
B5	9.8	14.3	2.19	n.s.	7.1	1.24	n.s.	8.9	0.20	n.s.	9.5	0.04	n.s.
B7	27.5	21.4	1.98	n.s.	30.4	0.60	n.s.	24.0	1.67	n.s.	25.4	1.15	n.s.
B13	4.2	7.9	3.32	n.s.	6.0	0.99	n.s.	6.4	2.89	n.s.	5.0	0.66	n.s.
B15	11.2	3.9	1.97	n.s.	17.4	5.92	<0.02	16.6	6.51	<0.02	15.2	5.40	0.02
B17	4.5	22.0	29.67	<0.001	9.2	7.40	<0.01	5.1	0.11	n.s.	7.8	10.13	<0.005
B18	5.6				7.6	0.98	n.s.	5.8	6.5×10^{6}	<0.005	6.4	0.43	n.s.
B27	8.4	7.9	0.0004	n.s.	13.6	5.31	<0.05	12.1	4.60	<0.05	11.7	6.79	<0.01
Bw35	12.5	15.1	0.53	n.s.	25.0	22.96	<0.001	16.3	3.40	n.s.	18.6	16.63	<0.001
B40	13.5	10.3	7.62	<0.01	9.2	2.38	n.s.	15.7	0.98	n.s.	12.7	0.23	n.s.

Table 6.8 Frequencies of selected HLA antigens in psoriatic patients without arthritis and in controls

Ref.	No. of patients	No. of controls	B13 Pat.	B13 Cont.	Bw16 Pat.	Bw16 Cont.	B17 Pat.	B17 Cont.	B27 Pat.	B27 Cont.	B37 Pat.	B37 Cont.	Bw38 Pat.	Bw38 Cont.	Cw6 Pat.	Cw6 Cont.	Dw11 Pat.	Dw11 Cont.
95	87	198	7	1			10	1	25	19								
96	24	200	16	5			21	6	33	9								
78	50	110	22	3	6	5	38	7	6	7								
97	32	160	13	8	3	11	28	11	13	9	0	0	0	7				
98	72	5046	19	6	13	3	25	8	6	8	6	2					22*	5†
99	61	204	20	3	7	3	46	10	7	7	4	2						
100	65	302	22	7	3	5	34	8	8	12	2	0						
76	10	326	10	8	20	12	60	4	0	14								
101	101	113	9	7	22	5	31	6	8	6								
102	25	100	8	15	4	5	24	5	20	14	0	3						
103	45	231	51	9			20	9										
104	45	1967	27	3							16	1						
105	44	89					23	9	14	10								
106	40	405													50	7		
107	110	231	13	4	9	5	22	4	7	10								
108	156	2103	18	4			32	8	8	8								
109	156	386	15	5			26	8	6	9								
110	125	233	7	5			50	6	12	8								

*n = 56   †n = 376

Table 6.9 Frequencies of selected HLA antigens in patients with psoriatic arthritis and in controls

Ref.	No. of patients	No. of controls	Antigen frequency (%)															
			B13		Bw16		B17		B27		B37		Bw38		Cw6		Dw11	
			Pat.	Cont.	Pat.	Cont.	Pat.	Cont.	Pat.	Cont.	Pat.	Cont.	Pat.	Cont.	Pat.	Cont.	Pat.	Cont.
74	60	300	12	5			12	6	38	7								
96	34	200	21	3			36	7	24	9								
78	67	110			1	5	28	8	24	7	0	0						
77	65	433					21	11	32	8								
97	28	160	7	8	39	11	19	6	21	9	7	2	37	7				
75	70	152	13	5			25	8	23	4	1	3	24	3				
100	60	302	18	7	7	5			27	12								
111	18								44									
76	36	326	25	8	11	12	8	4	42	14								
112	82	1000	7	4			20	6	28	8								
102	25	100	0	15	12	5	20	5	48	14	12	3						
73	40	256	7	4	17	6	22	9	28	6								
113	44	2103	12	4	12	5	29	8	21	8								

Greenberg et al.[67] that lymphocytes of B5 carriers respond better in vitro to some streptococcal antigens than do lymphocytes of non-carriers, was not observed.

A family study[35] showed a higher incidence of shared antigens in parents of patients with rheumatic fever (75% of 28 couples) compared with parents of unaffected children (32% of 22 couples)—whereas 79% of normal individuals have three or four different antigens at the HLA-A and B loci, only 56% of patients do so. This suggests an association between rheumatic fever and HLA homozygosity, and ought to be further investigated.

Berning et al.[31] found no significant C locus associations in 21 rheumatic heart disease patients while possible D and DR associations apparently remain to be investigated.

Among non-Europeans, Gorodezky et al.[68] reported a significant absence of A3 and a barely significant deviation of Bw22 in Mexican (mestizo) rheumatic heart disease patients. Caughey et al.[66] investigated Maori patients with rheumatic fever or rheumatic heart disease. Increases of A3 and B8 and a decrease in A10 were found, but these differences were not significant after correction for the number of tests done. Read et al. in a study of East Indian families living in Trinidad[69] found an increased incidence of B5 among the mothers of children with rheumatic fever.

Psoriatic arthritis

Psoriatic arthritis is an inflammatory arthritis distinguished from rheumatoid arthritis by the criteria of Moll and Wright[70]. The fact that the histology of

Table 6.10 Some HLA antigen frequencies in psoriasis and psoriatic arthritis—combined results from Tables 6.8 and 6.9

| Antigen | Frequency (%) | | χ^2 | p | Relative risk |
	Patients	Controls			
PSORIASIS ALONE					
B13	15	6	224.07	≪0.001	1.50
Bw16	10	4	37.52	≪0.001	1.48
B17	30	8	911.70	≪0.001	1.83
B27	11	9	7.12	<0.01	1.05
B37	5	1	15.86	<0.001	1.70
Bw38	0	7	4.43	<0.02	
Cw6	50	7	65.82	≪0.001	2.51
Dw11	22	5	34.82	≪0.001	1.81
PSORIATIC ARTHRITIS					
B13	13	4	93.02	≪0.001	1.84
Bw16	12	6	13.58	<0.001	1.38
B17	18	7	83.88	≪0.001	1.54
B27	37	9	405.38	≪0.001	1.97
B37	3	2	4.0×10^6	n.s.	1.21
Bw38	28	5	49.98	≪0.001	1.97

joints in psoriatic arthritis is similar to that of RA while IgG rheumatoid factor can be isolated from these joints has led to the suggestion that the two diseases may have a common pathogenesis[71, 72]. Sacroiliitis and/or ankylosing spondylitis is common in psoriatic arthritis, being as high as 58% in one series[73].

Several HLA antigens have been found to be increased in frequency in psoriasis uncomplicated by arthritis—Cw6, Dw11, B13, Bw16, B17, B37 (Table 6.8). These increases, though definite, are not dramatic and may represent different aetiologies of psoriasis or linkage relationships to *Ir* genes. Where psoriasis occurs with arthritis these HLA antigen frequencies appear to be similarly increased, as are two other antigens—B27 and Bw38 (Table 6.9)[31]. Relative risks from the combined data are given in Table 6.10.

There is a suggestion that both B27 and Bw38 may be involved in peripheral rather than central arthropathy[74–76]. More recently, B27 has been strongly implicated in arthritis with distal interphalangeal joint involvement[77, 78].

CONCLUSIONS

At first sight there appears to be some discrepancy between the different types of evidence. On the one hand, clinical genetics fails to find any clear evidence of simple Mendelian inheritance for any of the rheumatological disorders here discussed; for example in ankylosing spondylitis only 4% of first-degree relatives develop it as compared with the 50% expected with single-gene inheritance. Instead, the clinical data fit well a multifactorial model of inheritance, in which the genetic component is polygenic. As judged by radiographic evidence of bilateral sacroiliitis, with or without other manifestations of ankylosing spondylitis[79], liability to develop AS has a high heritability of $72.5 \pm 10.2\%$. On the other hand, those working on HLA associations look more to single-gene inheritance and attribute the associations to loci linked with HLA and immune response genes, and the lack of completeness of association, to breakdown of the necessary linkage disequilibrium. Certainly, the latter is far too simple, for with known rates of crossing-over relatively few generations would be required for the associations to disappear, unless there was intense selection for the linkage disequilibrium and this appears very unlikely in the rheumatic disorders. Both views can be reconciled, however, if among the battery of polygenes influencing the liability to develop the condition are some of major effect. For this there is good evidence; for example, the pronounced effect of HLA alleles in the ankylosing spondylitis group, the much less pronounced but positive effect of the A and B blood-group genes in rheumatic heart disease and the negative effect of the secretor gene in rheumatic fever. Such major genes act in the same way as other members of the battery of polygenes, except that the effect of each is correspondingly greater and therefore is open to selection. On this hypothesis, if some such major genes are located in the major histocompatibility region, it is not necessary to postulate an individual gene for susceptibility to a given disorder located in that region.

In addition, however, the HLA associations, whatever the mechanism by which their effect is brought about, have done much to change thinking on rheumatological disorders. They have suggested aetiological similarities, particularly in the ankylosing spondylitis group. They have suggested heterogeneity in other conditions. For example, in reactive arthritis B27 frequency appears to be increased when *Yersinia* or *Salmonella* is involved, but not in meningococcal arthritis; similarly, in juvenile arthritis the B27 antigen frequency is apparently increased when the spine is involved but not otherwise, while in psoriasis B27 appears to be associated with the development of arthritis. Moreover, patients suffering from a particular disorder with or without the appropriate antigen appear to differ in the nature of the disorder; in *Yersinia* arthritis patients without the B27 antigen usually have a mild or otherwise atypical disease[49].

In view of these advances made since immunogenetic mechanisms have been considered in rheumatology, there is obviously a great deal more to be learned. There is still considerable scope for investigations of possible associations between HLA-D and DR loci antigens and rheumatoid disease. Nevertheless, such associations have been clearly shown to exist in adult RA and Still's disease, and the B-locus associations found in other rheumatoid conditions indicate that D/DR antigens, in linkage disequilibrium with the B antigens, are likely to be involved here also. All forms of rheumatoid disease seem to be characterized by immunological abnormalities and thus may involve specific *Ir* genes, for which certain D/DR antigens are markers. An alternative hypothesis is that HLA molecules may be directly involved in the immunological response, different molecules having, for example, different abilities for displaying antigenic determinants for T cells[80, 81]. At present, however, the nature and mode of action of the genetic traits leading to the development of rheumatic disease is unknown.

Acknowledgments

The original Newcastle laboratory investigations incorporated in some of the tables of HLA associations were made possible by the support of the Wellcome Foundation, for which acknowledgment is gratefully made.

References

1. Milstein, C. and Munro, A. J. (1973). Genetics of immunoglobulins and of the immune response. In Porter, R. R. (ed.) *Defence and Recognition*, pp. 199–228 (London: Butterworth)

2. Grubb, R. (1970). *The Genetic Markers of Human Immunoglobulins*. (London: Chapman and Hall)

3. Billewicz, W. Z., McGregor, I. A., Roberts, D. F., Rowe, D. S. and Wilson, R. J. M. (1974). Family studies in immunoglobulin levels. *Clin. Exp. Immunol.*, **16**, 13

4. Grundbacher, F. J. (1972). Genetic aspects of selective immunoglobulin. A deficiency. *J. Med. Genet.*, **9**, 344

5. Ketch, R. P., Franklin, M. and Schmickel, R. D. (1971). Group D deletion syndrome. *J. Med. Genet.*, **8**, 341

6. Grundbacher, F. J. (1972). Human X chromosome carries quantitative genes for immunoglobulin M. *Science*, **178**, 311

7. Waldmann, T. A., Broder, S., Krakauer, R., Durm, M., Meade, B. and Goldman, C. (1976). Defects in immunoglobulin A secretion and in immunoglobulin A specific suppressor cells in patients with isolated immunoglobulin A deficiency. *Clin. Res.*, **24**, 483A

8. Tomkin, G. H., Mawhinney, M. and Nevin, N. C. (1971). Isolated absence of IgA with autosomal dominant inheritance. *Lancet*, **2**, 124

9. Day, N. K., Geiger, H., Stroud, R., De Bracco, M., Mancado, B., Windhorst, D. B. and Good, R. A. (1972). C′3 deficiency: an inborn error associated with cutaneous and renal disease. *J. Clin. Invest.*, **51**, 1102

10. Klemperer, M. R., Woodworth, H. C., Rosen, F. S. and Austen, K. F. (1966). Hereditary deficiency of 2nd component of complement in man. *J. Clin. Invest.*, **45**, 880

11. Polley, M. J. (1968). Inherited C′2 deficiency in man. *Science*, **161**, 1149

12. Leddy, J. P., Frank, M. M., Gaither, T., Baum, J. and Klemperer, M. R. (1974). Hereditary deficiency of the 6th component of complement in man. I. *J. Clin. Invest.*, **53**, 544

13. Boyer, J. T., Gall, E. P., Norman, M. E., Nilsson, U. R. and Zimmerman, T. S. (1975). Hereditary deficiency of the seventh component of complement. *J. Clin. Invest.*, **56**, 905

14. Landsteiner, K. (1901). Uber Agglutinationserscheinungen normalen menschlichen Blutes. *Wien. Klin. Wochenschr.*, **14**, 1132

15. Bodmer, W. F., Bodmer, J. G., Batchelor, J. R., Festenstein, H. and Morris, P. (eds.) (1978). *Histocompatibility Testing 1977*. (Copenhagen: Munksgaard)

16. *Bulletin, World Health Organization* (1975). **52**, 261

17. Grubb, R. (1956). Agglutination of erythrocytes coated with incomplete anti-Rh by certain rheumatoid arthritic sera and some other sera. The existence of human serum groups. *Acta Pathol. Microbiol. Scand.*, **39**, 195

18. Putnam, F. W. (1974). Comparative structural study of human IgM, IgA and IgG immunoglobulins. In Brent, L. and Holborow, J. (eds.) *Progress in Immunology, II*. Vol. 1. (Amsterdam: North Holland)

19. Dick, W. C. (1972). *An Introduction to Clinical Rheumatology*. (London and Edinburgh: Churchill Livingstone)

20. Astorga, G. P. and Williams, R. C. Jr. (1969). Altered reactivity in mixed lymphocyte culture of lymphocytes from patients with rheumatoid arthritis. *Arthr. Rheum.*, **12**, 547

21. Hedberg, H., Kallen, B., Low, B. and Nilsson, O. (1971). Impaired mixed leucocyte reaction in some different diseases, notably multiple sclerosis and various arthritides. *Clin. Exp. Immunol.*, **9**, 201

22. Wee, S. L. and Daymond, T. J. (1978). Diminished mixed lymphocyte response in ankylosing spondylitis. *Tiss. Antigens*, **11**, 409

23. Zabriskie, J. B., Hsu, K. C. and Seegal, B. C. (1970). Heart reactive antibody associated with rheumatic fever characterization and diagnostic significance. *Clin. Exp. Immunol.*, **7**, 147

24. Wilson, M. G. and Schweitzer, M. D. (1954). Pattern of hereditary susceptibility in rheumatic fever. *Circulation*, **10**, 699

25. Wilson, M. G., Schweitzer, M. D. and Lubschez, R. (1943). The familiar epidemiology of rheumatic fever: genetic and epidemiological studies: genetic studies. *J. Pediatr.*, **22**, 468

26. Gray, F. G., Quinn, R. W. and Quinn, J. P. (1952). A longterm survey of rheumatoid and non-rheumatoid families—with particular reference to environment and heredity. *Am. J. Med.*, **13**, 400

27. Stevenson, A. C. and Cheeseman, E. A. (1953). Heredity and rheumatoid factor. A study of 462 families ascertained by an affected child and 51 families ascertained by an affected mother. *Ann. Eugen. Lond.*, **17**, 177

28. Uchida, I. A. (1953). Possible genetic factors in the etiology of rheumatic fever. *Am. J. Hum. Genet.*, **5**, 61

29. Taranta, A., Torosday, S., Matrakos, J. D., Jegier, W. and Uchida, I. (1959): Rheumatic fever in monozygotic and dizygotic twins. *Circulation*, **20**, 773

30. Brewerton, D. A., Caffrey, M., Hart, F. D., James, D. C. O., Nicholls, A. and Sturrock, R. D. (1973). Ankylosing spondylitis and HLA-B27. *Lancet*, **1**, 904

31. HLA and Disease Registry. (1979). *Third Report.* (Copenhagen: Munksgaard)

32. Ivaskova, E., Dostal, C., Sajdlova, H., Macurova, H., Bartfield, R. and Hronkova, J. (1978). Rheumatoid arthritis. In *Histocompatibility Testing 1977*, p. 429. (Copenhagen: Munksgaard)

33. Panayi, G. S. and Wooley, P. H. (1977). B lymphocyte alloantigens in the study of the genetic basis of rheumatoid arthritis. *Ann. Rheum. Dis.*, **36**, 365

34. Stastny, P. (1978). Association of the B-cell alloantigen DRw4 with rheumatoid arthritis. *N. Engl. J. Med.*, **298**, 869

35. Falk, J. A., Fleischman, J. L., Zabriskie, J. B. and Falk, R. E. (1973). A study of HL-A antigen phenotypes in rheumatic fever and rheumatic heart disease patients. *Tiss. Antigens*, **3**, 173

36. Terasaki, P. I. and Mickey, R. R. (1975). HL-A haplotypes of 32 diseases. *Transplant. Rev.*, **22**, 105

37. Nikbin, D., Davatchi, F. and Ala, F. (1977). HLA A9-B5 haplotype in rheumatoid arthritis. *J. Rheumatol.* (Suppl.) 3, 111

38. Roitt, I. M., Corbett, M., Festenstein, H. and Jaraquemada, D. (1978). HL-A, DRw4 and prognosis in rheumatoid arthritis. *Lancet*, **1**, 990

39. Engelman, E. G., Sponzilli, E. E., Batey, M. E., Ramcharam, S. and McDevitt, H. O. (1978). Mixed lymphocyte reaction in healthy women with rheumatoid factor. *Arthr. Rheum.*, **21**, 690

40. Panayi, G. S., Wooley, P. and Batchelor, J. R. (1978). Genetic basis of rheumatoid disease: HLA antigens, disease manifestation and toxic reactions to drugs. *Br. Med. J.*, **2**, 1326

41. Schlosstein, L., Terasaki, P. J., Bluestone, R. and Pearson, C. M. (1973). High association of HL-A antigen W27 with ankylosing spondylitis. *N. Engl. J. Med.*, **288**, 704

42. Julkunen, H. (1962). Rheumatoid spondylitis. *Acta Rheum. Scand.* (Suppl.) 4, 30

43. Batchelor, J. R. and Morris, P. J. (eds.) (1978). Joint Report—HLA and Disease. In *Histocompatibility Testing 1977*, p. 205. (Copenhagen: Munksgaard)

44. Cleland, L. G., Hay, J. A. R. and Milazzo, S. G. (1975). The relation of HL-A27 to disease pattern in seronegative rheumatoid arthritis. *Scand. J. Rheumatol.*, **4** (Suppl.) 8, Abs. 30–20

45. Keats, A. C. and Barnes, R. M. (1976). HL-A27 associated arthritis. *Rheum. Rehabil.*, **15**, 87

46. Pasternack, A. and Tiilikainen, A. (1977). HLA-B27 in rheumatoid arthritis and amyloidosis. *Tiss. Antigens*, **9**, 80

47. Thomsen, M., Morling, N., Snorrason, E., Svejgaard, A. and Sorensen, S. F. (1979). HLA-Dw4 and rheumatoid arthritis. *Tiss. Antigens*, **13**, 56

48. Collin, C., Wentzel, J. and Roberts, D. F. (1979). HLA in families with rheumatoid arthritis (unpublished observations)

49. Aho, K., Ahvonen, P., Lassus, A., Sievers, K. and Tiilikainen, A. (1974). HL-A27 in reactive arthritis. A study of *Yersinia* arthritis and Reiter's disease. *Arthr. Rheum.*, **17**, 521

50. Leirisalo, M., Laitinen, O. and Tiilikainen, A. (1977). HLA phenotypes in patients with rheumatic fever, rheumatic heart disease and *Yersinia* arthritis. *J. Rheumatol.* (Suppl.) 3, 78

51. Dick, H. M., Sturrock, R. D., Dick, W. C. and Buchanan, W. W. (1974). Inheritance of ankylosing spondylitis and HL-A antigen W27. *Lancet*, **2**, 24

52. Toyoda, K., Saito, S., Naito, S., Konomi, K., Yamamoto, H., Nobunaga, M., Nomoto, K. and Takeya, K. (1977). HLA antigens in classical and malignant rheumatoid arthritis in Japanese population. *Tiss. Antigens*, **10**, 56

53. Veys, E. M., Coigne, E., Mielants, H. and Verbruggen, A. (1976). HLA and juvenile chronic polyarthritis. *Tiss. Antigens*, **8**, 61

54. Gershwin, M. E., Opelz, G., Terasaki, P. I., Castles, J. J. and Gorman, T. A. (1977). Frequency of HLA-Dw3 in juvenile rheumatoid arthritis. *Tiss. Antigens*, **10**, 330

55. Buc, M., Nyulassy, S., Stefanovik, J., Michalko, J. and Mozolova, D. (1974). HL-A system and juvenile rheumatoid arthritis. *Tiss. Antigens*, **4**, 395

56. Edmonds, J., Morris, R. I., Metzgar, A. L., Bluestone, R., Terasaki, P. I., Ansell, B. and Bywaters, E. G. L. (1974). Follow-up study of juvenile chronic polyarthritis with particular reference to histocompatibility antigen w27. *Ann. Rheum. Dis.*, **33**, 289

57. Macurova, H., Isaskova, E., Havelka, S. and Ivanyi, P. (1976). HLA antigens in juvenile rheumatoid arthritis. *J. Immunogenet.*, **3**, 229

58. Schaller, J. G., Ochs, H. D., Thomas, E. D., Nisperos, Feigl, P. and Wedgewood, R. J. (1976). Histocompatibility antigens in childhood-onset arthritis. *J. Pediatr.*, **88**, 926

59. Ansell, B. (1969). Still's disease followed into adult life. *Proc. R. Soc. Med.*, **62**, 49

60. Havelka, S., Macurova, H., Ivanyi, P., Hoza, J., Houstkova, H. and Bardfield, R. (1975). HL-A antigens in juvenile rheumatoid arthritis. *Scand. J. Rheumatol. 4*, (Suppl.) 8, Abs. 30–16

61. Gibson, D. J., Carpenter, C. B., Stillman, J. S. and Schur, P. H. (1975). Re-examination of histocompatibility antigens found in patients with juvenile rheumatoid arthritis. *N. Engl. J. Med.*, **293**, 636

62. Hall, M. A., Ansell, B. M., James, D. C. O. and Zylinski, P. (1975). HL-A antigens in juvenile chronic polyarthritis (Still's disease). *Ann. Rheum. Dis.*, **34** (Suppl.), 36

63. Mitsui, H., Juji, T. and Sonozaki, H. (1977). Juvenile ankylosing spondylitis, its clinical features and HLA-B27. *Arch. Orthop. Unfall-Chir.*, **87**, 31

64. Joysey, V. C., Roger, J. H., Ashworth, F., Bullman, W., Hazleman, B. L. and Lachmann, L. M. (1977). Parallel studies of HLA antigens in patients with rheumatic heart disease and scleritis: comparisons with three control populations. *J. Rheumatol.*, (Suppl.) 3, 84

65. Ward, C., Gelsthorpe, K., Doughty, R. W. and Hardisty, C. A. (1976). HLA antigens and acquired valvular heart disease. *Tiss. Antigens*, **7**, 227

66. Caughey, D. E., Douglas, R., Wilson, W. and Hassell, I. B. (1975). HL-A antigens in Europeans and Maoris with rheumatic fever and rheumatic heart disease. *J. Rheumatol.*, **2**, 319

67. Greenberg, L. J., Gray, E. D. and Yunis, E. J. (1975). Association of HL-A5 and immune responsiveness *in vitro* to streptococcal antigens. *J. Exp. Med.*, **141**, 935

68. Gorodezky, C., Ulloa-L. S. and Escobar-Gutierrez, A. (1977). HLA antigens and rheumatic heart disease in Mexico. *J. Rheumatol.* (Suppl.) 3, 112

69. Read, S. E., Reid, H., Poon-King, T., Fischett, A., Zabriskie, J. B. and Rapaport, F. T. (1977). HLA and predisposition to the non-suppurative sequelae of Group A streptococcal infections. *Transplant. Proc.*, **9**, 543

70. Moll, J. M. H. and Wright, V. (1973). Psoriatic arthritis. *Seminars in Arthritis and Rheumatism*, **3**, 55

71. Wright, V. (1978). In Scott, T. J. (ed.) *Copeman's Textbook of the Rheumatic Diseases*, 5th Edn., p. 538. (Edinburgh: Churchill Livingstone)

72. Howell, F. A., Chamberlain, M. A., Perry, R. A., Torrigiani, G. and Roitt, I. M. (1972). IgG antiglobulin levels in patients with psoriatic arthropathy, ankylosing spondylitis and gout. *Ann. Rheum. Dis.*, **31**, 129

73. Metzgar, A. L., Morris, R. I., Bluestone, R. and Terasaki, P. I. (1975). HL-Aw27 in psoriatic arthropathy. *Arthr. Rheum.*, **18**, 111
74. Brewerton, D. A., Caffrey, M., Walters, D. and James, D. C. O. (1974). HLA-B27 and arthropathies associated with ulcerative colitis and psoriasis. *Lancet*, **1**, 956
75. Feldman, J.-L., Amor, B., Cazalis, P., Dryll, A., Hors, J. and Hacquart, B. (1976). Antigènes HLA chez les malades atteints du rhumatisme psoriatique. *Nouv. Presse Med.*, **5**, 477
76. Karvonen, J., Lassus, A. and Tiilikainen, A. (1974). HLA antigens in psoriatic arthritis. *Ann. Clin. Res.*, **6**, 304
77. Eastmond, C. J. and Woodrow, J. C. (1977). The HLA system and the arthropathies associated with psoriasis. *Ann. Rheum. Dis.*, **36**, 112
78. Daymond, T. J. and Wentzel, J. (1980). Histocompatibility antigens in psoriasis and psoriatic arthritis (unpublished observations)
79. Emery, A. E. H. and Lawrence, J. S. (1967). Genetics of ankylosing spondylitis. *J. Med. Genet.*, **4**, 239
80. Thorsby, E. (1978). Biological function of HLA. *Tiss. Antigens*, **11**, 321
81. Zingernagel, R. M. and Doherty, P. C. (1977). Possible mechanisms of disease susceptibility association with major transplantation antigens. In *HLA and Disease*, p. 256. (Copenhagen: Munksgaard)
82. Brautbar, C., Porat, S., Nelken, D., Gabriel, K. R. and Cohen, T. (1977). HLA B27 and ankylosing spondylitis in the Israeli population. *J. Rheumatol.* (Suppl.) 3, 24
83. Calin, A., Grahame, R., Tudor, M. and Kennedy, L. (1974). Ankylosing rheumatoid arthritis, ankylosing spondylitis and HL-A antigens. *Lancet*, **1**, 874
84. Isomake, H., Koota, K., Martio, J., Nissila, M. and Tiilikaimen, A. (1975). HL-A27 and arthritis. *Ann. Clin. Res.*, **7**, 138
85. Kueppers, F., Brackertz, D. and Mueller-Eckhardt, Ch. (1972). HL-A antigens in sarcoidosis and rheumatoid arthritis. *Lancet*, **2**, 1425
86. Lies, R. B., Messner, R. P. and Troup, G. M. (1972). Histocompatibility antigens and rheumatoid arthritis. *Arthr. Rheum.*, **15**, 524
87. Marcolongo, R. and Contu, L. (1974). Les antigenes HL-A dans la polyarthrite chronique rhumatismale et la spondylarthrite ankylosante en Sardaigne. *Nouv. Presse Med.*, **3**, 2023
88. Matej, H., Sotnik, D. and MacKiewicz, S. (1977). HLA antigens and rheumatoid arthritis. *Arch. Immunol. Ther. Exp.*, **25**, 493
89. McMichael, A. J., Sasazuki, T., McDevitt, H. O. and Payne, R. O. (1977). Increased frequency of HLA-Cw3 and HLA-Dw4 in rheumatoid arthritis. *Arthr. Rheum.*, **20**, 1037
90. Morris, P. J., Vaughan, H., Tait, B. D. and Mackey, I. R. (1977). Histocompatibility antigens (HLA): association with immunopathic diseases and with responses to microbial antigens. *Aust. N.Z. J. Med.*, **7**, 616
91. Seignalet, J., Clot, J., Sany, J. and Serre, H. (1972). HL-A antigens in rheumatoid arthritis. *Vox Sang.*, **23**, 468
92. Nissila, M., Elomaa, L. and Tiilikainen, A. (1975). HL-A antigens in juvenile rheumatoid arthritis. *N. Engl. J. Med.*, **292**, 430
93. Rachelefsky, G. S., Terasaki, P. I., Katz, R. and Stiehm, E. R. (1974). Increased prevalence of W27 in juvenile rheumatoid arthritis. *N. Engl. J. Med.*, **290**, 892
94. Sturrock, R. D. and Dick, H. M. (1974). Association of HL-A27 and AJ in juvenile rheumatoid arthritis and ankylosing spondylitis. *J. Rheumatol.*, **1**, 269
95. Beckman, L., Bronnestam, R., Cedergren, B. and Linden, S. (1974). HL-A antigens, blood groups, serum groups and red cell enzyme types in psoriasis. *Hum. Hered.*, **24**, 496
96. Buchanan, R., Kraag, G., Rosenthal, D. and Singal, D. P. (1977). HLA antigens and psoriatic arthritis. *Transplant. Proc.*, **9**, 1873
97. Espinoza, J.-L., Amor, B., Cazalis, P., Dryll, A., Hors, J. and Hacquart, B. (1976). Antigenes HLA chez les malades atteints du rhumatisme psoriatique. *Nouv. Presse Med.*, **5**, 477

98. Grosse-Wilde, H., Wustner, H., Albert, E. D., Kuntz, B., Scholz, S. and Braun-Falco, O. (1978). HLA-D typing in 72 psoriasis vulgaris patients and distribution of seven HLA-D alleles. *Tiss. Antigens*, **11**, 427
99. Gunn, I., Leheny, W., Lakshmipathi, T., Lamont, M. A. and Faed, M. (1979). HLA antigens in a Scottish psoriatic population. *Tiss. Antigens*, **14**, 157
100. Jajic, I., Kastelan, A., Brnobic, A., Kerhin, V. and Brkljacic, L. (1977). HLA antigens in psoriatic arthritis and psoriasis. *Arch. Dermatol.*, **113**, 1724
101. Krulig, L., Farber, E. M., Grumet, C. and Payne, R. O. (1975). Histocompatibility (HLA) antigens in psoriasis. *Arch. Dermatol.*, **111**, 857
102. Marcusson, J., Moller, E. and Thyresson, N. (1975). HL-A antigens (17, 27, UPS) in psoriasis with special reference to patients with arthritis lesions. *Acta Derm. Venereol.*, **55**, 297
103. Majsky, A. and Novotny, F. (1977). HL-A antigens in psoriasis vulgaris and patient's siblings. *Tiss. Antigens*, **9**, 131
104. Nyfors, A. and Svejgaard, A. (1976). The relation of HL-A antigens to liver histology in methotrexate-treated psoriatics. *Acta Derm. Venereol.*, **56**. 235
105. Russell, T. J., Schultes, L. M. and Kuban, D. J. (1972). Histocompatibility (HLA) antigens associated with psoriasis. *N. Engl. J. Med.*, **287**, 738
106. Scandinavian Regional Report (1978). *Histocompatibility Testing 1977*, p. 499. (Copenhagen: Munksgaard)
107. Seignalet, J., Clot, J., Guilhou, J. J., Duntze, F., Meynadier, J. and Robinet-Levy, M. (1974). HL-A antigens and some immunological parameters in psoriasis. *Tiss. Antigens*, **4**, 59
108. Svejgaard, A., Staub-Nielsen, L., Svejgaard, E., Kissmeyer-Nielsen, F., Hjortshoj, A. and Zachariae, H. (1974). HLA in psoriasis vulgaris and in pustular psoriasis: population and family studies. *Br. J. Dermatol.*, **91**, 145
109. White, S. H., Newcomer, V. D., Mickey, M. R. and Terasaki, P. I. (1972). Disturbance of HL-A antigen frequencies in psoriasis. *N. Engl. J. Med.*, **287**, 740
110. Woodrow, J. C. (1975). The HL-A system and psoriasis. *Br. J. Dermatol.*, **92**, 427
111. Joliat, G., Ferro, M., Jeannet, M. and Ott, H. (1976). HLA-B27 antigen in diagnosis of atypical seronegative inflammatory arthropathy. *Ann. Rheum. Dis.*, **35**, 531
112. Lambert, J. R., Wright, V., Rajah, S. M. and Moll, J. M. H. (1976). Histocompatibility antigens in psoriatic arthritis. *Ann. Rheum. Dis.*, **35**, 526
113. Zachariae, H., Hjortshøj, A., Kissmeyer-Nielsen, F., Svejgaard, A., Svejgaard, E. and Zachariae, E. (1975). HL-A antigens and psoriatic arthritis. *Acta Derm. Venereol.*, **54**, 443

7
Polymorphonuclear Leukocytes (PMN)—Origins, Functions and Roles in the Rheumatic Diseases

G. B. HOWE and J. N. FORDHAM

INTRODUCTION

It is over 200 years since the English surgeon, William Hewson[1], first described the white blood cells. A little more than 100 years were to pass before Elie Metchnikoff, the famous Russian biologist working in France, observed and appreciated that the phagocytic white cell is capable of intracellular killing of bacteria. He realized that this was done by intracellular cytases (lysomal enzymes) and he felt that these cytases might also be capable of provoking inflammation[2]; however, he thought that they were mainly released by dead and dying cells. It was not until the last 15 years or so that the molecular basis for these events began to be understood. In recent years the volume of literature in this area of physiology has grown exponentially. This review will therefore not aim to be an exhaustive examination of all available literature but will attempt to summarize areas where a general consensus has been reached and to provide an overview of current thoughts on the role of the polymorph in the pathophysiology of some of the rheumatic diseases.

ORIGINS (GRANULOPOIESIS)

Kinetics

The kinetics of granulopoiesis have been reasonably well worked out over the last 20 years, using various radioisotopic techniques. The most widely used isotopes have been diisopropylfluorophosphatase-^{32}P (DF^{32}P), ^{51}Cr[chromium], tritiated thymidine (^{3}HTdR) and ^{99}Tc^m[technetium]. The most accurate estimate[3] of the size and kinetics of the various granulocyte pools are obtained using ^{3}HTdR.

Granulocytes are produced in the bone marrow from a stem cell pool. The stem cell is believed to be pluripotential, the common ancestor, also, of erythrocytes and platelets[4-8]. Its morphology is not known, but it may be similar to bone marrow lymphocytes[9-13]. From the stem cell, the committed granulocyte precursor enters a proliferative and maturative phase, passing through the morphologically recognizable stages of myeloblast, promyelocyte and myelocyte. It has been estimated that the number of cell divisions occurring in this phase is between three and seven[14]. This proliferative phase has been estimated to be 135 h (approx. $5\frac{1}{2}$ days)[15].

The transition from myelocyte to metamyelocyte marks the end of proliferation but the granulocyte continues to mature in the bone marrow, passing from metamyelocyte to band form to segmented neutrophil (PMN). This phase has been estimated to last between 130 and 158 h ($5\frac{1}{2}$–6 days)[15-17]. Thus the evolution from stem cell to mature blood PMN takes approximately 11–12 days. Movement through these proliferative and maturative phases is on a 'first-in, first-out' basis[3], under normal conditions.

Once mature PMNs reach the peripheral blood, they become randomly distributed between a circulating pool and a marginated pool of roughly equal dimensions[17,18]. The marginated pool consists of PMNs 'adhering' to the walls of small venules and possibly also in the spleen[19]. PMNs leave the peripheral blood randomly and this half-life in the peripheral blood is 6–7 h[3,17]. Having migrated into the tissues, they do not return to the blood[20]. It is primarily in the tissues that the PMN is destined to fulfil its functional role, and it is here that the PMN ultimately dies after 4–5 days. Thus, from birth to senescence, the total life-span of a PMN is of the order of 15 days.

Regulation

The rapid turnover of the PMN population means that any alteration of the *status quo* may have profound consequences. Obviously the production and release of PMNs must be a closely regulated process. The mechanism of this regulation is less well understood than the kinetics. There is evidence that both positive and negative feedback mechanisms may be operating; involving 'granulopoietin' (possibly colony-stimulating factor), various inhibitory substances including chalones, and perhaps even the number of mature PMNs circulating through the bone marrow.

Colony-stimulating factor (CSF) is now thought to be produced by the monocyte–macrophage system[21-24]. The physical properties of granulocyte CSF have been investigated by Stanley et al.[25-30]. It is a heat-labile glycoprotein with an estimated molecular weight of 45 000 and migrates electrophoretically in the α-globulin range. The mechanism of action of CSF is unclear. It does not act as a mere trigger to proliferation but is required for cellular division[31]. Factors controlling the production or release of CSF are not known. Although the cyclic nature of its production indicates that CSF may have a physiological role, the temporal relationship to granulopoiesis and its significance, if any, to the control of this process remains unclear.

A variety of inhibitory substances have been described[32-41]. Supernatant solutions from human granulocyte cultures have been shown to contain potent inhibitors of growth and ³[H]thymidine uptake of several proliferating haematopoietic cells. However, variations in experimental design and methodology make interpretations of these data difficult, especially with regard to the existence of 'chalones' (a product of mature granulocytes which inhibits the replication of granulocytic progenitors). This inhibitor is specific for the granulocyte cell series, but is not species-specific. It is apparent that mature granulocytes are capable of producing potent (non-lethal) inhibitors[41] of cell replication that are not necessarily primarily active against granulocyte precursors. The nature, subcellular source and mechanism of action of these inhibitors are unknown.

Mature PMNs in the marrow constitute a granulocyte reserve pool which can be stimulated to leave the marrow and enter the peripheral blood by a fall in the concentration of PMNs in the blood perfusing the marrow[42, 43].

Other mechanisms which have been implicated in the release of mature PMNs from the bone marrow in the steady state are a leukocytosis-inducing factor in the serum[44] (not CSF[45]) and perhaps also intramedullary nerve pathways[46]. In the non-steady state, a PMN leukocytosis can be induced by exercise and adrenaline (mobilizing marginated cells)[18], corticosteroids (increased marrow release and decreased efflux of PMNs from the blood)[47], bacterial endotoxin (increase in the rate of release of PMN from the marrow)[18] and etiocholanolone (release of stored PMNs from the marrow)[48].

FUNCTIONS

Migration

Adhesion

To achieve the ultimate function of ingestion and digestion of noxious substances (bacteria, immune complexes, etc.), the PMN must (in most cases) first adhere to the endothelial cells lining small blood vessels, emigrate between endothelial cells and then migrate in a directed fashion (chemotactically) towards the stimulus before phagocytosing and digesting the source of the chemotactic stimulus. Phagocytosis can also occur in free circulation.

The PMN has a selective preference for adhering to endothelial cells[49, 50]. Under physiological conditions, circulating PMNs flow freely through blood vessels, adhering transiently to the endothelial wall. The mechanism of adhesion is not known precisely. It involves both net surface negative charges[49, 51, 52] and physical contact, probably by microfilaments[53, 54], with the substrate. The cell surface charge may be important in allowing cells to approach one another sufficiently closely so that microfilament attachment can occur. Initial studies (personal observation in conjunction with Dr K. A. Brown) suggest that there is a direct correlation between the more adherent population of circulating PMNs and electrophoretic mobility in normal subjects and in rheumatoid arthritis.

Adhesion to a surface is necessary for PMN locomotion. The two functions are closely related since several chemotactic factors (N-formyl-methionyl-leucyl-phenylalanine, C5a, endotoxin, and zymosan-activated serum[49, 55]) have been shown to increase adhesiveness both to endothelial cells and to nylon fibre. This is probably because microfilaments are involved in both processes[53, 54]. In support of this is the observation that cytochalasin B impairs both adhesion and locomotion. One of the actions of this drug is to impair microfilament function. This subject (adhesion) has been extensively reviewed recently[56, 57].

Locomotion

The mechanism of PMN locomotion is not fully understood (in common with all motile cells); certainly not at a molecular level. Three types of locomotion are recognized: *random locomotion* (which occurs in the absence of any stimulus to motility); *activated random locomotion*, or *chemokinesis* (which occurs when chemotactically active molecules are present in uniform concentration without a gradient); and *directed locomotion*, or *chemotaxis* (which occurs when chemotactically active molecules are present in a concentration gradient). Much of the information concerning the ultrastructural events that occur during locomotion has been obtained by studying more technically suitable cell types, such as the chick fibroblast, where structures such as microfilaments are more easily detected. However, in recent years sufficient evidence has been accumulating, from work on PMNs, to suggest that extrapolations in general are not unreasonable.

In an elegant electronmicroscopic study of human PMN ultrastructure under conditions of random locomotion, chemokinesis and chemotaxis, Malech *et al.*[53] used small-pore Micropore filters (0.45 μm pore size) to impede migration whilst allowing pseudopod penetration of the filter matrix. They were able to demonstrate that, under conditions of random locomotion, the PMNs as a population tended to be rounded on the surface of the filter, without evidence of pseudopod formation. The nucleus tends to occupy a central position within the cell and there is no evidence of polarization of internal structures. There was almost no penetration by pseudopods into the filter.

When exposed to a chemotactic gradient, a polarization of intracellular structures occurred that was virtually uniform for the whole population of cells studied. The result gave the appearance of an actively migrating cell even though actual migration was impeded by a physical barrier. There was an increase of microfilaments at the leading end, with restriction of pseudopod formation to the leading end and toward the chemoattractant. There also tended to be focal concentrations of microfilaments at sites of contact with the filter matrix. The microtubular system is radially arranged throughout the cell, centred upon the centriole. With the induction of chemotaxis the nucleus is shifted to the rear of the cell and the centriole moves to the side of the nucleus toward the chemoattractant. When the chemotactic gradient is reversed suddenly, there is an initial movement of the centriole away from the new source of the gradient, possibly reflecting inertial forces, followed by a reversal of the previously described orientation of nucleus and centriole. It is not until this reorientation has occurred that an increase in microfilaments, and the formation of pseudopods in the side of the cell closest to the chemoattractant, is observed. Only then does migration begin towards the new chemotactic source.

Under conditions of chemokinesis there was an increase in the numbers of cells with locomotory morphology but with a random orientation. Thus with the induction of chemotaxis and chemokinesis, there is an orientation of specific cellular structures and a change in cell shape, rather than the appearance of new structures.

The functional roles of microfilaments and microtubules were studied further by using cytochalasin B (which disrupts microfilaments) and colchicine (which binds to, and disrupts, microtubules). Disruption of the microfilaments prevented migration and pseudopod penetration of the filter, but permitted normal orientation and internal polarization to occur. Disruption of the microtubular assembly prevented orientation of cells within a gradient and internal polarization. It also impaired pseudopod formation where a substrate was not present. Random migration was not affected, chemokinesis was slightly impaired and chemotaxis was markedly inhibited. Thus 'microfilaments are necessary for locomotion, and intact microtubules are essential for normal pseudopod formation and orientation, and maximal undirectional migration during chemotaxis'[53].

The metabolic events that occur during these processes and their controlling factors are largely unknown. Calcium and magnesium ions are involved[58, 59]. The mechanics of locomotion are also unknown. This subject has been extensively reviewed recently[56, 57, 60].

Phagocytosis and secretory function

Phagocytosis is the act of internalization and subsequent sequestration into phagosomes of extracellular particulate matter. This process is accompanied by profound metabolic changes in the cell designed to digest, or render inert, the ingested material.

Over recent years it has been appreciated that exocytosis—that is the fusion of specific granules or lysosomes with the cell membrane and subsequent release of their contents into the surrounding medium—occurs in response to certain triggering factors, e.g. bound immune complexes[61-63] and endotoxins. This appears to be a true secretory event sharing features in common with endocrine organs and the secretory functions of mast cells and platelets. Thus this process appears to be under adrenergic (inhibitory), and cholinergic (stimulatory) control[64,65]. It is an active process and is accompanied by metabolic sequelae associated with phagocytosis. This aspect of polymorphonuclear function is of particular relevance from the standpoint of the mediation of tissue injury in the rheumatic diseases.

Phagocytosis can be considered as a sequence of events[66], though each step interdigitates with the preceding and subsequent stage.

Recognition and surface attachment

Most phagocytosed particles are taken up following a process of opsonization, usually by IgG or the complement product C3b[67]. Sometimes binding of immunoglobulin to the phagocytosable particle results in release of chemotactic factors, via C3a and C5a, attracting the PMN to the site of its 'meal'. This appears to happen in the case of staphylococci[68] though other bacteria release chemotactic factors of their own. Surface binding of C3b enables the PMN to bind to the particle[69]. This binding is mediated by specific surface membrane receptors and is the so-called 'immune adherence phenomenon'. Immunofluorescence studies have shown PMNs to possess Fc and C3b surface receptors[70]. Uptake of appropriately opsonized material is specifically related to such binding sites. Thus Griffin et al.[71] showed that the uptake of IgG-coated red blood cells halted when the partially taken-up RBCs were exposed to trypsin. This suggested that uptake of such particles depends on the sequential recognition by the PMN of the IgG surface coating. Other such specific binding sites on the PMN surface membrane include receptors for antigenic determinants, phospholipase[72] and neurohormones[64].

Some particles adhere by non-specific receptor binding. Knowledge about such binding is limited. Presumably surface charge and hydrophobic interactions are involved. Latex particles are such an example, though such uptake is markedly increased by opsonization with IgG[73].

Surface binding of particulate matter induces a profound change in the metabolic activity of the cell. This is manifest by an increase in oxygen consumption of 500–600% over basal rates. Similarly, carbon dioxide production increases between 1000 and 2000% over resting levels[74,75]. This 'oxidative burst' is associated with the production of the oxygen derivatives, O_2^- (superoxide anion), $^1O_2$ (singlet oxygen) and OH. It probably occurs at the cell membrane secondary to increased activity of the flavoprotein NADPH oxidase[76]. Spontaneous, and dismutase-assisted, transformation of super-oxide anion into H_2O_2 occurs. The latter appears to act as a triggering mechanism, inducing a marked increase in the hexose monophosphate shunt activity. Internalization of the phagocytosable material is not a necessary prerequisite for this metabolic burst[77]. Metabolic activation occurs in PMNs adherent to concavalin A attached to Sepharose beads[78] or in response to immune complexes bound to filters[79]. Antileukocyte antibodies, circulating immune complexes, endotoxins[80], complement products (C5a[81], $\overline{C567}$[82], C3b[83]), fatty acids, phospholipase[72] and kallikrein are all capable of inducing a similar metabolic response.

The 'purpose' behind the production of these toxic products from oxygen appears to be a direct bactericidal mixture. An indirect mechanism employing myeloperoxidase and halogens, together with these oxygen derivatives, also operates resulting in a bactericidal effect. A system of detoxifying substances within each cell serves to protect against possible damage. These include superoxide dismutase, catalase and various scavenging substances.

The acute-phase copper-containing protein, caeruloplasmin, serves as a similar extracellular defence mechanism in inhibiting the superoxide anion[84].

The nature of the trigger or transducer mechanism, which signals to the cell a call for the metabolic burst, is incompletely understood. Studies using tritiated triphenylmethyl phosphonium[85] indicate that the initial detectable change in the phagocytosing cell is a transient hyperpolarization of the surface membrane, occurring between 10 and 15 s after surface stimulation. Super-oxide generation occurs 30–40 s after surface stimulation. Experimental evidence from the use of ionophores suggests that cations, and particularly calcium, when displaced from the cell membrane, are able to induce the characteristic respiratory burst[86].

Engulfment of particulate matter

Together with the metabolic events outlined, surface stimulation induces assembly of microtubules in the centriolar and peripheral regions of the cell. Assembly of microfilaments occurs in the sub-plasmalemal region adjacent to the stimulated membrane. Such filaments are made up of actin (which constitutes 10% of cell protein) and myosin. The assembly and disassembly of microtubules and microfilaments is governed by interplay between the cyclic nucleotides cAMP and cGMP and Ca^{2+} (see references 86–92). Elevation of intracellular cAMP induces disassembly and, conversely, elevation of cGMP and Ca^{2+} induces assembly of α and β tubulins to form microtubules. Ca^{2+} similarly induces assembly of actomyosin. A protein cofactor also appears necessary for actin–myosin interaction. Actomyosin, thus formed, becomes bound to actin binding protein (ABP)[93,94]. This appears to be an integral part of the cell membrane and appears to transmit the surface contact by phagocytosable particles into a 'muscular' response by the cell, manifest by pseudopod formation around the particle and subsequent 'pinching off' to form a phagosome. ABP appears to be directly involved in the process of inducing polymerization of actin, as well as acting as an anchorage site for the contractile protein complex[94].

Fusion of lysosomal granules with phagosomes

Following its formation, the phagosome becomes drawn towards the cell centre and fusion occurs with one of the vacuoles to form a phagolysosome. This contains a potent fungicidal, bactericidal, and viricidal mixture of lysosomes, proteolytic enzymes, hydrolytic enzymes, and lactoferrin together with the toxic oxygen derivatives.

Lysosomal enzyme release is intimately related to the assembly of microtubules and cannot take place in the absence of extracellular Ca^{2+} (see reference 95). Microtubular disrupting agents, such as colchicine and vinblastine[96], reduce lysosomal enzyme release. Cytochalasin B, which impairs binding of ABP to acromyosin, transforms the phagocytic cell into a true secretory cell[96]. Normal closure of the phagosome does not occur, and this results in the extracellular release of lysosomal enzyme.

Changes in intracellular concentration of cAMP and cGMP have opposing effects on lysosomal enzymes release (Yin-Yang hypothesis[97])—elevation of cAMP impairing release and elevation of cGMP promoting release.

The stable prostaglandins PGE_2 and PGF_2 are generated during phagocytosis. These are not in themselves important as mediators of inflammation and it has been shown that such substances, through receptor interactions at the cell surface, have an inhibiting effect on lysosomal enzyme release[96]. This effect is likely to be mediated by an elevation of intracellular cAMP. Potent inflammatory mediators such as thromboxane A_2 are also released during phagocytosis[65]—as are potent chemotactic factors (either directly by an effect of superoxide anion on arachidonic acid[98] or due to the action of C5 cleaving enzyme release[81]). It appears, therefore, that there are opposing effects of these products of arachidonic acid metabolism produced during phagocytosis. This possibly represents a self-regulating mechanism designed to curtail the inflammatory response induced during phagocytosis.

ROLE IN RHEUMATIC DISEASES

Histopathological considerations

Although histologically the polymorphonuclear leukocyte is not present in great numbers in the pannus of rheumatoid arthritis[99] or the synovial lining tissue in such diseases as systemic lupus erythematosus[100], it is the commonest cell in the synovial fluid. It has been suggested that PMN infiltration at the pannus–cartilage border in rheumatoid arthritis is scanty[101]. However, one histochemical study showed PMNs to be present in high numbers at this site[102]. These cells were frequently seen in clefts in the cartilage, suggesting active participation in cartilage destruction. The focal accumulation of such cells may have accounted for the previously held views. In Behçet's syndrome, PMNs are a prominent component of the cellular infiltration in the synovium as well as being present in the synovial fluid[103]. A similar situation to rheumatoid arthritis obtains in the synovial lining tissue of most of the seronegative spondyloarthritides. In addition, the vascular lesions of malignant arteritis in rheumatoid arthritis, systemic lupus erythematosus, and the necrotizing arteritides show dense PMN infiltration within the vessel walls[104]. This is not to deny the importance of the cellular and hormonal immune responses resulting in the production of immune complexes, soluble or insoluble. However, the latter, *per se*, do not appear to be directly responsible for tissue damage in the connective tissue diseases.

Experimental models—PMN and tissue injury

The Arthus reaction

Injection of the immunizing antigen into the skin of a previously immunized animal possessing high titres of circulating antibodies to that antigen results in a vascular reaction characterized by haemorrhage, necrosis and blockage of post-capillary venules by thrombosis—the Arthus reaction. Immune complexes, neutrophils and platelets are deposited in the vessel walls[105, 106]. Binding of immune complexes to vessel walls is associated with the generation of the chemotactic factors $\overline{C567}$ and C5a. Animals rendered neutropenic do not manifest an Arthus reaction[107]. Similarly, decomplemented animals fail to show aggregation of PMNs in the vessel walls[108].

Immune complex disease (serum sickness)

Experimental animals which are only moderate producers of antibody react to injected antigen by producing antigen–antibody complexes in slight antigen excess. Poor clearance of such circulating complexes results in their persistence for several days. This results in the syndrome of arthritis, glomerulonephritis and arteritis[109]. Rendering the animals neutropenic results in partial suppression of the arteritis[110].

Other experimental models, such as systemic aggregate anaphylaxis adjuvant disease in the rat, implicate PMNs as important in the mediation of tissue damage[110].

Immune complex-mediated PMN activation

The synovitis of rheumatoid arthritis is characterized by the presence of soluble or insoluble IgG complexes in the synovial fluid[112, 113]. It is believed that it is the presence of such complexes which causes the characteristic decreased complement levels[114] and the associated presence of cleavage products C3a, C3b, and C5a[115], the latter being a chemotactic factor for PMNs.

Immune complexes are actively phagocytosed and uptake is associated with the characteristic metabolic burst[116] at the cell membrane and the production of toxic oxygen derivatives. Soluble immune complexes are not able to trigger the metabolic burst. The subsequent formation of a phagolysosome may be associated with the regurgitation of some of the constituents, consisting of hydrolytic and proteolytic enzymes and oxygen-derived radicals together with the newly formed arachidonic acid derivatives (the latter including prostacyclin, endoperoxides, thromboxanes and stable prostaglandins)[117]. Stable prostaglandins have potential for both amplifying and reducing the inflammatory response (see the section 'Fusion of lysosomal granules with phagosomes'). It has been shown that lysates of human neutrophil lysosomes generate C5a from the 5th component of complement[81]. It has also been shown that activated neutrophils have a mitogenic effect on B lymphocytes, probably mediated through neutral proteinases[118].

Recent work[119] has suggested that children with rheumatoid arthritis show reduced superoxide dismutase activity in their PMNs. Oxygen-derived radicals may therefore be free to exhibit a toxic effect on either the PMN or joint tissues.

In vivo and *in vitro* studies have shown that bound immune complexes are capable of triggering the active extrusion of lysosomal enzymes[63, 120] ('reversed endocytosis' or 'frustrated phagocytosis'). In one such study[121], it was shown that immune complex-stimulated PMNs actively invaded cartilage, being seen well below the superficial surface of cartilage. In a series of elegant experiments employing liposomes, Weissman and colleagues have produced evidence to suggest that hydrophobic sites in the Fc portion of aggregated immunoglobulins are the sites of engagement with the cell membrane[98].

Crystal-induced PMN activation

The work of McCarty and co-workers demonstrated the inflammatory effects of intrasynovial crystals[122], and furthermore, that this was dependent on the presence of neutrophils in the joint space. Monosodium urate and calcium pyrophosphate have been the most completely studied. It is now appreciated that both of these are potent activators of the classic complement pathway, particularly if immunoglobulin-coated[123]. Intrasynovial immune complexes, as detected by C1q assay, have been identified in gout and pseudogout[124]. The release of chemotactic products of complement activation (mainly C3a and C5a) serve to attract the PMN to the crystals[123]. Phagocytosis occurs and is probably increased if the crystal is coated with immunoglobulin[125]. The PMN then synthesizes and secretes a glycoprotein (molecular weight 8400) which is chemotactic for both PMNs and monocytes[126, 127]. This crystal-induced chemotactic factor (CCF) is capable of inducing a profound arthritis in rabbits, following intra-articular injection of purified CCF[128]. This arthritis is histologically identical with that produced by urate crystal injection. Following the formation of a phagolysosome, digestion of the plasma-protein/immunoglobulin coating occurs. Urate crystals appear to have a disruptive effect on the cholesterol-rich membrane with the consequence that lysis of the phagosomal membrane occurs with disastrous effects on the cell. The resultant death of the phagocytosing cell causes release of intracyto-plasmic enzymes into the synovial fluid together with the full complement of lysosomal enzymes, prostaglandin derivatives and unstable oxygen deriva-tives. The raised plasma urate in gout appears to have an inhibitory effect on the normal protective coating of albumin on both lysosomal membrane and crystal[129].

The amplifying effect of the release of CCF, the contents of the phagolyso-somes and the cytoplasmic constituents is manifest by the further recruitment of PMNs to the joint space. Experimental evidence[121] suggests that intra-synovial urate crystals result in the avid adherence of PMNs to cartilage surface.

PMN and cartilage degradation

The synovial fluid in active osteoarthrosis, the inflammatory arthropathies, crystal-induced and infective arthropathies is characterized by the presence of PMNs. Also present, often in high concentration, are the enzymatic contents of lysosomes and azurophilic granules of these cells[130-132]. The various mech-anisms for the release of these substances have been described above. The pannus macrophages and chondrocytes[133] are also important sources of acid cathepsins and neutral proteases. The relative importance of each of these sources in the production of articular damage in any of the arthropathies has not been settled. However, there is no doubt that PMN-derived enzymes are capable of inducing chronic arthropathies in experimental models. For example, the repeated injection of PMN granular lysates into the joint spaces of experimental animals induces an acute and chronic arthropathy. It has been calculated that approximately 8 mg of the PMN neutral protease, elastase, is released into a typical rheumatoid knee each day. Unneutralized, this would be sufficient to release the total proteoglycan content of the joint together with 10–20% of the collagen content every 24 h[134]. Whatever the contribution to joint destruction from the two other sources mentioned, it seems likely that PMN leukocyte enzymes will be proved to be an important part of the process.

One must be cautious in applying *in vitro* data on enzyme activity to the *in vivo* situation where, in the pericellular region, conventional enzyme kinetics may not apply[129].

However, the likeliest candidates for cartilage damage in the physico-chemical conditions prevailing in synovial fluid are the neutral proteases, cathepsin G and elastase, although the acid proteases and cathepsin D may be active in the pericellular environment where a lower pH may prevail. Both elastase and cathepsin G have been shown to be active in the release of the protective proteoglycans[134,135], keratin sulphate and chondroitin sulphate, leaving the collagen infrastructure open to further attack from the same enzymes. They appear to have a solubilizing effect on type II collagen by attacking at the cross-linkage region[131]. This renders collagen fibrils available for direct phagocytic engulfment by synovial lining cells[136] and enzymatic attack from the specific collagenases[137]. The loss of the proteoglycan 'packing material' renders cartilage susceptible to tensile and compressive stress[138] in the face of inadequate repair of proteoglycan loss. The subsequent denaturation of collagen is the irreversible step in the loss of functional and physical integrity of cartilage.

PMN collagenase appears unlikely to play a major role in collagen breakdown[134]. It probably has some effect on solubilization in conjunction with the serine proteinases; the latter and the specific collagenase being the prime mediators of collagen destruction.

The extracellular inhibitors of PMN neutral enzymes, α_1 antitrypsin, α_2 macroglobulin and α_1 plasmin inhibitor are unlikely to be present in sufficient concentration at the site of enzyme release to affect enzyme activity, particularly when high substrate availability means that ready binding of released enzyme renders them immune from such neutralization[129]. It has been suggested that the activity of collagenase, secreted in various tissue and cell cultures, may be governed by inactivation of the inhibitor of the enzyme which is attached to it—proteolytic attack releasing the active enzyme[139]. There exists the intriguing possibility that the abundant proteases present in synovial fluid of the inflammatory arthropathies may activate collagenase of pannus origin through this mechanism. Pharmacological control of the inhibitors of enzyme activity represents a possible lever in the moderation of enzymatic tissue damage in rheumatic diseases.

Drug treatment and PMN function

Studies of the effects of drugs on the various aspects of PMN function in rheumatic diseases have largely centred on the symptomatic, or quick-acting drugs. These drugs have a non-specific effect on inflammatory responses without any effect on the underlying disease progress. Some of the specific antirheumatics, such as gold, have also been closely studied and the more recently developed drugs such as D-penicillamine and levamisole to a lesser degree. Interpretation of a good deal of the work to date is made difficult by the tendency of research workers to use experimental animals as the source of cellular material and by the use of high, non-pharmacological, and *in vitro* drug concentrations.

Symptomatic drugs

With the discovery that drugs in this group blocked prostaglandin (PG) synthesis from a wide range of biological systems[140, 141] (or in some cases also blocked cell receptor sites, e.g. fenemates), it was assumed that the potency of these drugs was related to this effect. However it soon became apparent that the degree of PG inhibition and the anti-inflammatory effects of the drugs did not always run hand in hand. The picture became further complicated with the demonstration that PGs had both inflammatory-inducing and inflammatory-reducing effects. Furthermore, it has been shown that aspirin, a weak *in vitro* inhibitor of PG synthesis, was able to completely suppress PG synthesis at low dosage in synovial membranes, whereas indomethacin, ibruprofen and naproxen (potent *in vitro* inhibitors of PG synthesis) incompletely impaired PG synthesis in the synovial tissue[142]. The sources of prostaglandin in the synovial fluid are likely to be PMN, platelets and synovial membrane. However, it has been suggested that the macrophage is the main source of local PG formation in both gout and rheumatoid arthritis[143].

Possibly as important as any effect on PG synthesis is the impairment of lysosomal enzyme release by drugs of this class, such as indomethacin[144]. Similarly, impairment of random motility, phagocytic ability[145], inhibition of neutral proteases[146], and reduced adhesion[147] have been variously described as important effects of these drugs.

It has also recently been shown that indomethacin, ibuprofen and phenylbutazone induce a dose-related reduction in superoxide production in neutrophils following stimulation by chemotactic factors[148].

The effects of colchicine have been extensively investigated from the point of view of elucidating PMN motility mechanisms (by an effect on microtubule assembly). A consistent finding in *in vitro* work has been an impairment of chemotaxis with no effect on random motility[149] (chemokinesis). Much of this work has been carried out using high, *in vitro*, concentrations of the drug and it remains to be proved if its almost specific effect in acute gout is related to impairment of motility, or whether decreased phagocytic ability[150], reduced lysosomal enzyme release, or reduced adhesion[147] are more important. Recent evidence[151] suggests that impairment of motility may be important. Ingestion of sodium urate crystals by PMNs induces the release, by PMNs, of a glycoprotein (CCF). CCF is a potent chemotactic factor both *in vivo* and *in vitro* (see the section 'Crystal-induced PMN activation'). At therapeutic levels colchicine inhibits either its production or release from PMNs.

Antirheumatic drugs (slow-acting)

Gold has been most extensively investigated and has been shown to impair the inflammatory cell responses of both macrophage and PMNs[152, 153], *in vitro* and *in vivo*. Inhibition of PGF_2 and PGE_2 synthesis and lysosomal enzyme activity have also been demonstrated, probably by a direct toxic effect of the drug localized at the lysosomal membrane[154, 155]. DNA and RNA synthesis is also impaired[156]. Taken together with the listed effects above, and the tendency of gold and all the slow-acting drugs in rheumatoid arthritis to cause neutropenia, this suggests that the mode of action of these superficially disparate drugs may be to produce a general functional impairment in phagocytic cells, notably macrophages and PMNs. Such cells would be less able to respond with the full battery of inflammatory mediators at their control to whatever the provoking stimulus in rheumatoid arthritis, infective or otherwise, ultimately proves to be.

Glucocorticosteroids

This class of drug appears to include the only drugs which reliably and markedly suppress rheumatoid inflammation. They have been shown to impair prostaglandin synthesis, probably by an effect on substrate availability[157]. Lysosomal enzyme release has been shown to be inhibited from circulating PMNs and the non-phagocytic release of lysosomal enzymes is also reduced[158]. This is probably due to inhibition of calcium influx into the PMN, removing the intracellular signal for cyclic GMP accumulation[159] (see the section 'Fusion of lysosomal granules with phagosomes'). Granulocyte egression[160] and adhesion[147] have similarly been shown to be reduced, so that an overall functional impairment of PMNs occurs similar to that with the specific antirheumatics.

It is not the purpose of this review to define the place of these agents in the various rheumatic diseases. In particular, the place of corticosteroids remains controversial, especially in rheumatoid arthritis.

Acknowledgments

The authors wish to thank Professors H. L. F. Currey, P. A. Castaldi and E. J. Holborow for their help in reviewing and criticizing this manuscript.

References

1. Gulliver, G. C. (1846). *The Works of William Hewson*. (Bartholomew Close, London: J. Adland)
2. Metchnikoff, E. (1905). *Immunity in Infective Diseases*, p. 70. (New York and London: Johnson Reprint Corp.)
3. Vincent, P. C. (1977). Granulocyte kinetics in health and disease. *Clin. Haematol.*, 6, 695
4. Rickard, K. A., Shadduck, R. K., Morley, A. and Stohlman, F. (1970). *In vitro* and *in vivo* colony technic in the study of granulopoiesis. In Stohlman, F. Jr. (ed.) *Hemopoietic Cellular Proliferation*. (New York: Grune and Stratton)
5. Rickard, K. A., Morley, A., Howard, D., Garrity, M. and Stohlman, F. Jr. (1971). Stem cell stimulatory properties *in vitro* of an agar colony-stimulating factor. *Proc. Soc. Exp. Biol. Med.*, **136**, 608

6. Dunn, C. D. R. (1971). The differentiation of haemopoietic stem cells. *Series Haematologica*, IV, **4**, 3

7. Greenberg, P. L., Nicholas, W. C. and Shrier, S. L. (1971). Granulopoiesis in acute myeloid leukaemia and pre-leukaemia. *N. Engl. J. Med.*, **284**, 1225

8. Vincent, P. C. (1974). Granulocytes and monocytes. In Hardisty, R. M. and Weatherall, D. (eds.) *Blood and Its Disorders*. (Oxford: Blackwell Scientific Publications)

9. Bohne, F., Hass, R. J., Fliedner, T. M. and Fache, I. (1970). The role of slowly proliferating cells in rat bone marrow during regeneration following hydroxyurea. *Br. J. Haematol.*, **19**, 533

10. Fliedner, T. M., Calvo, W., Haas, R., Forteza, J. and Bohne, F. (1970). Morphologic and cytokinetic aspects of bone marrow stroma. In Stohlman, F. Jr. (ed.) *Haemopoietic Cellular Proliferation*. (New York: Grune and Stratton)

11. Haas, R. J., Bohne, F. and Fliedner, T. M. (1969). On the development of slowly-turning-over cell types in neonatal rat bone marrow. *Blood*, **34**, 791

12. Haas, R. J., Bohne, F. and Fliedner, T. M. (1971). Cytokinetic analysis of slowly proliferating bone marrow cells during recovery from radiation injury. *Cell Tissue Kinet.*, **4**, 31

13. Dickie, K. A., van Noord, M. J., Maat, B., Schaefer, V. W. and van Bekkum, D. W. (1973). Identification of cells in primate bone marrow resembling the haemopoietic stem cell in the mouse. *Blood*, **42**, 195

14. Craddock, C. G. (1972). Granulocyte kinetics. In Williams, W. J., Beutler, E., Erslev, A. J. and Rundles, R. W. (eds.) *Haematology*, p. 593. (New York: McGraw-Hill)

15. Cronkite, E. P. and Vincent, P. C. (1969). Granulocytopoiesis. *Series Haematologica*, II, **4**, 3

16. Donohue, D. M., Reiff, R. H., Hanson, M. L., Betson, Y. and Finch, C. A. (1958). Quantitative measurement of the erythrocytic and granulocytic cells of the marrow and blood. *J. Clin. Invest.*, **37**, 1571

17. Dancey, J. T., Deubelbeiss, K. A., Harker, L. A. and Finch, C. A. (1976). Neutrophil kinetics in man. *J. Clin. Invest.*, **58**, 705

18. Athens, J. W., Raab, S. O., Haab, O. P., Mauer, A. M., Ashenbrucker, H., Cartwright, G. E. and Wintrobe, M. M. (1961). Leukokinetic studies. IV. *J. Clin. Invest.*, **40**, 989

19. McMillan, R. and Scott, J. L. (1968). Leucocyte labelling with ^{51}chromium. I. Technic and results in normal subjects. *Blood*, **32**, 738

20. Boggs, D. R., Athens, J. W., Haab, O. P., Raab, S. O., Cartwright, G. E. and Wintrobe, M. M. (1964). Leukokinetic studies. VIII. *Proc. Soc. Exp. Biol. Med.*, **115**, 792

21. Chervenick, P. A. and Lo Buglio, A. F. (1972). Stimulators of granulocyte and mononuclear colony formation *in vitro*. *Science*, **178**, 164

22. Golde, D. W. and Cline, M. J. (1972). Identification of the colony stimulating cell in human peripheral blood. *J. Clin. Invest.*, **51**, 2981

23. Golde, D. W., Finley, T. M. and Cline, M. J. (1972). Production of colony-stimulating factor by human macrophages. *Lancet*, **2**, 1397

24. Moore, M. A. S. and Williams, N. (1972). Physical separation of colony-stimulating cells from *in vitro* colony forming cells in hemopoietic tissues. *J. Cell. Physiol.*, **80**, 195

25. Stanley, E. R., Robinson, W. A. and Ada, G. L. (1968). Properties of the colony-stimulating factor in leukaemic and normal mouse serum. *Aust. J. Exp. Biol. Med. Sci.*, **46**, 715

26. Stanley, E. R. and Metcalf, D. (1969). Partial purification and some properties of the factor in normal and leukaemic human urine stimulating mouse bone marrow colony growth *in vitro*. *Aust. J. Exp. Biol. Med. Sci.*, **47**, 467

27. Stanley, E. R. and Metcalf, D. (1971). Enzyme treatment of colony-stimulating factor: evidence for a peptide component. *Aust. J. Exp. Biol. Med. Sci.*, **49**, 281

28. Stanley, E. R., Bradley, T. R. and Sumner, M. H. (1971). Properties of the mouse embryo conditioned medium factor(s) stimulating colony formation by mouse bone marrow cells *in vitro*. *J. Cell Physiol.*, **78**, 301

29. Stanley, E. R. and Metcalf, D. (1971). The molecular weight of colony-stimulating factor (CSF). *Proc. Soc. Exp. Biol. Med.*, **137**, 1029

30. Stanley, E. R. and Metcalf, D. (1972). Purification and properties of human urinary colony-stimulating factor (CSF). *Cell Diff.*, **18**, 272

31. Metcalf, D. (1970). Studies on colony formation *in vitro* by mouse bone marrow cells. II. Action of colony-stimulating factor. *J. Cell Physiol.*, **76**, 89

32. Granstroem, M., Wahren, B., Gahrton, G. *et al.* (1972). Inhibitors of the bone marrow colony formation in serum of patients with leukaemia. *Int. J. Cancer*, **10**, 482

33. Haskill, J. S., McKnight, R. D. and Galbraith, P. R. (1972). Cell–cell interaction *in vitro*: studied by density separation of colony forming, stimulating, and inhibiting cells from human bone marrow. *Blood*, **40**, 394

34. Metcalf, D. (1971). Inhibition of bone marrow colony formation *in vitro* by dialysable products of normal and neoplastic haemopoietic cells. *Aust. J. Exp. Biol. Med. Sci.*, **49**, 351

35. Metcalf, D., Chan, S. J., Gunz, F. W. *et al.* (1971). Colony-stimulating factor and inhibitor levels in acute granulocytic leukaemia. *Blood*, **38**, 143

36. Rytomaa, T. and Kiviniemi, K. (1968). Control of granulocyte production. I and II. *Cell Tissue Kinet.*, **1**, 329

37. Paukovits, W. R. (1971). Control of granulocyte production: separation and chemical identification of a specific inhibitor (chalone). *Cell Tissue Kinet.*, **4**, 539

38. Broxmeyer, H. F., Moore, M. A. S. and Ralph, P. (1977). Cell free granulocyte inhibiting activity derived from human polymorphonuclear neutrophils. *Exp. Haematol.*, **5**, 87

39. Heit, W., Kern, P., Heimpel, H. and Kubanek, B. (1977). The role of granulocytes in colony stimulation by human white blood cells in agar cultures. Enhancement and inhibition of CSA. *Scand. J. Haematol.*, **18**, 105

40. Lord, B. I., Testa, N. G., Wright, E. G. and Banerjee, R. K. (1977). Lack of effect of a granulocyte proliferation inhibitor on their committed precursor cells. *Biomedicine*, **26**, 163

41. Herman, S. P., Golde, D. W. and Cline, M. J. (1978). Neutrophil products that inhibit cell proliferation: relation to granulocytic 'chalone'. *Blood*, **51**, 207

42. Dornfest, B. S., Lo Bue, J., Handler, E. S., Gordon, A. S. and Quastler, H. (1962). Mechanisms of leukocyte production and release. I. *Acta Haematol.*, **28**, 42

43. Dornfest, B. S., Lo Bue, J., Handler, E. S., Gordon, A. J. and Quastler, H. (1962). Mechanisms of leukocyte production and release. II. *J. Lab. Clin. Med.*, **60**, 777

44. Gordon, A. S., Neri, R. O., Siegel, C. D., Dornfest, B. S., Handler, E. S., Lo Bue, J. and Eister, M. (1960). Evidence for a leukocytosis-inducing factor. *Acta Haematol.*, **23**, 323

45. Broxmeyer, H., Zant, G. V., Zucali, J. R., Lo Bue, J. and Gordon, A. S. (1974). Mechanisms of leukocyte production and release. XII. *Proc. Soc. Exp. Biol. Med.*, **145**, 1262

46. Fliedner, T. M., Calvo, W., Haas, R., Forteza, J. and Bohne, F. (1970). Morphologic and cytokinetic aspects of bone marrow stroma. In Stohlman, F. Jr. (ed.) *Hemopoietic Cellular Proliferation.* (New York: Grune and Stratton)

47. Bishop, C. R., Athens, J. W., Boggs, D. R., Warner, H. R., Cartwright, G. E. and Wintrobe, M. M. (1968). Leukokinetic studies. XIII. A non-steady-state kinetic evaluation of the mechanism of cortisone-induced granulocytosis. *J. Clin. Invest.*, **47**, 249

48. Godwin, H. A., Zimmerman, T. S., Kimball, H. Y., Wolff, S. M. and Perry, S. (1968). The effect of etiocholanolone on the entry of granulocytes into the peripheral blood. *Blood*, **31**, 461

49. Hoover, R. L., Briggs, R. T. and Karnovsky, M. J. (1978). The adhesive interaction between polymorphonuclear leukocytes and endothelial cells *in vitro*. *Cell*. **14**, 423

50. MacGregor, R. R., Macarak, E. J. and Kefalides, N. A. (1978). Comparative adherence of granulocytes to endothelial monolayers and nylon fibre. *J. Clin. Invest.*, **61**, 697

51. Atherton, A. and Born, G. V. R. (1973). Effects of neuraminidase and N-acetyl neuraminic acid on the adhesion of circulating granulocytes and platelets in venules. *J. Physiol.*, **234**, 66P

52. Atherton, A. and Born, G. V. R. (1972). Quantitative investigations of the adhesiveness of circulating polymorphonuclear leucocytes to blood vessel walls. *J. Physiol.*, **222**, 447

53. Malech, H. L., Root, R. K. and Gallin, J. I. (1977). Structural analysis of human neutrophil migration. *J. Cell Biol.*, **75**, 666

54. Heath, J. P. and Dunn, G. A. (1978). Cell to substratum contacts of chick fibroblasts and their relation to the microfilament system. A correlated interference-reflexion and high-voltage electron-microscope study. *J. Cell. Sci.*, **29**, 197

55. O'Flaherty, J. T., Kreutzer, D. L. and Ward, P. A. (1978). The influence of chemotactic factors on neutrophil adhesiveness. *Inflammation*, **3**, 37

56. Stossel, T. P. (1978). The mechanism of leucocyte locomotion. In Gallin, J. I. and Quie, P. G. (eds.) *Leucocyte Chemotaxis.* (New York: Raven Press)

57. Wilkinson, P. C. and Lackie, J. M. (1979). The adhesion, migration and chemotaxis of leucocytes in inflammation. In Movat, H. Z. (ed.) *Current Topics in Pathology—Inflammatory Reaction*, **68**, 48–88 (Berlin, Heidelberg, New York: Springer-Verlag)

58. Gallin, J. I. and Rosenthal, A. S. (1974). The regulatory role of divalent cations in human granulocyte chemotaxis; evidence for an association between calcium exchanges and microtubule assembly. *J. Cell Biol.*, **62**, 594

59. Naccache, P. J., Showell, H. J., Becker, E. L. and Sha'afi, R. I. (1977). Transport of sodium. potassium, and calcium across rabbit polymorphonuclear leukocyte membranes. Effect of chemotactic factor. *J. Cell Biol.*, **73**, 428

60. Gallin, J. I., Gallin, E. K., Malech, H. L. and Cramer, E. B. (1978). Structural and ionic events during leukocyte chemotaxis. In Gallin, J. I. and Quie, P. G. (eds.) *Leucocyte Chemotaxis.* (New York: Raven Press)

61. Hawkins, D. (1971). Biopolymer membrane. A model system for the study of the neutrophilic leukocyte response to immune complexes. *J. Immunol.*, **107**, 344

62. Henson, P. M. (1971). The immunologic release of constituents from neutrophil leukocytes. I. The role of antibody and complement on non-phagocytosable surfaces or phagocytosable particles. *J. Immunol.*, **107**, 1535

63. Henson, P. M. (1971). The immunologic release of constituents from neutrophil leukocytes. II. The mechanisms of release during phagocytosis and adherence to non-phagocytosable surfaces. *J. Immunol.*, **107**, 1547

64. Ignarro, L. J. and George, W. J. (1974). Hormonal control of lysosomal enzyme release from human neutrophils: elevation of cyclic nucleotide levels by autonomic neurohormones. *Proc. Natl. Acad. Sci. USA*, **71**, 2027

65. Goldstein, I. M., Malmsten, C. L., Kindahl, H., Kaplan, H. B., Radmark, O., Samuelson, B. and Weissman, G. (1978). Thromboxane generation by human peripheral blood polymorphonuclear leukocytes. *J. Exp. Med.*, **148**, 787

66. Stossel, T. P. (1974). Phagocytosis. *N. Engl. J. Med.*, **290**, 717, 774, 833

67. Gigli, I. and Nelson, R. A. (1968). Complement-dependent immune phagocytosis. I. Requirements for C1, C4, C2, C3. *Exp. Cell Res.*, **51**, 45

68. Russell, R. J., Wilkinson, P. C., McInroy, R. J., McKay, S., McCartney, A. C. and Arbathnott, J. P. (1976). Effects of staphylococcal products on locomotion and chemotaxis of human blood neutrophils and monocytes. *J. Med. Microbiol.*, **9**, 433

69. Lay, W. J. and Nussenzweig, V. (1968). Receptors of complement on leukocytes. *J. Exp. Med.*, **128**, 991

70. Sajaani, A. N., Ranadive, N. S. and Movat, H. Z. (1976). Redistribution of immunoglobulin receptors on human neutrophils and its relationship to the release of lysosomal enzymes. *Lab. Invest.*, **35**, 143

71. Griffin, F. M. Jr., Griffin, J. A., Leider, J. E. and Silverstein, S. C. (1975). Studies on the mechanisms of phagocytosis. I. Requirements for circumferential attachment of particle-bound ligands to specific receptors on the macrophage plasma membrane. *J. Exp. Med.*, **142**, 1263

72. Patriaria, P., Cramer, R., Marussi, M., Moncalvo, S. and Rossi, F. (1971). Phospholipid splitting and metabolic stimulation in polymorphonuclear leucocytes. *J. Reticuloendotheliol. Soc.*, **10**, 251

73. Hallgren, R., Jansson, L. and Venge, P. (1977). Kinetic studies of phagocytosis of IgG-coated latex particles with a thrombocyte counter. *J. Lab. Clin. Med.*, **80**, 786

74. Rossi, F. and Zatti, M. (1964). Changes in the metabolic pattern of polymorphonuclear phagocytes during phagocytosis. *Br. J. Exp. Pathol.*, **45**, 548

75. Rossi, F. and Zatti, M. (1966). Effects of phagocytosis on the carbohydrate metabolism of polymorphonuclear leucocytes. *Biochem. Biophys. Acta.* **121**, 110

76. Patriaria, P., Cramer, R., Moncalvo, S., Rossie, F. and Roneo, D. (1971). Enzymatic basis of metabolic stimulation in leucocytes during phagocytosis: the role of activated NADPH oxidase. *Arch. Biochem. Biophys.*, **145**, 255

77. Hawkins, D. (1972). Neutrophilic leucocytes in immunologic reactions: evidence for the release of lysosomal contents. *J. Immunol.*, **108**, 310

78. Romeo, D., Jag, M., Zabacchi, G. and Rossi, F. (1974). Perturbation of leukocyte metabolism by non-phagocytosable concanavalin A-coupled beads. *FEBS Lett.*, **42**

79. Hawkins, D. (1971). Biopolymer membrane: a model system for the study of the neutrophilic leukocyte response to immune complexes. *J. Immunol.*, **107**, 344

80. Karnovsky, M. L. (1962). Metabolic basis of phagocytic activity. *Physiol. Rev.*, **42**, 143

81. Goldstein, I. M. and Weissman, G. (1974). Generation of C5-derived lysosomal enzyme releasing activity (C5a) by lysates of leukocyte lysosomes. *J. Immunol.*, **113**, 1583

82. Tedesco, F., Trani, S., Saranzo, M. R. and Patriaria, P. (1975). Stimulation of glucose oxidation in human polymorphonuclear leukocytes by C3-sepharose and soluble C567. *FEBS Lett.*, **51**, 232

83. Goetzl, E. J. and Austen, K. F. (1974). Stimulation of human neutrophil leukocyte aerobic glucose metabolism by purified chemotactic factors. *J. Clin. Invest.*, **53**, 591

84. Goldstein, I. M., Kaplan, H. B., Edelson, H. S. and Weissman, G. (1979). Caeruloplasmin: a scavenger of superoxide anion radicals. *J. Biol. Chem.*, **254**, 4040

85. Karchak, H. M. and Weissman, G. (1978). Changes in membrane potential of human granulocytes antecede the metabolic responses to surface stimulation. *Proc. Natl. Acad. Sci. USA*, **75**, 3818

86. Schell-Frederick, E. (1974). Stimulation of the oxidative metabolism of polymorphonuclear leukocytes by the calcium ionophore A23187. *FEBS Lett.*, **48**, 371

87. Hoffstein, S. T. (1979). Ultrastructural demonstration of calcium loss from local regions of the plasma membrane of surface-treated human granulocytes. *J. Immunol.*, **123**, 1395

88. Hoffstein, S. and Weissman, G. (1978). Microfilaments and microtubules in calcium ionophore-induced secretion of lysosomal enzymes from human polymorphonuclear leukocytes. *J. Cell Biol.*, **78**, 769

89. Parker, C. W. (1976). The role of cAMP in immunologic inflammation. *J. Invest. Dermatol.*, **67**, 638

90. Parker, C. W., Sullivan, T. J. and Wedner, H. J. (1974). cAMP and the immune response. In Greengard, P. and Robison, G. A. (eds.) *Advances in Cyclic Nucleotide Research*, Vol. 4. (New York: Raven Press)

91. Rassmussen, H. and Goodman, D. B. P. (1975). Calcium and cAMP as interrelated intracellular messengers. In Soifer, D. (ed.) *The Biology of Cytoplasmic Microtubules (Ann. NY Acad. Sci.*, **253**, 789*)*

92. Rassmussen, H., Jensen, P., Lake, W., Friedman, N. and Goodman, D. P. P. (1975). Cyclic nucleotides and cellular calcium metabolism. In Drummond, G. I., Greengard, P. and Robison, G. A. (eds.) *Advances in Cyclic Nucleotide Research*. Vol. 5, p. 375. (New York: Raven Press)

93. Boxer, L. A. and Richardson, S. (1976). Identification of actin-binding protein in membrane of PMN leukocytes. *Nature (London)*, **263**, 249

94. Stossel, T. P. and Hartwig, J. H. (1976). Interaction of actin, myosin, and a new actin-binding protein of rabbit pulmonary macrophages. II. Role in cytoplasmic movement and phagocytosis. *J. Cell. Biol.*, **68**, 602

95. Ignarro, L. J. and Cech, S. Y. (1975). Lysosomal enzyme secretion from human neutrophils mediated by cGMP: inhibition of cGMP, accumulation and neutrophil function by gluco-corticosteroids. *J. Cyclic Nucl. Res.*, **1**, 283

96. Zurier, R. B., Weissman, G., Hoffstein, S., Kammerman, S. and Tsai, H. H. (1974). Mechanisms of lysosomal enzyme release from human leukocytes. II. Effects of cAMP and cGMP autonomic agonists, and agents which affect microtubule function. *J. Clin. Invest.*, **53**, 297

97. Goldberg, N. D., Haddox, M. K., Teilig, C. E., Nicol, S. E., Acott, T. S. and Glaso, D. B. (1976). Cyclic GMP, cyclic AMP and the Yin–Yang hypothesis of biologic regulation. *J. Invest. Dermatol.*, **67**, 641

98. Weissman, G. (1979). Mediators of tissue damage in rheumatoid arthritis: phagocytes as secretory organs of rheumatoid inflammation. *Triangle Sandoz J. Med. Sci.*, **18**, 45

99. Harris, E. D., Faulkner, C. S. and Brown, F. E. (1975). Collagenolytic systems in rheumatoid arthritis. *Clin. Orthop. Rel. Res.*, **110**, 303

100. Cruikshank, B. (1959). Lesions of joints and tendon sheaths in systemic lupus erythematosus. *Ann. Rheum. Dis.*, **18**, 111

101. Pearson, C. M., Paulus, H. H. and Machleder, H. I. (1975). The role of the lymphocyte and its products in the propagation of joint disease. *Ann. NY Acad. Sci.*, **256**, 150

102. Mohr, W. and Weissinghage, D. (1978). The relationship between polymorphonuclear granulocytes and cartilage destruction in rheumatoid arthritis. *Z. Rheumatol.*, **37**, 126

103. Vernon-Roberts, B., Barnes, C. G. and Revell, P. A. (1978). Synovial pathology in Behçet's syndrome. *Ann. Rheum. Dis.*, **37**, 139

104. Ball, J. (1954). Rheumatoid arthritis and polyarteritis nodosa. *Ann. Rheum. Dis.*, **13**, 277

105. Uriuhara, T. and Movat, H. Z. (1964). Allergic inflammation. IV. The vascular changes during development and progression of the direct active and passive Arthus reactions. *Lab. Invest.*, **13**, 1057

106. Uriuhara, T. and Movat, H. Z. (1964). The role of the PMN leucocyte lysosomes in tissue injury, inflammation and hypersensitivity. I. The vascular changes and the role of PMN leucocytes in the reversed passive Arthus reaction. *Exp. Mol. Pathol.*, **5**, 539

107. Stetson, C. A. (1951). Similarities in the mechanisms determining the Arthus and Schwartzman phenomenon. *J. Exp. Med.*, **94**, 347

108. Ward, P. A. and Cochrane, C. G. (1965). Bound complement and immunologic injury of blood vessels. *J. Exp. Med.*, **121**, 215

109. Dixon, F. J., Vazquez, J. J., Weigle, W. O. and Cochrane, C. G. (1958). The pathogenesis of serum sickness. *Ann. Med. Assoc. Arch. Pathol.*, **65**, 18

110. Kniker, W. T. and Cochrane, C. G. (1965). Pathogenetic factors in vascular lesions of experimental serum sickness. *J. Exp. Med.*, **122**, 83

111. Leber, P. D. and McCluskey, R. T. (1974). Immune complex diseases. In Zweifach, B. W., Grant, L. and McCluskey, R. T. (eds.) *The Inflammatory Process*. Vol. III, p. 401. (New York: Academic Press)

112. Hollander, J. L., McCarty, D. J. and Asturga, G. (1965). Studies on the pathogenesis of rheumatoid joint inflammation. *Ann. Intern. Med.*, **62**, 271

113. Winchester, R. J. (1975). Characterization of IgG complexes in patients with rheumatoid arthritis. *Ann. NY Acad. Sci.*, **256**, 73

114. Winchester, R. J., Agnello, V. and Kunkel, H. G. (1969). The joint-fluid γ-globulin complexes and their relationship to intra-articular complement diminution. *Ann. NY Acad. Sci.*, **168**, 195

115. Zvaifler, N. J. (1969). Breakdown products of C3 in human synovial fluids. *J. Clin. Invest.*, **48**, 1532

168   IMMUNOLOGICAL ASPECTS OF RHEUMATOLOGY

116. Turner, R., Mashburn, R., Collins, L., Dechatelet, L. and Kaufmann, T. (1977). Rheuma-
     toid factor—immunoglobulin G complex precipitation and neutrophil stimulation: an *in
     vitro* model for rheumatoid inflammation. In Willoughby, D. A., *et al.* (eds.) *Perspectives in
     Inflammation*, p. 39. (Lancaster: MTP Press)
117. Weissmann, G., Goldstein, I. M., Hoffstein, S., Chavet, G. and Robineaux, R. (1975).
     Yin–Yang modulation of lysosomal enzyme release from polymorphonuclear leukocytes by
     cyclic nucleotides. IV. Role of inflammatory cells in the destruction of synovial tissues. *Ann.
     NY Acad. Sci.*, **256**, 222
118. Baggiolini, M. (1979). Inflammatory phagocytes: their properties and their involvement in
     rheumatoid arthritis. *Triangle*, **18**, 53
119. Rister, M., Bauermeister, K., Gravert, V. and Gladtke, E. (1979). Superoxide dismutase and
     glutathione peroxidose in polymorphonuclear leukocytes. *Eur. J. Pediatr.*, **130**, 127
120. Henson, P. M. (1974). Mechanisms of mediator release from inflammatory cells. In Weiss-
     mann, G. (ed.) *Mediators of Inflammation*, p. 9. (New York and London: Plenum Press)
121. Ugai, K., Ziff, M. and Jasin, H. E. (1979). Interaction of polymorphonuclear leukocytes
     with immune complexes trapped in joint collageneous tissue. *Arth. Rheum.*, **22**, 353
122. McCarty, D. J. (1965). The inflammatory reaction to microcrystalline sodium urate. *Arth.
     Rheum.*, **8**, 726
123. Hasselbacher, P. (1979). C3 activation by monosodium urate monohydrate and other
     crystalline material. *Arth. Rheum.*, **22**, 571
124. Zubler, R. H., Nydegger, U., Perrin, L. H., Fehr, K., McCormick, T., Lambert, P. H. and
     Mescher, P. A. (1976). Circulating and intra-articular immune complexes in patients with
     rheumatoid arthritis. Correlation of ^{125}I-Clq binding activity with clinical and biological
     features of the disease. *J. Clin. Invest.*, **57**, 1308
125. Skosey, J. L., Kozin, F., Chow, D. C. and May, J. (1976). Differential responses of human
     neutrophils to monosodium urate crystals and MSU coated with gammaglobulin. *Clin.
     Res.*, **24**, 111A
126. Phelps, P. (1969). Polymorphonuclear leukocytes motility *in vitro*. III. Possible release of a
     chemotactic substance following phagocytosis of urate crystals by polymorphonuclear
     leukocytes. *Arth. Rheum.*, **12**, 197
127. Spilberg, I., Gallacher, A., Mehta, J. M. and Mandell, B. (1976). Urate crystal-induced
     chemotactic factor. Isolation and partial characterization. *J. Clin. Invest.*, **58**, 815
128. Spilberg, I., Rosenberg, D. and Mandell, B. (1977). Induction of arthritis by purified cell-
     derived chemotactic factor. *J. Clin. Invest.*, **59**, 582
129. Malawista, S. E., Van Blaricon, G., Cretella, S. B. and Schwatz, M. L. (1979). The phlogistic
     potential of urate in solution: studies of the phagocytic process in human leukocytes. *Arth.
     Rheum.*, **22**, 728
130. Weissmann, G., Zurier, R. B., Speiler, P. J. and Goldstein, I. M. (1971). Mechanisms of
     lysosomal enzyme release from leukocytes exposed to immune complexes and other par-
     ticles. *J. Exp. Med.*, **134**, 149
131. Henson, P. (1971). Interaction of cells with immune complexes. Adherence, release of
     constituents and tissue injury. *J. Exp. Med.*, **134**, 114
132. Werb, Z. and Dingle, J. T. (1976). Lysosomes as modulators of cellular functions. Influence
     on the synthesis and secretion of non-lysosomal materials. In Dingle, J. T. and Dean, R. T.
     (eds.) *Lysosomes in Biology and Pathology*. Vol. 5, p. 127. (Amsterdam: North Holland Pub.
     Co.)
133. Dingle, J. T. (1979). Recent studies on the control of joint damage: the contribution of
     the Strangeways Research Laboratory. (Heberden oration, 1978.) *Ann. Rheum. Dis.*, **38**,
     201
134. Barrett, A. J. (1978). The possible role of neutrophil proteinases in damage to articular
     cartilage. *Agents and Actions*, **8**, 11
135. Dingle, J. T., Blow, A. M. J., Barrett, A. J. and Martin, P. E. N. (1977). Proteoglycan

degrading enzymes. A radiochemical assay method and the detection of a new enzyme, cathepsin F. *Biochem. J.*, **167**, 775

136. Harris, E. D., Glauert, A. M. and Murley, A. H. G. (1977). Intracellular collagen fibres at the pannus–cartilage junction in rheumatoid arthritis. *Arth. Rheum.*, **20**, 657

137. Harris, E. D. and Krane, S. M. (1974). Collagenases. *N. Engl. J. Med.*, **291**, 605

138. Kempson, G. E., Tuke, M. A., Dingle, J. T., Barrett, A. J. and Horsfield, P. M. (1976). The effects of proteolytic enzymes on the mechanical properties of adult articular cartilage. *Biochem. Biophys. Acta*, **428**, 741

139. Horwitz, A. L., Kelman, J. A. and Crystal, R. G. (1976). Activation of alveolar macrophage collagenase by a neutral protease secreted by the same cell. *Nature (London)*, **264**, 772

140. Ferreira, S. H., Moncada, S. and Vane, J. R. (1974). Prostaglandins and signs and symptoms of inflammation. In Robinson, H. D. and Vane, J. R. (eds.) *Prostaglandin Synthetase Inhibitors; their Effect on Physiological Functions and Pathological States*, p. 175. (New York: Raven Press)

141. Vane, J. R. (1971). Inhibition of prostaglandin synthesis as a mechanism of action for aspirin-like drugs. *Nature New Biol.*, **231**, 232

142. Crook, D., Collins, A. J., Bacon, P. A. and Chan, R. (1976). Prostaglandin synthetase activity from human rheumatoid synovial microsomes. Effects of 'aspirin-like' drug therapy. *Ann. Rheum. Dis.*, **35**, 327

143. Sturge, R. A., Yates, D. B., Gordon, D., Franco, M., Paul, W., Bray, A. and Morley, J. (1978). Prostaglandin production in arthritis. *Ann. Rheum. Dis.*, **37**, 315

144. Northover, B. J. (1977). Effect of indomethacin and related drugs on the calcium ion dependent secretion of lysosomal and other enzymes by neutrophil polymorphonuclear leukocytes *in vitro*. *Br. J. Pharmacol.*, **59**, 253

145. Robinson, B. V. (1978). The pharmacology of phagocytosis. Supplement to *Rheumatology and Rehabilitation*, pp. 37–46

146. Kruze, D., Fehr, K., Menninger, H. and Boni, A. (1976). Effects of antirheumatic drugs on neutral protease from human leucocyte granules. *Z. Rheumatol.*, **35**, 337

147. MacGregor, R. R. (1976). The effect of anti-inflammatory agents and inflammation on granulocyte adherence. Evidence for regulation by plasma factors. *Am. J. Med.*, **61**, 597

148. Simchowitz, L., Mehta, J. and Spilberg, I. (1979). Chemotactic factor induced generation of superoxide radicals by human neutrophils. *Arth. Rheum.*, **22**, 755

149. Ward, P. A. (1971). Leukotactic factors in health and disease. *Am. J. Pathol.*, **64**, 521

150. Stossel, T. P., Mason, R. J., Hartwig, J. and Vaughan, M. (1972). Quantitative studies of phagocytosis by polymorphonuclear leukocytes: use of emulsion to measure the initial rate of phagocytosis. *J. Clin. Invest.*, **51**, 615

151. Spilberg, I., Mandell, B., Mehta, J., Simchowitz, L. and Rosenberg, D. (1979). Mechanism of action of colchicine in acute urate crystal-induced arthritis. *J. Clin. Invest.*, **64**, 775

152. Vernon-Roberts, B., Jessop, J. D. and Dore, J. L. (1973). Effects of gold salts and prednisolone on inflammatory cells. II. Suppression of inflammation and phagocytosis in the rat. *Ann. Rheum. Dis.*, **32**, 301

153. Clarke, A. K., Vernon-Roberts, B. and Currey, H. L. F. (1975). Assessment of anti-inflammatory drugs in the rat using subcutaneous implants of polyurethane foam impregnated with dead tubercle bacilli. *Ann. Rheum. Dis.*, **34**, 326

154. Ennis, R. S., Granda, J. L. and Posner, A. S. (1968). Effect of gold salts and other drugs on the release and activity of lysosomal hydrolases. *Arth. Rheum.*, **11**, 756

155. Chadially, F. N., Oryschak, A. B. and Mitchell, D. M. (1978). Ultrastructural changes produced in rheumatoid synovial membrane by chrysotherapy. *Ann Rheum. Dis.*, **37**, 57

156. Westwich, W. J., Allsop, J., Gumpel, J. D. *et al.* (1974). Studies on pyrimidine biosynthesis in the granulocytes of patients receiving gold therapy for rheumatoid arthritis. *Q. J. Med.*, **170**, 231

157. Floman, C. T. and Zor, U. (1976). Mechanism of steroid action in inflammation: inhibition of prostaglandin synthesis and release. *Prostaglandins*, **12**, 403
158. Ignarro, L. J. (1977). Glucocorticosteroid inhibition of non-phagocytic discharge of lysosomal enzymes from human neutrophils. *Arth. Rheum.*, **20**, 73
159. Ignarro, L. J. (1978). Interference with stimulus-secretion coupling by glucocorticosteroids. *Adv. Cyclic Nucl. Res.*, **9**, 677
160. Senn, H. J. and Jungi, W. F. (1975). Neutrophil migration in health and disease. *Sem. Haematol.*, **12**, 27

8
Eosinophils and the Connective Tissue Diseases

P. DAVIS

INTRODUCTION

> The addition of some coloring agent such as iodine or eosine is of assistance
> in searching for them.
>
> A. Flint, Princ. Med. (1880), p. 866

The rapidly increasing information on the structure and function of the cellular components of blood has considerably improved our understanding of the pathogenesis of a number of diseases. In the connective tissue diseases, research on the role of neutrophils in the mediation of the inflammatory process and of lymphocytes and their interaction in the modulation of the immune response has been particularly valuable. Relatively little is known, however, on the role of the eosinophil in the pathogenesis of the connective tissue diseases although this cell is of considerable importance in the mediation of other diseases, particularly those involving immediate hypersensitivity reactions and host responses against parasitic infection. This may be an indication that the cell has little part to play in the pathogenesis of the rheumatic diseases although this need not necessarily be the case, there being some experimental evidence that eosinophils are involved in immune complex-mediated, complement-mediated and certain delayed hypersensitivity reactions.

This chapter will attempt to outline some of the current information on the structure and function of the eosinophil and will then review in more detail the evidence available that eosinophils have a part to play in some aspects of the pathogenesis of the connective tissue diseases. For more in-depth information on the structure and function of eosinophils the reader is referred to the excellent monograph on the subject by Beeson and Bass[1].

STRUCTURE

Mature eosinophils are generally bilobed nucleated phagocytic leukocytes, slightly larger than neutrophils although structurally very similar. Histologically, under standard techniques, eosinophils contain eosinophilic staining cytoplasmic granules. The staining characteristics of these granules are the major histological features which differentiate the eosinophil from other polymorphonuclear cells. The granules are of various sizes with the smaller granules containing arylsulphatase and acid phosphatases and larger granules containing a variety of hydrolytic enzymes. The contents of these granules are directly related to eosinophil function and are therefore worthy of specific note. Many contain peroxidases, although these are chemically and antigenically different from those found in neutrophils. Acid phosphatases are also present but, in contrast to the neutrophil, there is a low content of alkaline phosphatases. Histaminases are present which inhibit histamine as well as arylsulphatase which inactivates the slow-reacting substance of anaphylaxis (SRS-A). Phospholipases are present which may inhibit platelet activation factors. Prostaglandins are also present within the eosinophil and these have been shown to specifically prevent basophil degranulation in addition to their other anti-inflammatory actions. These substances will individually or in combination have specific modulatory effects on the inflammatory response.

One characteristic of the eosinophil is a high zinc concentration. This is also of significance in relation to eosinophil function as zinc is known to inhibit mast cell histamine release, platelet aggregation, macrophage migration, phagocytosis, superoxide dismutase and a number of lysosomal enzymes. The high zinc concentration, therefore, will also have some significance in the modulation of the inflammatory response. One characteristic of eosinophils which is occasionally seen, particularly in exudates with high eosinophil concentrations, is the Charcot–Leyden crystal. Although the function of this histologically unique feature is not clearly determined, it appears to originate from within activated eosinophils as a condensation of eosinophil granules with a high zinc concentration.

The cell membrane of the eosinophil is similar to other neutrophils. Electron-microscopic studies demonstrate a characteristic membrane with microvilli which have receptors for both C3b and immunoglobulin.

Despite the histologically similar characteristics between the eosinophil and neutrophils, it is erroneous to believe that the eosinophil is necessarily similar in function. In particular, there are major differences between eosinophils and other neutrophils worthy of comment. As discussed later, eosinophil numbers increase in response to antigenic challenge and in contrast to the neutrophil some of their functions are T-cell dependent. Their response to adrenocorticotrophic hormone (ACTH) and stress is a marked fall which is different to the rise seen with other neutrophils. In the tissues, neutrophils are detected at sites of pyogenic inflammation where there is enhanced phagocytic activity. In contrast, the eosinophil appears at other inflammatory sites where it functions as a modulator of immediate hypersensitivity reactions. The significantly different hydrolytic enzymes found within the granules of the two cells would also appear to be of major importance in regard to their different functions.

KINETICS

Eosinophils are derived in the bone marrow although the cell of origin is unknown. Experimental evidence exists, however, to suggest that this precursor cell is different from that of the neutrophil. Maturation also occurs in the bone marrow with subsequent release into the marginated pool. Unlike the information available on the neutrophil, however, the size of the marginated eosinophil pool is not known. Eosinophils are subsequently released into the circulation where they have a half-life of approximately 3–8 h. This is followed by a migration into the tissues, particularly the skin, mucous membranes, the respiratory and gastrointestinal tract and connective tissues. The tissue half-life may be as long as 3 days. It is important to remember, however, that in contrast to the neutrophil, the eosinophil is a cell whose importance and function lies primarily in its migratory ability into the tissues. It is unlikely that circulating blood eosinophils are functionally important. Migration into the tissues occurs between the endothelial cells by pseudopod formation. Experimentally, eosinophils can be shown to be attracted to sites of antigen deposition and sites of immediate hypersensitivity reactions. Histologically, this is usually associated with presence of both lymphocytes and macrophages.

A number of substances are known to influence the migration of eosinophils into these sites. Probably the most important is the eosinophil chemotactic factor of anaphylaxis (ECF-A). This substance has been shown to be released by activated mast cells and basophils and may be detected both in the nasal secretions and serum of patients at the time of acute immediate hypersensitivity reactions. This substance is a well characterized preformed tetrapeptide whose function, both experimentally and *in vivo*, appears to be in no doubt.

Some controversy exists as to the relative importance of other substances in the attraction and migration of eosinophils into sites of immediate hypersensitivity reactions. There is some evidence to suggest that histamine itself may attract eosinophils although serotonin and bradykinin have been shown to have no such effect. The association between eosinophils and T lymphocytes within the tissues has led to the possibility that eosinophil chemotactic lymphokines exist which are released by activated T lymphocytes. For example, T lymphocytes sensitized to trichinella antigen have been shown to produce a soluble factor which will not only attract eosinophils but will also stimulate bone marrow production. In addition, experimental data suggest that eosinophils are attracted to sites of antigen–antibody complex deposition and complement activation. In particular, the release of C5a, and to a lesser extent C3a and C$\overline{567}$, may induce eosinophil chemotaxis.

Tissue eosinophilia is occasionally a feature of certain neoplastic diseases. Experimental evidence currently exists indicating that some tumours will actively produce polypeptides which are structurally and functionally indistinguishable from ECF-A. In addition, the supernatant of activated Hodgkin's lymphoma cells has been shown to contain a substance which has eosinophilochemotactic properties.

BLOOD EOSINOPHILS

Eosinophils account for approximately 4% of the total white blood cells detectable in the circulation. Absolute eosinophil counts are of significantly more value and eosinophils are usually found in concentrations of up to 350/mm³. A diurnal variation exists with an increased eosinophil count at night. There also appears to be some relation to the menstrual cycle with a decreased count at the time of ovulation and an increase during menstruation. Total blood eosinophil counts represent a dynamic state between eosinophil production and tissue demands. Increased tissue demands at the time of immediate hypersensitivity reactions will lead to increased bone marrow production although this need not necessarily be reflected by an increased total blood eosinophil count. Increased eosinophil production is at least in part T-cell dependent. Experimentally, T-cell obliteration by thoracic duct drainage or irradiation results in a decreased production in eosinophils despite increasing demands. This is reversible with subsequent reinfusion of T lymphocytes. Under some circumstances increased tissue demands and increased production lead to blood eosinophilia. However, it is important to remember that eosinophilia itself is a relatively poor reflection of total body numbers and eosinophil activation. Blood eosinophilia without increased tissue concentrations is uncommon.

Total circulating eosinophil counts may be influenced by a number of other factors. In particular, eosinophil counts fall during times of stress probably in relation to increased ACTH release and steroid production. In addition, total eosinophil counts fall in acute inflammatory states possibly due to increased margination of the eosinophils or migration to inflammatory sites.

Hormonal control of eosinophil production appears to be influenced both by steroids and epinephrine, which reduce total numbers of circulating eosinophils. The relationship between total eosinophil numbers and production and oestrogens appears to be less clear.

FUNCTION

Considerable information is available on the function of eosinophils both experimentally and *in vivo*.

Phagocytosis

Eosinophils have the ability to phagocytose bacteria, immune complexes, denatured immunoglobulin and mast-cell granules. It would appear that they have enhanced capabilities of phagocytosing immune complexes and mast-cell granules compared with polymorphoneutrophils but will less readily phagocytose bacteria and denatured immunoglobulin. Despite this functional capacity which can readily be demonstrated *in vitro*, it is not clear to what extent this is an important function *in vivo*. Phagocytosis by eosinophils leads to a metabolic burst within the cells leading to the generation of superoxide radicals and chemiluminescence. Although this is greater than in neutrophils, phagocytic efficiency is less *in vitro*, resulting in an overall reduced bacterial kill rate.

Exocytosis

Probably the most important function of eosinophils is degranulation and release of the active hydrolytic enzymes present within cytoplasmic granules. This is of particular importance in relation to the function of eosinophils in the inactivation of the chemical mediators of immediate hypersensitivity. The factors leading to eosinophil degranulation are not clearly understood but in some instances may be due to activation of cell membrane receptors, both for C3b and immunoglobulin.

Microbicidal

Eosinophils have been shown to be capable of killing ingested bacteria and fungi. However, this action appears to be relatively poor and may have little *in vivo* significance. In particular, eosinophils do not present an adequate host resistance to pyogenic infection as witnessed by their inability to control infection in patients suffering from neutropenia despite adequate numbers of eosinophils. Eosinophils, as well as neutrophils, are defective in chronic granulomatous disease. In contrast, eosinophils appear to have particular importance in the host responses to protozoal infection and in particular, those protozoal infestations where tissue invasion is a characteristic feature. They have been shown to adhere to protozoa within the tissues and have an important role in the mediation of both antibody dependent cell-mediated cytotoxicity (ADCC) and direct cell-mediated immune responses (CMI). In this regard, they appear to have a complicated relationship with both mast cell and T-cell host responses as absence of eosinophils will significantly reduce host responses to protozoal tissue invasion. In particular, the eosinophil has a unique role as the effector cell in ADCC responses with K-cell activity, a function which is usually associated only with neutrophils or macrophages.

Immunological involvement

One of the prime functions of the eosinophil is as the homeostatic cell of immediate hypersensitivity reactions. Thus, characteristically, both blood and tissue eosinophilia may be seen in patients suffering with asthma, allergic rhinitis, drug hypersensitivity and anaphylaxis. Tissue deposition of allergen leads to the stimulation and activation of homocytotropic antibody (IgE) with fixation of this antibody both to mast cells and basophils. Degranulation occurs with the release of the chemical mediators of immediate hypersensitivity such as histamine and SRS-A. In addition, ECF-A is released, which leads to increased tissue migration of eosinophils and subsequently increased eosinophil production, leading to eosinophilia. The activation of eosinophils within the tissue results in the release of their hydrolytic enzymes and other chemical mediators such as prostaglandins which inhibit further mast-cell degranulation and both histaminases and arylsulphatases which inhibit histamine and SRS-A.

The involvement of eosinophils in immune complex-mediated reactions remains controversial. Experimentally, eosinophils have been shown to ingest antigen–antibody complexes and do this with greater efficiency than other neutrophils. They will not ingest antigen or antibody alone. It is not clear to what extent these findings have *in vivo* significance, as the eosinophil is not a characteristic cell, histologically, of immune complex-mediated reactions. In general, it is probably not the interaction of antigen and antibody *per se* which results in eosinophil functional activity but more the events which surround such interaction. In particular, the release of a soluble factor from antigen-activated T lymphocytes and the activation of the complement system with subsequent release of C5a may be of more importance.

The relationship between the eosinophil and IgE antibody is often confused. In general, any relationship which exists is primarily through the association of homocytotropic antibody with mast cells and basophils and the subsequent release by these cells of ECF-A and the subsequent tissue migration of eosinophils. No direct relationship exists between the two. For instance, IgE does not have the ability to induce eosinophilia *per se*, e.g. eosinophils are normal in numbers in cases of IgE myeloma; nor do eosinophils have any direct relationship with IgE antibody, which is not elevated in hypereosinophilic syndromes.

DISEASES IN WHICH EOSINOPHILS PLAY A MAJOR ROLE

It is beyond the scope of this chapter to discuss in detail those conditions where eosinophils are known to play a major role in the pathogenesis of the disease. However, certain general points can be learned from these conditions. Tissue and blood eosinophilia are particular features of those conditions involving Type 1 hypersensitivity responses where a known or punitive antigen becomes tissue-bound, particularly in the mucous membranes of the upper or lower respiratory tract, skin or gastrointestinal tract. Thus, many allergic or atopic states such as hay fever, angio-oedema and asthma are associated with tissue infiltration by eosinophils and subsequently may be associated with blood eosinophilia or a high content of eosinophils in secretions. Secondly, tissue invasion by eosinophils is a characteristic feature of parasitic infection. The important factor appears to be the invasion of these parasites into the tissues themselves. Thus, eosinophils are not usually seen nor are they a major host response in those parasitic infections that are localized to the lumen of the gastrointestinal tract. Invasion of the tissues, however extensive and however complicated the life cycle of the parasite, appears to be the factor which initiates involvement of eosinophils in the host response. Finally, eosinophils play a major role in the pathogenesis of some forms of drug hypersensitivity reactions; usually those associated with increased levels of IgE antibody and giving rise to anaphylactic reactions, e.g. penicillin hypersensitivity. In general, therefore, it can be assumed that in all those conditions where eosinophils play a major role in pathogenesis of the disease, a Type 1 hypersensitivity reaction is often involved. This, however, by no means entirely explains their role. As already mentioned, eosinophils may have a complicated interaction with macrophages and T lymphocytes in the mediation of ADCC and CMI host responses to parasitic invasion. As far as is known, they are not necessarily involved in the mediation of CMI responses under other circumstances. In addition, the presence of eosinophils in the tissues and the generation of blood eosinophilia may have other causes. Although these are not as clearly defined, they include conditions which involve the deposition of antigen–antibody complexes, the activation of the complement pathway and, as in the case of some neoplastic diseases, e.g. Hodgkin's disease, the release of eosinophil chemotactic factors.

EOSINOPHILS IN THE CONNECTIVE TISSUE DISEASES

The connective tissue diseases, in general, are not usually characterized by tissue invasion by eosinophils or subsequent blood eosinophilia. For this reason relatively little is known about the role of the eosinophils in the common rheumatic diseases although, as outlined later, clinical eosinophilia may be a feature of a number of connective tissue diseases. It would not be unreasonable to assume that this is a manifestation of increased tissue demands although the presence of eosinophils within the tissues is not a major feature of the rheumatic diseases histologically nor are Type 1 hypersensitivity responses generally regarded as playing anything but a minor role in the pathogenesis of these conditions. In general, therefore, information on eosinophils in the connective tissue diseases revolves around the clinical observations of eosinophilia in certain clinical syndromes and at the present time we are left to speculate as to the possible significance of these clinical findings.

EOSINOPHILIC FASCIITIS (SCHULMAN'S SYNDROME)

Until recently, no connective tissue disease was known to be associated with eosinophilia with any frequency. The recent description of eosinophilic fasciitis by Schulman[2,3] appears to be a notable exception. In the original cases, Shulman described a new syndrome characterized by inflammation and thickening of the fascial planes leading to oedema and skin induration. The particularly interesting features of this condition were a characteristic marked eosinophilia, increased levels of IgG and an absence of Raynaud's phenomenon and evidence of systemic involvement. Histologically, most cases have marked thickening of the fascial planes with fibrosis and cellular infiltration by plasma cells and lymphocytes. In the majority of cases reported, eosinophils have also been detected not only in the fascial planes but also in the surrounding dermis, fat tissues and occasionally in adjacent muscle. In general, responses to prednisone have been good and the condition was thought to have a relatively benign prognosis until the recent follow-up of Shulman's original cases[4]. The aetiology of this condition is completely unknown but acute onset of the disease does appear in many cases to be associated with trauma or unaccustomed physical exertion. Since the original reports other cases have been added to the literature with similar clinical and histological findings[5,6]. The condition has also been reported in childhood[7]. Almost uniformly, the cases reported have been associated with eosinophilia often in excess of several thousand per cubic millimetre. In most reports, eosinophils have been a histological feature of the disease although this is not universally the case. As the aetiology of the disease is at present unknown the exact role of the eosinophil in the mediation of the condition is unclear.

At the present time, however, there appears little evidence that this is mediated by a Type 1 hypersensitivity reaction, and information on the possible association with IgE antibody is not available. This condition is therefore of considerable interest as not only is it relatively unique in the connective tissue diseases in its association with the eosinophil, but also it does not appear to resemble the clinical or histological features of any of the other non-connective tissue diseases with which eosinophilia is so closely associated.

MORPHEA AND SCLERODERMA

Some of the clinical features of eosinophilic fasciitis so resemble scleroderma that some authors have regarded this as merely a variant of scleroderma and related diseases[8]. Some studies have reported the presence of eosinophilia in morphea and scleroderma[9] but in these cases the association is not as strong, nor the extent of the eosinophilia so great. Some authors would dispute the association of eosinophilia with scleroderma[10], however, although linear scleroderma would appear to be a possible exception[11]. A review of the literature would certainly suggest that eosinophilia and tissue invasion by eosinophils is an inconstant and relatively unimportant association with scleroderma and related conditions. However, as both eosinophilic fasciitis and scleroderma appear to have similar histological changes at different tissue levels, and as scleroderma is known to be biochemically associated with a defect in collagen production and degradation, it remains to be seen whether an as yet unknown stimulus for these changes or some component of collagen synthesis may be related to the generation of tissue eosinophils and subsequent eosinophilia.

RHEUMATOID ARTHRITIS

It has been known for many years that some patients with rheumatoid arthritis have an associated eosinophilia[12], although eosinophils do not appear to be a feature of the histological appearances of the chronic rheumatoid synovium or rheumatoid synovial fluid. In two recent studies[13, 14] eosinophilia was noted to be a particular feature of patients with extra-articular manifestations of rheumatoid disease. In both studies patients with marked eosinophilia had associated high titres of rheumatoid factor, cutaneous vasculitis, pericarditis, pulmonary fibrosis, rheumatoid nodules and depressed serum C3 levels. In some cases, the eosinophilia was associated with Felty's syndrome. The role of the eosinophil in rheumatoid arthritis, particularly in those with extra-articular manifestations of the disease, is not without theoretical interest. Recent studies have clearly shown that such patients, and those suffering from Felty's syndrome, have high levels of detectable circulating immune complexes within the serum, a feature which is not prominent in patients with less severe disease[15, 16]. In addition, there is increasing evidence that rheumatoid disease is associated with defects in cell-mediated immune responses[17]. From experimental work, eosinophils are known to be associated with both immune complex deposition and in some cases T-cell-mediated responses. Thus eosinophils are attracted to the site of antigen–antibody deposition by the activation of the complement pathway and may themselves be dependent upon modulation by T lymphocytes. A direct cause and relationship between these considerations and the eosinophilia seen in some patients with rheumatoid disease remains to be proven.

POLYARTERITIS NODOSA

Although eosinophilia is often listed as a common association with polyarteritis nodosa, this usually occurs only in patients with pulmonary involvement. In such cases, patients have clinical signs and symptoms of bronchial asthma and obvious pulmonary involvement on chest X-ray. In a study of 111 cases of polyarteritis nodosa reported in 1957[18], 14 cases had pulmonary involvement and eight of these had significant eosinophilia. None of the remaining 97 cases without pulmonary involvement had elevated eosinophil counts. This study supplements a previous report[19] where almost all patients with eosinophilia in association with polyarteritis nodosa had evidence of pulmonary involvement at some stage during their illness. The significance of this strong association between the eosinophil, pulmonary involvement and polyarteritis nodosa is not yet clear. It is apparent, however, that the polyarteritis nodosa syndrome may be a response to exposure to a number of different antigens of which the hepatitis B antigen appears to be the most clearly defined. As pulmonary involvement is not a manifestation of all cases of polyarteritis nodosa, it remains to be seen whether exposure to an antigen through the respiratory tract may be the initiating factor in those patients with this clinical presentation.

Eosinophilia in other forms of vasculitis is rare with the exception of patients with Wegener's granulomatosis[20]. As this condition is primarily a disease involving the upper and lower respiratory tracts in association with a glomerulonephritis it remains theoretically possible that the eosinophil may have a similar role in Wegener's granulomatosis to that seen in patients with polyarteritis nodosa and pulmonary involvement.

SYSTEMIC LUPUS ERYTHEMATOSUS (SLE)

This condition is often quoted as a classical example of an immune complex-mediated disease with the deposition of immune complexes leading to complement activation and initiation of an inflammatory response. Eosinophilia is not a common laboratory feature of patients with SLE. Dubois's review of the condition[21] reports its occurrence in less than 2% of cases. This negative association between eosinophilia and SLE is of theoretical interest. As already mentioned, eosinophils are attracted to the site of antigen–antibody deposition and have the ability to phagocytose immune complexes *in vitro*. These experimental and *in vitro* observations might suggest that, in an immune complex-mediated disease such as SLE, eosinophilia would be a prevalent feature. The fact that this is not the case suggests that these *in vitro* eosinophil functions do not necessarily have *in vivo* significance.

DRUG HYPERSENSITIVITY

A number of drugs producing Type 1 hypersensitivity reactions are associated with eosinophilia, e.g. penicillin hypersensitivity. In the case of drugs used in the treatment of the rheumatic diseases, two are of particular interest. Hypersensitivity reactions to aspirin are commonly associated with eosinophilia.

This association, however, does not appear to have any direct relationship to the underlying connective tissue disease but more to an unrelated idiosyncratic reaction by the patient. Those with an atopic diathesis and nasal polyps are particularly prone to aspirin intolerance resulting in asthmatic attacks[22]. In such patients, eosinophilia is commonly an associated feature.

Hepatotoxicity secondary to salicylate ingestion is a subject of recent interest. This condition is particularly seen in patients with juvenile rheumatoid arthritis and patients with SLE receiving salicylates. In one study, all six patients reported with salicylate hepatotoxicity had eosinophilia[23]. This preceded the evidence of liver disease in four of the patients. It appears to be a relatively benign condition which histologically is characterized by nonspecific periportal collections of inflammatory cells and is associated biochemically with rises in serum transaminase levels. The association with eosinophilia in the initial reports would certainly suggest that this is a hypersensitivity reaction which in most cases resolves on stopping the medication. Other reports, however[24, 25], dispute the presence of eosinophilia in this condition. The similar clinical situation seen in some patients with SLE exposed to salicylates in not associated with eosinophilia[26].

Chrysotherapy is the commonest medication associated with eosinophilia in the treatment of rheumatoid arthritis. Two studies[27, 28] have reported a similar prevalence of eosinophilia in association with such treatment which may be as high as 40%. This haematological association with chrysotherapy is not necessarily associated with other side-effects of the medication, although nearly half the patients with eosinophilia also had a dermatological reaction. In some cases the eosinophilia spontaneously disappears after a period of several weeks with no adverse effect being experienced by the patient. One of these studies has also reported an association between the eosinophilia and increased levels of IgE antibody. This association has led to the suggestion that eosinophilia in association with chrysotherapy represents a Type 1 hypersensitivity reaction to the drug[29]. The presence of elevated IgE levels in such patients, however, is controversial. This interesting association still requires clarification although the presence of eosinophilia during chrysotherapy is not regarded as an indication for stopping treatment.

References

1. Beeson, P. B. and Bass, D. A. (1977). *The Eosinophil*. (London: W. B. Saunders Co.)
2. Shulman, L. E. (1974). Diffuse fasciitis with hypergammaglobulinaemia and eosinophilia: a new syndrome? *J. Rheumatol.*, **1** (Suppl.), 82
3. Shulman, L. E. (1977). Diffuse fasciitis with eosinophilia: a new syndrome? *Arth. Rheum.*, **20** (Suppl.), 205
4. Shulman, L. E., Hoffman, R., Adelman, H. M. and Lawless, O. J. (1979). Aplastic anaemia and thrombocytopenic purpura in eosinophilic fasciitis. Presented at the *9th European Congress of Rheumatology*. 2–8 September. Wiesbaden

5. Rodnan, G. P., DiBartolomeo, A., Medsger, T. A. and Banes, E. L. (1975). Eosinophilic fasciitis: report of seven cases of a newly recognized scleroderma-like syndrome. *Arth. Rheum.*, **18**, 422

6. Bennett, R. M., Herron, A. and Keogh, L. (1977). Eosinophilic fasciitis. *Ann. Rheum. Dis.*, **36**, 354

7. Ansell, B. M., Nasseh, G. A. and Bywaters, E. G. L. (1976). Scleroderma in childhood. *Ann. Rheum. Dis.*, **35**, 189

8. Caperton, E. M., Hathaway, D. E. and Dehner, L. P. (1976). Morphoea, fasciitis and scleroderma with eosinophilia: a broad spectrum disease. *Arth. Rheum.*, **19**, 792

9. Flieschmajer, R., Jacotot, B., Shore, S. and Binnick, S. (1978). Scleroderma, eosinophilia and diffuse fasciitis. *Arch. Dermatol.*, **114**, 1320

10. Rodnan, G. P. (1979). *Progressive Systemic Sclerosis*, p. 246. (London: W. B. Saunders Co.)

11. Rodnan, G. P., Lipinski, E., Rabin, B. S. and Reichlin, M. (1977). Eosinophilia and serologic abnormalities in linear localized scleroderma. *Arth. Rheum.*, **20**, 133

12. Short, C. L., Bauer, W. and Reynolds, W. E. (1957). *Rheumatoid Arthritis*. (Cambridge, Mass.: Harvard University Press)

13. Panush, R. S., Franco, A. E. and Schur, P. M. (1971). Rheumatoid arthritis associated with eosinophilia. *Ann. Intern. Med.*, **75**, 199

14. Winchester, R. J., Litwin, S. D., Koffler, D. and Kunkel, M. G. (1971). Observations on the eosinophilia of certain patients with rheumatoid arthritis. *Arth. Rheum.*, **14**, 650

15. Halla, J. T., Volanakis, J. E. and Schrohenloher, R. E. (1979). Immune complexes in rheumatoid arthritis sera and synovial fluids. *Arth. Rheum.*, **22**, 440

16. Hurd, E. R., Chubick, A., Jasin, H. E. and Ziff, M. (1979). Increased Clq binding immune complexes in Felty's syndrome. *Arth. Rheum.*, **22**, 697

17. Yu, D. T. and Peter, J. B. (1974). Cellular immunological aspects on rheumatoid arthritis. *Sem. Arth. Rheum.*, **4**, 25

18. Rose, G. A. and Spencer, H. (1957). Polyarteritis nodosa. *Q. J. Med.*, **26**, 43

19. Wilson, K. S. and Alexander, H. L. (1945). The association of periarteritis nodosa, bronchial asthma and hypereosinophilia. *J. Lab. Clin. Med.*, **30**, 361

20. Walton, E. W. (1958). Giant cell granuloma of the respiratory tract (Wegener's granulomatosis). *Br. Med. J.*, **2**, 265

21. Dubois, E. L. (1974). *Lupus erythematosus*, 2nd Edn, p. 366 (University of Southern California Press)

22. Samter, M. and Beers, R. F. (1968). Intolerance to aspirin. *Ann. Intern. Med.*, **68**, 975

23. Rich, R. R. and Johnson, J. S. (1973). Salicylate hepatotoxicity in patients with juvenile rheumatoid arthritis. *Arth. Rheum.*, **16**, 1

24. Athreya, B. H., Moser, G., Cecil, H. S. and Myers, A. R. (1975). Aspirin induced hepatotoxicity in juvenile rheumatoid arthritis. *Arth. Rheum.*, **18**, 347

25. Barone, R., Chase, P. H. and Wallace, S. L. (1976). Salicylate induced hepatic injury. *Arth. Rheum.*, **19**, 964

26. Seaman, W. E., Ishak, K. G. and Poltz, P. M. (1974). Aspirin induced hepatoxicity in patients with systemic lupus erythematosus. *Ann. Intern. Med.*, **80**, 1

27. Davis, P. and Hughes, G. R. V. (1974). Significance of eosinophilia during gold therapy. *Arth. Rheum.*, **17**, 964

28. Jessop, J. D., Dippy, J., Turnbull, A. and Bright, M. (1974). Eosinophilia during gold therapy. *Rheum. Rehab.*, **13**, 75

29. Davis, P., Ezeoke, A., Munro, J., Hobbs, J. R. and Hughes, G. R. V. (1973). Immunological studies on the mechanism of gold hypersensitivity reactions. *Br. Med. J.*, **3**, 678

9
The Macrophage—Origins, Functions and Role in the Rheumatic Diseases

N. HURST and G. NUKI

INTRODUCTION

Metchnikoff[1] recognized the importance of the macrophage in host defence and in mounting inflammatory responses in the nineteenth century; indeed it formed the cornerstone for his cellular theory of immunity. A vast amount of subsequent work has confirmed that mononuclear phagocytes participate in all types of inflammation, tending to play a dominant part wherever the inflammatory process becomes chronic[2]. Recent research has revealed that cells of the mononuclear series may play a key role in the initiation[3, 4], and genetic regulation[5] of the immune response as well as being an important source of inflammatory mediators and destructive enzymes. Yet these cells have been little studied in rheumatoid arthritis (RA) and other inflammatory connective tissue disorders.

Over the years studies of the immunopathogenesis of these diseases have emphasized in turn:

(1) infection and antigen persistence;
(2) autoimmunity and humoral autoantibodies;
(3) immune-complex formation and activation of the complement system;
(4) the role of neutrophil polymorphonuclear phagocytes (PMN) as the source of proteolytic enzymes and amplification factors;
(5) the role of lymphocytes as the source of lymphokines mediating stimulation and suppression of cellular subpopulations;
(6) the role of lymphocytes in the genetic regulation of the immune response.

183

At each and every phase the potential role of the macrophage has been largely ignored.

This chapter reviews some of the important facets of the anatomy and cell biology of monocyte macrophages as well as current knowledge of their role in immune responses and their secretory and biochemical activities with the overall aim of relating these to the pathogenesis of rheumatic diseases.

SYNOVIOCYTES AND THE MONONUCLEAR PHAGOCYTE SYSTEM

The blood monocyte is derived from a bone marrow precursor, the pro-monocyte, and after release from the marrow persists in the peripheral blood for up to 3–4 days before leaving randomly to enter the tissues where it matures into the tissue macrophage. The peripheral blood monocyte is a large cell about 10 μm or larger in diameter with a kidney-shaped nucleus and abundant pale-staining cytoplasm. There may be some difficulty distinguishing monocytes and large lymphocytes using conventional stains. For more accurate identification cytochemical methods demonstrating peroxidase, lysozyme or non-specific esterase may be used. The electronmicroscopic appearance of the mononuclear phagocyte is characteristic (Figure 9.1)—the cytoplasm contains numerous granules, prominent secretory apparatus, mito-chondria and occasional phagosomes. The lysosomal granules are hetero-

Table 9.1   Tissue distribution of the bone-marrow derived monocyte–macrophage system

Tissue site	Name
Blood	monocyte
Connective tissue	histiocyte
Brain	microglial cells
Liver	Kupffer cells[108]
Bone	osteoclasts[109]
Lung	alveolar macrophages[12]
Synovium	synovial A cells (? B cells)[18,79]
	multinucleate giant cells[110,111]
Synovial fluid	macrophages
	multinucleate giant cells[112,113]
Granulomata	epithelioid cells
	multinucleate giant cells[114,115]
Spleen	macrophages

geneous in content—some staining for peroxidase, others for enzymes such as acid phosphatase and aryl sulphatase. With maturation into the larger tissue macrophage the peroxidase content diminishes but phagocytic vacuoles become more evident[6]. Granule discharge into these vacuoles after phago-

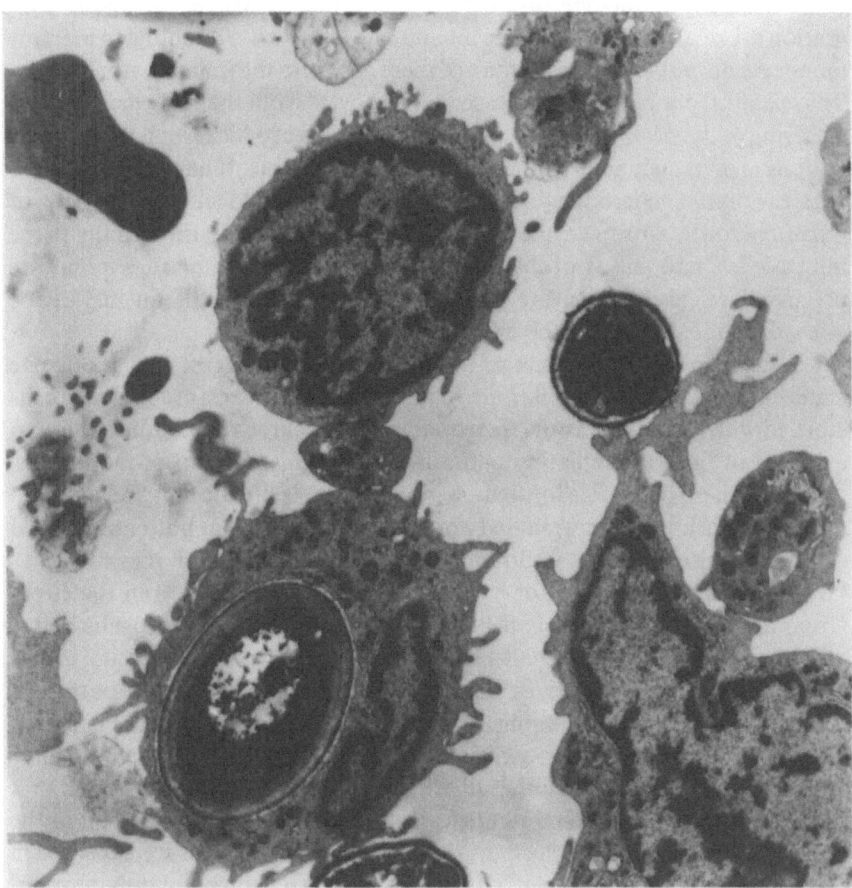

Figure 9.1 Electronmicrograph of blood monocyte containing an ingested yeast particle (×5600). Note the intact phagosome membrane, cytoplasmic granules, mitochondria and filipodia

cytosis can be shown using cytochemical techniques. The mononuclear phagocyte membrane carries specific receptors for C3b, C3d[7] and the Fc component of IgG1 and IgG3. These can be readily demonstrated using rosette techniques with suitably coated red cells or by the rapid phagocytosis of material coated with these opsonins.

Various eponyms are given to tissue macrophages according to the site in which they are found (Table 9.1). Isotope-labelling experiments, however, have confirmed that blood monocytes are the common source of these anatomically scattered but functionally homogeneous tissue macrophages[8,9].

The kinetics of turnover of promonocytes, monocytes and tissue macrophages have been studied with isotope-labelling techniques in animals with inflammatory lesions and in normal controls[9-15]. These studies show that while normally monocyte production in the bone marrow and tissue emigration are relatively slow, during inflammation there is a doubling in marrow monocyte output and a large efflux of these cells into the inflammatory lesion. This results from premature release of monocytes from the bone marrow and a halving of the promonocyte cell cycle time; an effect which can be blocked by inhibitors of nucleic acid synthesis such as azathioprine. It has been suggested that the tissue macrophage is capable of dividing locally at the site of inflammation[11]. However, the contribution of local cell division to the tissue infiltrate is small and is probably due to the arrival of immature monocyte precursors released prematurely from the marrow which subsequently divide once, or at most twice, at the inflammatory focus[12, 13].

Limited studies[14, 15] of human monocyte kinetics suggest that monocyte traffic is qualitatively similar in man. Using autotransfused blood cells labelled with [³H]di-isopropyl fluorophosphate Meuret and Hoffman[14] found evidence of both a circulating and a larger marginated pool of monocytes. However, these two pools formed essentially a single kinetic unit and the ratio of the circulating and marginated pools was about 1:3.5 in both normal and diseased subjects. There is doubt as to the significance of these findings however, since the half-life of 8.4 h for their disappearance from the circulation approximates to the half-life of 6 h for neutrophil polymorphs and is very much shorter than the half-life of 71 h found by Whitelaw[15] using *in vivo* pulse labelling with [³H]thymidine. Whitelaw calculated a daily output of 9.4×10^8 cells/24 h and demonstrated a 13–26 h delay before labelled cells emerged from the bone marrow, giving some indication of the cell cycle time. In monocyte distribution studies in the rat Whitelaw and Batho[16] found that there were 25 times more mononuclear phagocytes in the tissues than in the peripheral blood and that the majority of tissue macrophages were located in the spleen and lungs. This is in contradistinction to neutrophil polymorphonuclear phagocytes of which the vast majority remain in circulation during health.

The factors regulating monocyte production in health, and the signals which stimulate the increase in monocyte production during inflammation, are not fully understood. There is good evidence for the existence of a humoral 'factor-inducing monocytopoiesis' (FIM), which is released both in early acute inflammation and during prolonged inflammation[13, 17]. This acts by reducing the promonocyte cell cycle time and by monoblast stimulation increases the number of promonocytes. FIM appears to be a thermolabile protein of molecular weight 18 000–24 000 which is produced by monocytes at the inflammatory site. With the subsidence of inflammation a monocyte-inhibiting factor slows monocytopoiesis by inhibiting proliferation of monoblasts.

The relationship of synovial cells to the mononuclear phagocyte system is an important issue which has not yet been completely clarified. Ultrastructural studies of the human synovium[18] demonstrate two types of synoviocyte, designated A and B cells. The more numerous A cells appear to be phagocytic and the B cells secretory in function. Recent work[19, 20] strongly suggests that A and B cells are in fact a single cell type engaged in different functions. The structural and functional features of the A cell type in particular suggests that it forms part of the mononuclear phagocyte system. Conclusive proof that A and B synoviocytes have a common origin from bone marrow monocytes must await *in vivo* labelling studies in humans.

CELL BIOLOGY OF THE MONONUCLEAR PHAGOCYTE

The cellular mechanisms which determine the ability of the monocyte to leave the circulation and move into an inflammatory focus in order to perform its phagocytic function are clearly fundamental to our understanding of the mononuclear phagocyte in inflammation.

Leukocyte locomotion depends on the ability of the cell to adhere reversibly to a substrate. There must be sufficient adhesion to allow traction, but not so much as to inhibit. During locomotion the cell becomes morphologically 'polarized' in the direction of movement, with the formation of a short uropod or tail and an anterior lamellipodium. The latter can be seen under phase contrast as a spreading veil of cytoplasm. Endocytosis also involves adherence followed by active movement of cytoplasm around the surface of the particle during engulfment. These three properties of the cell—spreading, locomotion and endocytosis—may have a common underlying mechanism.

In order for any cell to move it must be able to distort its shape. For this to occur, it must have an internal 'fulcrum' or skeleton on which contractile or motile elements can act. It is thought that the microtubules of the cell cytoplasm form this 'cytoskeleton' and that the microfilaments found in the clear peripheral zone of the cell cytoplasm are the contractile elements which act upon it. The microfilament system has been shown to consist of three components: actin, the contractile protein; actin-binding protein, which cross-links actin filaments; and myosin, the energy-transducing protein of skeletal muscle.

Actin-binding protein serves to convert the actin filaments from a low-viscosity 'sol' of individual polymer molecules to a more rigid 'gel' structure in which cross-linking of the molecules has occurred. Contraction of the actin gel is activated by myosin with the utilization of ATP (Figure 9.2).

The microtubular cytoskeleton connects with the microfilament system and contraction of a segment of the peripheral microfilaments leads to distortion of the overlying membrane. The basic alteration of cell shape necessary for movement is thus attained.

Two pharmacological probes, cytochalasin B and colchicine, have provided insight into the separate components of this system. Colchicine binds reversibly to microtubules[21], and interferes with their structural properties, causing loss of cell 'polarity' and directional cell movement. Endocytosis may still occur in the presence of colchicine but the directional movement of vacuoles and granules within the cytoplasm is lost resulting in failure of degranulation following phagocytosis. Low concentrations of cytochalasin B, on the other hand, cause dissolution of the microfilament gel by preventing the binding of actin-binding protein to the actin polymer. Intense focal aggregation and

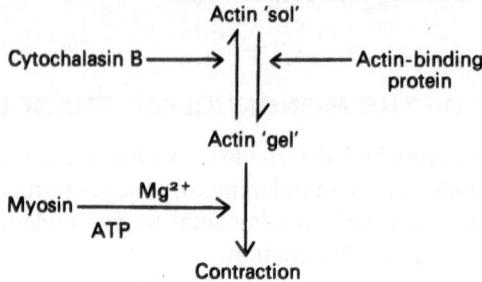

Figure 9.2   The sequence of events leading to contraction of actin

contraction of microfilaments occurs resulting in failure of endocytosis, cell membrane ruffling and movement[21-23]. These events are also related to 'capping' of surface receptors. During capping, surface receptors and contractile microfilaments are simultaneously translocated to the uropod[24].

The precise mechanism by which the microfilament system produces cell movements is not clear. However, there is evidence that at least one component of this process involves local gelation of actin brought about by actin-binding protein and myosin. It is suggested that membrane activation in the advancing pseudopodia causes translocation of actin-binding protein and myosin with secondary gelation and contraction of actin within the pseudopodia. The tension thus produced results in membrane ruffling, and increased contact with the substrate[22].

The signals for the activation and modulation of these functional activities appear to involve changes in cAMP and cGMP levels. These two cyclic nucleotides have been shown to depress and enhance microtubule formation respectively, their effects probably being mediated via protein kinases. Agents known to stimulate the formation of these nucleotides are illustrated in Figure 9.3.

The effect on phagocytosis, either of modulation of cyclic nucleotides or direct disruption of microtubules by colchicine, has not yet been clarified. Some studies have shown inhibition[25, 26] but others no effect[27]. These differences may be methodological and perhaps reflect secondary effects of microtubule disruption on microfilament function in certain experimental systems. It is of interest that the immunostimulant levamisole has cholinergic actions and may restore depressed T-cell and macrophage function in anergic states by elevating cGMP levels.

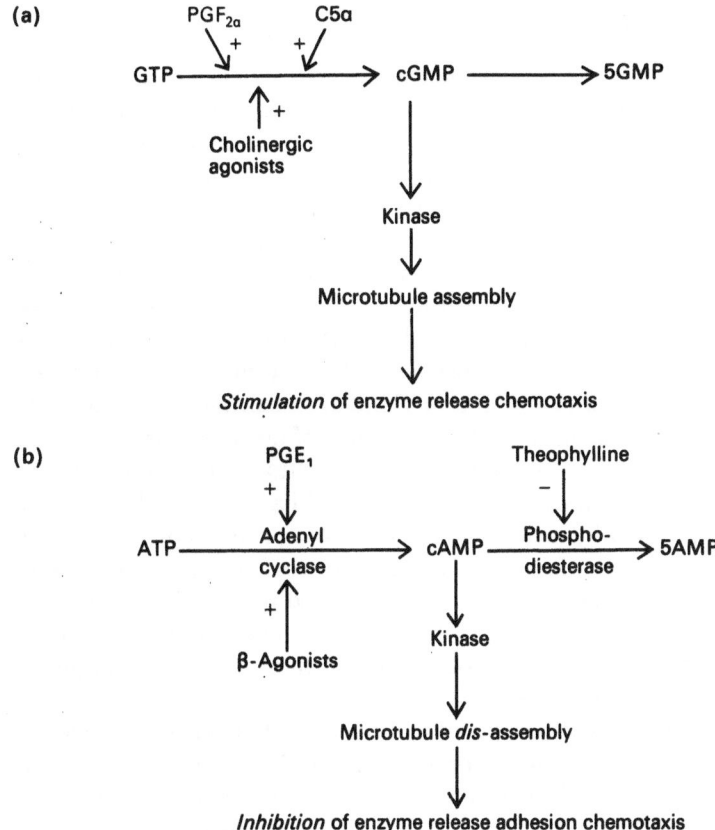

Figure 9.3 The sequence of events leading to microtubular (a) assembly and (b) disassembly

Two clinical conditions, malakoplakia and Chediak–Higashi syndrome, illustrate the importance of cyclic nucleotides in maintaining an intact microtubule system and emphasize their role in post-phagocytic lysosomal degranulation. Malakoplakia is an uncommon condition characterized clinically by recurrent inflammatory granulatoma and failure to digest certain Gramnegative bacteria. The pathological defect, confined to the monocyte, is expressed as low levels of intracellular cGMP, large intracytoplasmic lysosomes and failure of lysosomal enzyme release. Phagocytosis and chemotaxis appear to be normal. Administration of cholinergic agonists *in vitro* and *in vivo* correct both the monocyte defect and the clinical abnormalities[28]. Both PMNs and monocytes from patients with Chediak–Higashi syndrome contain large cytoplasmic lysosomes, show defective post-phagocytic degranulation and, in certain test systems, impaired chemotaxis—these defects are associated with impaired intracellular killing of bacteria, elevated cAMP levels and defective microtubule assembly—all of which can be corrected by agents which raise levels of cGMP or by ascorbic acid[29].

Membrane receptors

It has long been accepted that, while endocytosis is a feature of many cell types, phagocytosis of opsonized material is peculiar to polymorphonuclear and mononuclear phagocytes which carry receptors for immunoglobulin and complement. Phagocytosis of hydrophobic charged particles occurs in the absence of opsonins, albeit less efficiently, but requires the presence of Ca^{2+}. Hydrophilic particles, such as pneumococci, however, are very poorly phagocytosed and must be opsonized before being engulfed. Coating with C3b was shown to reduce the requirement for divalent cations and may even allow phagocytosis to occur in the presence of EDTA. Studies with $^{45}Ca^{2+}$ show that the mechanism is truly independent of extracellular Ca^{2+} and that complement does not simply enhance the binding of calcium to the particle[30]. Monocyte receptors recognize the Fc component of IgG1 and IgG3 as well as C3b and C3d[7,31]. Uptake of material coated with these moieties is rapid once contact is made. Experiments by Griffin et al.[32] have shown that there is sequential recognition by membrane receptors of opsonin molecules on the particle being engulfed. Using immunoglobulin-coated red cells they were able to demonstrate that ingestion could be halted if the red cell surface is partially denuded of opsonin after contact has been made. Other studies have shown that particle uptake is also local and segmental, and does not signal a generalized membrane response[33].

There is a wide range of agents which influence cell movement. Some are chemotactic, while others enhance or inhibit random movements and modulate the response of cells to chemotactic agents. The composite effect of a variety of different leucoattractants and modulators determine the composition of the cellular infiltrate to be found in different pathological situations. For example eosinophils are a major feature of immediate hypersensitivity, neutrophils of acute/subacute inflammation and macrophages of chronic inflammation. Some of the more important leucoattractants and their cellular specificity are shown in Table 9.2.

The effect of leucoattractants is often complex. For example histamine, which is strongly chemotactic for eosinophils, is less so for neutrophils and not for monocytes[34]. It can, however, modulate the response both of eosinophils and neutrophils to other chemotaxins such as C5a. In low dose it enhances, while in high dose it inhibits, both chemotaxis and random migration of eosinophils. Experiments with histamine antagonists suggest that the low- and high-dose effects exerted on eosinophils are mediated by H1 and H2 receptors respectively. In neutrophils H1 agonists enhance and H2 agonists inhibit chemotaxis to C5a while both stimuli enhance random migration.

The cell receptors for many of these agents are not clearly defined but a considerable amount of information has recently been obtained from the study of small synthetic peptide leucoattractants. The discovery that formylmethionyl peptides are extremely potent cellular chemoattractants followed

Table 9.2 Chemotactic agents and their cellular targets

	Mononuclear phagocytes	Neutrophils	Eosinophils
C5a	++	++	++
C567 C3B	?	++	+
Fibronopeptide B	++	++	?
Kallikrein	++	++	+
Lymphokines			
LDCF	++	0	?
LIF	0	—	?
MIF	—	0	?
NCF	0	++	?
Neutrophil-derived			
NIF	0	—	
Mast-cell derived			
Histamine—high dose	?	0	$-H_2$
low dose	?	0	$++H_1$
Low MW ECF (tetra peptide)	0	+	++
High MW NCF	0	++	+
Lipids			
Thromboxane B_2	?	++	?
HETE	?	++	++
Synthetic peptides			
F-Met-Leu-Phe	+	++	++
Methyl ester of F-Met-Leu-Phe	++	+	?

LDCF = lymphocyte-derived chemotactic factor
LIF = leucocyte inhibitory factor
MIF = macrophage inhibitory factor
NCF = neutrophil chemotactic factor
NIF = neutrophil inhibitory factor
ECF = eosinophil chemotactic factor
MW = molecular weight

from work on leucoattractants produced by bacteria. Studies of structure activity relationships[35] showed that the F-Met-Leu Phe peptide was several orders of magnitude more potent than other related peptides and stimulated chemotaxis at concentrations around 10^{-11} mol/l. Affinity studies showed highly specific binding sites on the phagocyte and about 10^5 receptors per cell. Additionally, a membrane-located esterase was demonstrated which hydrolyses the peptide after contact with the receptor, thereby releasing the receptor for further stimuli—a situation analogous to the well-known acetylcholine esterase system at the motor endplates of skeletal muscle. A further point of interest is that while F-Met-Leu-Phe is much less chemotactic for monocytes than polymorphs, if the peptide is esterified to the methyl ester the situation is reversed and the peptide becomes several orders of magnitude more chemoattractive for monocytes than polymorphs[36]. In addition to revealing a new and important membrane receptor these studies are ı important landmark in the quest for understanding the stereochemical structure–function relationships of membrane receptors.

Clinical studies

There are relatively few clinical studies of the cellular activity of monocytes in patients with rheumatic diseases and many unanswered questions remain.

Skin window techniques have been used to measure phagocytosis of carbon particles by exudate cells in patients with rheumatoid arthritis[37]. Jessop and his colleagues found that phagocytic activity of macrophages and neutrophil polymorphs was increased in rheumatoid arthritis and suppressed during treatment with gold and prednisolone. Parallel experiments with rats confirmed the effects of gold and prednisolone and also showed a gross inhibitory effect of these drugs on both the fluid and cellular components of the inflammatory response[38]. While these studies may provide a useful overall view of the inflammatory response in rheumatoid arthritis, individual components such as neutrophil polymorph and monocyte chemotaxis, adherence, spreading and phagocytosis and the net effect of *humoral* inflammatory mediators alone cannot be separated in any detail. In addition to phagocytosis of carbon particles the method reflects the cells' ability to adhere, spread and move about on the coverslip and also their ability to remain attached to the glass after phagocytosis. *In vitro* studies[39] using adherent synovial cells from excised synovial membrane have shown similar increases in phagocytic activity in rheumatoid arthritis with suppression by gold, but again the coverslip technique does not allow one to distinguish the phenomena of spreading and movement from phagocytosis. Further work on the kinetics of phagocytosis and the role of opsonins are clearly required and may well be relevant in determining rates of clearance of immune complexes.

Another study examined the phagocytic function of peripheral blood monocytes from patients with RA and SLE[40]. Function was depressed in SLE but normal in RA. The impairment seen in SLE was restored to normal by levamisole and accompanied by a fall in circulating immune complexes. Fc receptors were assayed using IgG-coated red cell rosette techniques and showed apparent enhancement of Fc receptor function in the SLE patients. The yeast particles used as substrate in the phagocytic test were coated with C3b and IgM so that the reduced phagocytic uptake in SLE could well be a reflection of impaired C3 receptor activity. These observations parallel those of Wilton et al.[41]. Using blood and synovial fluid PMN from RA patients they demonstrated defective phagocytosis in a number of subjects which correlated with impaired C3b receptor function.

Landry[42] also found reduced chemotaxis and phagocytosis of both peripheral blood PMN and monocytes from patients with untreated SLE and depressed delayed type hypersensitivity (DTH) skin reactions but normal T and B cell function and concluded that the impairment of CMI seen was secondary to defective monocyte and PMN function.

Another approach to phagocytosis is to measure rates of clearance of particulate material administered intravenously. Williams et al.[43] demonstrated impaired clearance of heat-damaged red cells in patients with active RA and an inverse relationship between the presence of immune complexes and clearance rates. Since clearance of heat-damaged red cells occurs in the spleen by non-immune mechanisms, it is clear that the impairment of phagocytosis cannot be attributed solely to the blockade of macrophage receptors, and must reflect a more fundamental defect of phagocytosis. Whether this defect is primary or secondary to the presence of circulating complexes is not clear.

A similar study[44] using IgG-coated red cells to study splenic Fc receptor function in patients with SLE showed a striking defect in clearance correlating both with disease activity and the presence of circulating complexes. However, in six of these patients with defective Fc function no abnormality of clearance was found using ^{125}I-aggregated albumin—the latter is cleared primarily by non-immune mechanisms in the liver and the failure to demonstrate any abnormality underlines the importance of defining the precise phagocytic pathway which is being tested.

Evidence that defective splenic clearance of red cells is secondary to the presence of circulating complexes rather than primary comes from studies of the effects of plasma exchange on clearance rates in patients with immune-complex disease[45]. Splenic clearance of IgG-coated red cells and heat-damaged red cells is reduced in patients with Wegener's granulomatosis, Goodpasture's syndrome and cutaneous vasculitis, and the defect can be reversed by plasma exchange.

The role of serum factors in monocyte phagocytosis has been studied in detail[46]. Phagocytosis of yeast by normal monocytes was reduced in the presence of sera from 51% of SLE patients, 16% of RA patients and 12% of other connective tissue diseases. Phagocytosis was normal in the presence of sera for 30 subjects with other chronic arthritides. The defect was correlated with cryoglobulinaemia, depressed C1q, C3 and C4 levels in the SLE group and depressed C4 and extra-articular manifestations in the RA group. Further studies on SLE patients showed a strong correlation of defective phagocytosis with clinical and immunological parameters of disease activity. Studies of sera containing cryoglobulins suggested that the phagocytic abnormality reflected defective yeast opsonization rather than a defect of the monocyte cell receptors. *In vitro* studies of monocyte phagocytosis in our laboratory (unpublished results) suggest, however, that a cellular defect may contribute to the persistence of circulating complexes. The kinetics of phagocytosis of opsonized yeast by blood monocytes in suspension were found to follow simple second-order kinetics:

$$\text{i.e. Rate of phagocytosis} = K \times [M\phi] \times [y]$$
$$[M\phi] = \text{number of monocytes/ml.}$$
$$[y] \ \ = \text{number of yeast/ml.}$$

and that the rate constant K could be easily derived and used as a measure of

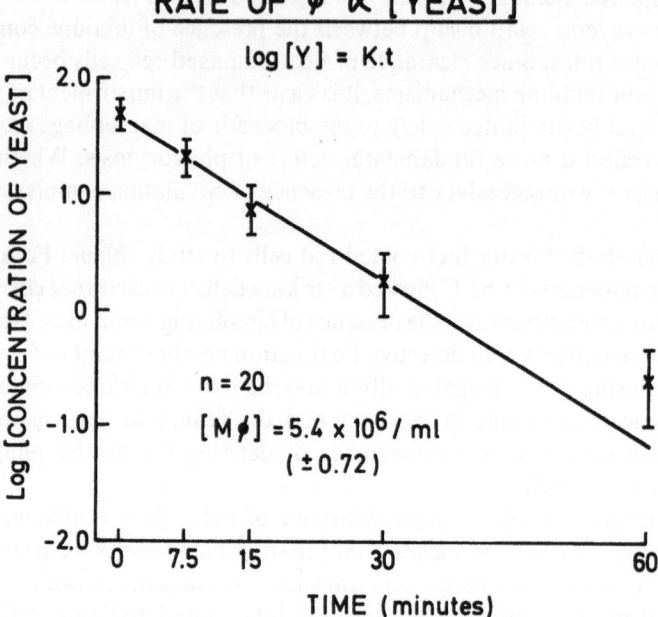

Figure 9.4 Rate of fall in concentration of yeast during phagocytosis is exponential; i.e. rate of phagocytosis α (concentration of yeast). Each point represents mean and 1 SD of 20 experiments. Monocyte concentration = 5.4 (± 0.72) × 10^6/ml; mean initial yeast concentration = 5.3 (± 0.86) × 10^6/ml

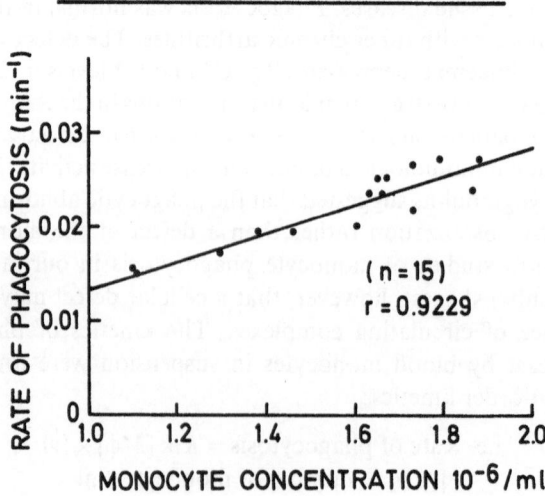

Figure 9.5 Rate of phagocytosis of yeast is proportional to the monocyte concentration. Each point represents the mean value of one experiment performed in quadruplicate

the efficiency of phagocytosis (Figures 9.4–9.6). Preliminary studies have shown that monocytes from patients with RA with evidence of vasculitis or circulating complexes have defective phagocytosis (Figure 9.6). Further studies are now in progress in which separate C3 and Fc receptor functions are being studied by measuring the uptake of either C3-coated or IgG-coated yeast. These studies will help to delineate the type of phagocytic defect present in patients with circulating complexes.

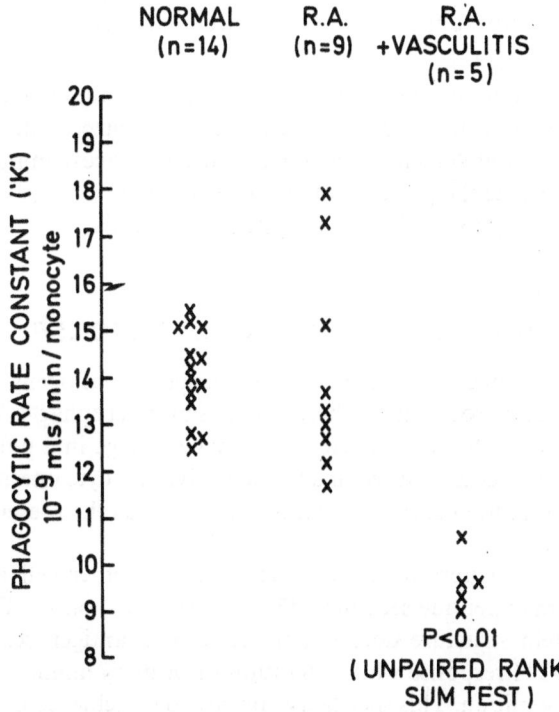

Figure 9.6 The phagocytic rate constant (K) in normal subjects and patients with rheumatoid arthritis with and without vasculitis. All five patients with vasculitis show depressed rates of phagocytosis compared with normal subjects and RA patients without vasculitis.

Overall the majority of studies have shown that there is a defect of phagocytosis by peripheral monocytes and fixed splenic macrophages which correlates with the presence of circulating complexes. The situation with respect to synovial macrophages remains to be clarified. A number of factors probably contribute to the defects demonstrated:

(1) A primary macrophage defect of phagocytosis may predispose to the persistence of circulating complexes.
(2) The phagocytic defect may be secondary to blockade either of Fc receptors by a large excess of complexes, or of C3 receptors by soluble unbound C3b generated during complement activation.

(3) The phagocytic defect may be a consequence of the biological nature of the complexes to which the monocyte is exposed. For example, small soluble complexes may be unable to trigger phagocytosis on contact with a membrane receptor. This could result in receptor blockade and persistent but ineffectual stimulation of the cell with secondary metabolic fatigue, and would explain the presence of a defect of both immune and non-immune phagocytosis[43]. It would also be consistent with the suggested mode of action of levamisole, which might act as a metabolic stimulus restoring the balance of intracellular cyclic nucleotides.

(4) Since no receptors for IgM and IgA are present on the mononuclear phagocyte, immune complexes containing these immunoglobulins will be poorly phagocytosed unless adequately opsonized with complement. Thus, hypocomplementaemic states induced by excess immune complexes will perpetuate the presence of immune complexes, as for example in the rheumatoid synovial fluid or in systemic vasculitis.

MACROPHAGES AND THE IMMUNE RESPONSE

An efficient immune response to thymus-dependent antigens requires both phagocytosis and processing of these antigens by macrophages. The antigen is then presented to the lymphocyte by the macrophage in a potent immunogenic form. This requires direct macrophage–lymphocyte interaction and the recognition of mutual surface alloantigens as well as the presence of specific antigen[5, 47, 48].

Delayed-type hypersensitivity (DTH) and T helper cell responses are specific for small peptide sequences (3–4 amino acids) only[48]. Destruction of tertiary protein structure does not interfere with antigen recognition in a secondary DTH response while alteration of primary amino acid sequences abolishes recognition. This specificity appears to be achieved by MHC-linked IR genes which, it is suggested, code for receptor sites on alloantigen molecules (the Ia antigens of mice) found on the B cell and macrophage membrane. These receptor sites are able to bind specified peptide sequences of three or four amino acids determined by the immune response gene. It is only when the antigen determinant is complexed to these alloantigen binding sites that it is recognized as antigenic by the responding lymphocyte; thus recognition can be blocked by antisera directed against the alloantigen (Ia molecule). Such a mechanism allows for a wide range of proteins to be recognized since the chances of any given peptide sequence being present will be inversely proportional to the size of the protein.

A number of animal studies have shown that, at least for certain antigens, immune response genes are expressed at the level of the macrophage and operate by specifying antigenic determinants for presentation to the lymphocyte[5, 49]. T helper cell–B cell interactions are also governed by histocompatibility restrictions[50] and it seems likely that the antigen–Ia molecule complex presented to the T cell by the macrophage must again be recognized on the B cell surface by the T cell for helper activity to occur.

In the human there is growing evidence that HLA-D antigens play a similar role to the Ia antigens of mice[51]. The secondary proliferative responses of monocyte-depleted T lymphocytes to PPD were restored only when monocytes sharing identical HLA-D alleles with the T cells were added, whether or not the monocytes were from the original or unrelated donor. Similar results were obtained using hapten-conjugated human mononuclear cells[52]. 'Ia-like', D region-determined alloantigens occurring on human monocytes and B cells can now be identified serologically. The original observation that patients with erosive seropositive rheumatoid arthritis had a higher incidence of the HLA-Dw4 haplotype as determined by the mixed leukocyte reaction[53] has now been correlated with the finding of serologically defined DRw4 alloantigen in a high proportion of such patients compared with controls[54]. The possibility that this haplotype is a genetic marker of defective antigen handling by macrophages must therefore be a serious possibility.

SECRETORY AND BIOCHEMICAL ACTIVITIES OF MONONUCLEAR PHAGOCYTES

Macrophages secrete a wide range of potentially destructive inflammatory agents and in contrast to the short-lived neutrophil polymorph are capable of sustaining secretion for long periods of time. These agents, which include acid hydrolases, neutral proteinases, complement components and prostaglandins, not only damage tissue directly but some also amplify their own secretion by positive feedback mechanisms operating on the monocyte. In addition, prostaglandins have important effects on lymphokine secretion, neutral proteinases may also enhance γ-globulin synthesis and significant amounts of potent oxidizing agents such as superoxide anion may be generated at the monocyte cell membrane with damaging consequences for other tissues.

Amplification of chronic inflammation by secretory products of mononuclear phagocytes

In vitro work has shown that many stimulants of chronic inflammation such as immune complexes, dental plaque, zymosan and mouldy hay dust have two properties in common. They activate the alternative complement pathway, with conversion of C3 to C3b, and stimulate prolonged lysosomal enzyme secretion from macrophages[55, 56]. These two effects appear to operate in parallel, are dose-dependent and are not associated with macrophage cell death. C3b itself also stimulates lysosomal enzyme release, thus amplifying the original inflammatory signal[57, 58].

There are further refinements to this amplification system. The macrophage is itself able to excrete a number of complement components (Factor B, C2, C3, C4 and [?] C5)[56, 59–61], and some of the lysosomal enzymes it secretes are themselves able to cleave complement components. For example, plasminogen activator, produced in large quantities by activated macrophages[62–64], converts plasminogen to plasmin, and the latter cleaves C3 to generate more C3b. Factor B can also combine with C3b, and the resulting C3bB complex also cleaves C3 to generate yet more C3b[56].

Production of chemotactic stimuli is a further consequence of macrophage lysosomal enzyme release. For example, C5a, a potent chemotactic agent, is produced by conversion of C5 by plasmin. Similarly, monocyte procoagulant activity (PCA) stimulates coagulation with subsequent conversion of fibrinogen into a number of products including the chemotaxin, fibrinopeptide B[65].

This kind of self-sustaining inflammatory system is a feature of the rheumatoid inflammatory process where there is evidence of immune complexes, complement-activation products, increased lysosomal enzyme activity and fibrinolysis.

The role of macrophage lysosomal enzymes in tissue damage

The evidence that macrophages in the synovium contribute directly to destruction of connective tissue by secreting damaging enzymes is supported by the presence of these cells in the synovium and inflammatory pannus, their ability to secrete the appropriate enzymes and finally the demonstration that intact synovium degrades cartilage proteoglycan and collagen.

In addition to housing an enlarged intimal cell population the inflamed synovium is heavily infiltrated with subsynovial lymphocytes and macrophages. Close anatomical proximity of synovial macrophages to erosion of cartilage has been demonstrated in electron-microscopic studies[66]. These show three kinds of pathological lesion: proliferation of small blood vessels with invasion of cartilage, direct invasion of cartilage by macrophages, and macrophage-containing pannus overlying cartilage. In each it is clear that the cellular infiltrate, which includes many macrophages, is closely related to the underlying erosion.

While acid hydrolases contained in macrophage lysosomes are probably mainly of importance in intracellular digestion, the neutral proteinases such as collagenase[67–69], elastase[70], plasminogen activator[62–64, 71] and certain cathepsins are probably of greater importance in degrading extracellular material. These proteinases are secreted in increased amounts by stimulated macrophages. Collagenase is secreted by rheumatoid synovium in inactive form prior to activation by plasminogen activator[72]. It degrades both Type 1 and Type 2 collagen[73]. The *in vivo* detection of these enzymes in synovial fluid is complicated by the presence of an excess of serum proteinase inhibitors such as α_2-macroglobulin and α_1-antitrypsin[74, 75]. While this might suggest that *in vivo* these enzymes are unimportant, there are a number of reasons for believing otherwise. The fact that collagenase is not bound by serum inhibitors until it has been converted to its active form and the close proximity of macrophages in the synovial pannus to the underlying cartilage[66] both diminish the potential effectiveness of serum proteinase inhibitors[72, 74]. Immunofluorescent studies have confirmed that active collagenase is present at the pannus cartilage junction but not elsewhere in the rheumatoid synovium[76]. Collagen destruction by mononuclear phagocytes in the inflamed joint may also follow macrophage phagocytosis of collagen fibrils and intracellular digestion[77] although this has not been demonstrated in man.

The ability of normal and rheumatoid synovium to degrade cartilage matrix was first shown in 1967[78]. The development of this work in recent years by Honor Fell and her colleagues[19, 20, 79–83] has confirmed that normal synovium in an organ culture system causes breakdown of cartilage. The initial changes are of rapid loss of metachromatic proteoglycan followed by a slower loss of collagen. There are also changes seen in the chondrocytes which become basophilic and subsequently divide, forming groups of cells within the cartilage; eventually these cells appear to leave the cartilage forming a layer of fibroblast-like cells. While these degradative changes are maximal when synovium is directly in contact with cartilage they also occur, although more slowly, when synovium and cartilage are not in direct contact. Furthermore, dead cartilage is less quickly degraded than live cartilage containing viable chondrocytes under these tissue culture conditions, and it seems likely that synovium releases soluble material which stimulates chondrocytes to degrade cartilage.

Other actions of macrophage-derived proteinases *in vivo* and *in vitro*

A number of other potentially important proteinase activities have been identified in addition to those already described. Several proteinases of different specificities (e.g. trypsin, plasmin, thrombin and elastase) are capable of stimulating lymphocytes. For example they stimulate increased γ-globulin synthesis by B cells[84] and substitute for T helper cell activity, thus behaving like thymus-independent antigens such as lipopolysaccharide[85]. It has also been suggested that the macrophage-derived lymphocyte-activating factor (LAF) which acts on T cells might also be a proteinase[86]. Proteinases also damage host proteins of both connective tissue and non-connective tissue origin, giving rise to exposure of new antigenic sites and autoantibody formation. For example cathepsin D and neutral proteinases partially degrade γ-globulins giving rise to agglutinating autoantibodies against the exposed antigenic sites[87], and similar activity may be responsible for the production of anticollagen antibodies[88].

Mononuclear phagocytes and prostaglandins

The production of prostaglandins by mononuclear phagocytes and their possible regulatory role has recently been well reviewed[89].

It is now clear that macrophages from a variety of sources including man[90,91] produce significantly larger amounts of E-type prostaglandins and thromboxane A2 than other leukocytes. Furthermore, prostaglandins from mononuclear phagocytes may have important regulatory effects on the immune system. Wahl *et al.*[92] showed that the stimulation of guinea-pig macrophages by lymphokines or endotoxin to produce collagenase could be blocked by indomethacin and that the blocked cultures could be reactivated by the addition of PGE_2. Conversely PGE_2 has inhibitory effects on lymphocytes— inhibition of antibody production[93] and lymphokine secretion[94] have both been demonstrated. In the latter study lymphokines stimulated macrophage production of PGE_2 while the latter suppressed lymphokine secretion thus providing a negative feedback control system. This regulatory effect could again be blocked by non-steroidal anti-inflammatory drugs (NSAID). Uncritical acceptance of the desirability of PG synthetase blockade as a therapeutic aim may therefore not be wise, particularly in view of the lack of correlation between clinical efficacy of NSAID and their ability to block PG synthesis *in vitro*.

Another potentially important activity of monocyte derived E-type prostaglandins is their ability to cause bone resorption. Prostaglandins in *in vitro* tissue culture systems cause bone resorption[95]. More recently monocyte-derived prostaglandin E was found to promote production of an osteoclast-activating factor, which results in bone resorption[96].

Mononuclear phagocytes and fibrosis

Fibrosis and collagen formation is a late feature of some chronic inflammatory diseases but in others (e.g. pulmonary fibrosis, systemic sclerosis, hepatic cirrhosis, etc.) it may be an early or prime feature of the disease. The role of mononuclear phagocytes in the fibrotic process has been shown in animal studies using a 'pneumoconiosis' type of model with silica as the provoking agent[97].

These experiments showed that macrophages, after ingesting silica, released soluble agents which stimulated fibroblastic proliferation and fibrosis. There was no evidence that macrophages, having ingested silica, transformed into fibroblasts or that silica could stimulate fibroblasts directly. Furthermore live macrophages were more fibrogenic, as high cytotoxic doses of silica were less efficient than low doses of silica in provoking a fibrotic reaction. Similar experiments[97] using spleen cells from unimmunized mice and mice immunized against *Babesia microti* showed that lymphocytes were also involved in the fibrotic response. Antigenic stimulation of immune lymphocytes resulted in the secretion of a soluble mediator which provoked macrophage and fibro-blastic infiltration resulting in an intense fibrogranulomatous reaction. No such stimulation was seen with non-immune lymphocytes.

Whether mononuclear phagocytes play a similar role in the rheumatic diseases remains unanswered but clearly this is an important possibility.

The respiratory burst and free radical formation

Membrane perturbation of both PMN and mononuclear phagocytes results in activation of a 'respiratory burst' which is manifest by increased oxygen consumption and increased hexose monophosphate (HMP) activity. This subject has recently been well reviewed[98, 99].

Respiratory burst activity (RBA) was first observed to accompany phago-cytosis and it was originally thought to provide energy for phagocytosis. However, it is now known that phagocytosis does not require oxygen and occurs quite normally even in an atmosphere of nitrogen[100].

A wide variety of stimuli can cause RBA, their common mode of action being membrane perturbation. Suitable agents include opsonized material, aggregated γ-globulin, C5a[101], latex particles[102], phorbol myristyl acetate[103], fluoride[104] and histamine bound to particulate material[105]. The function of this system is to reduce oxygen to a number of highly reactive intermediate species including superoxide anion O_2^- hydrogen peroxide H_2O_2, singlet oxygen $^1O_2$ and hydroxyl radical $OH^{\cdot}$ which may participate in microbial killing. One of the consequences of RBA is the oxidation of NADPH to $NADP^+$ both in the conversion of O_2 to O_2^- and in the scavenging of cytoplasmic H_2O_2 by the glutathione system. The hexose-monophosphate shunt (HMP) is controlled by supplies of $NADP^+$ and its activity is therefore increased in parallel with RBA, regenerating NADPH from $NADP^+$ (Figure 9.7).

Before discussing the relevance of these pathways to inflammatory disease brief mention should be made of the recognized enzyme deficiencies which can occur in this system. The first is a defect of the initial NADPH oxidase, manifested phenotypically as chronic granulomatous disease. In these patients there is complete absence of RBA and they are severely affected by infection with catalase-positive organisms such as *Staphylococcus aureus* and *Escherichia coli*. They are not troubled, however, by catalase-negative organisms such as streptococci which, in common with other catalase-negative organisms, pro-duce but cannot destroy H_2O_2. After phagocytosis they provide the defective white cell with H_2O_2 which is converted to microbicidal agents such as $^1O_2$, O_2^- and $OH^{\cdot}$. Severe G6PD deficiency is clinically very similar to chronic granulo-matous disease and is also associated with recurrent infection by catalase-positive organisms. The biochemical defect is at the start of the HMP shunt pathway with resulting inability to provide NADPH for O_2 production. The third well-characterized defect, 'myeloperoxidase deficiency', is clinically much less obvious since it does not usually result in recurrent infections; but it can

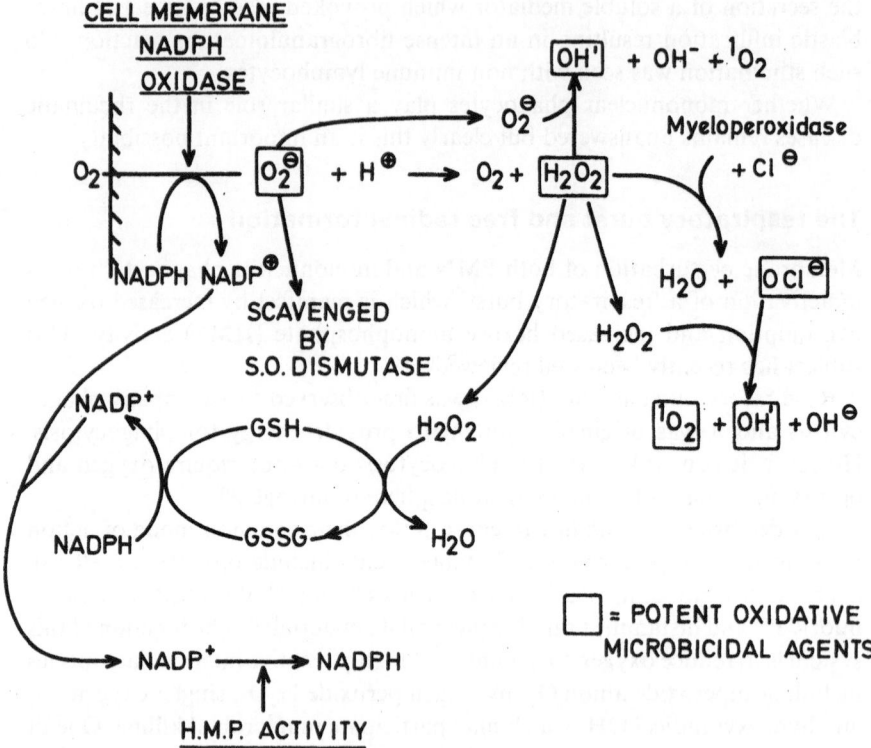

Figure 9.7 The leukocyte 'respiratory burst'. Membrane perturbation by a variety of agents results in activation of a burst of respiratory enzyme activity and production of a number of potent microbicidal species

be detected *in vitro* by slower killing of organisms by white cells from these patients, and by a more prolonged rise in superoxide anion levels compared with normal white cells. The latter is attributed to reduced conversion of O_2^- to H_2O_2 in the absence of myeloperoxidase.

There are a number of reasons for believing these pathways to be relevant to the chronic inflammatory process. For example the appropriate stimuli for activating RBA are present in chronic inflammatory disease (e.g. immune complexes, activated complement) and the reactive oxygen species produced could be important agents of host tissue damage. *In vitro* work[106] has shown that superoxide anion participates in cellular cytotoxicity. Furthermore one of the features of chronic inflammatory disease is that there are fewer available reduced thiol groups and this might be a consequence of oxidation by these reactive oxygen species. The possibility that inherited defects in these enzyme systems might contribute to chronic inflammatory disease must be considered. No systematic search among patients with rheumatic disease has yet been made for defects such as myeloperoxidase deficiency which might cause delayed bacterial killing and thus result in prolonged stimulation of mono-nuclear phagocytes and the immune system. Susceptibility to chronic inflam-mation could also result from a failure of control of RBA with overproduction of highly reactive, partially reduced oxygen species.

One final point of interest is that certain non-steroidal anti-inflammatory drugs (indomethacin, phenylbutazone and ibuprofen) cause dose-dependent inhibition of O_2^- production by neutrophils at levels approximating to the therapeutic range in humans[107], suggesting a further anti-inflammatory action of these drugs. Phenylbutazone *in vitro* inhibits intracellular bacterial killing, presumably through its effect on these pathways.

CONCLUSIONS

This brief review of some aspects of the origin, cell biology, secretory and biochemical activity of macrophages emphasizes the crucial role of mono-nuclear phagocytes as initiators, regulators and effectors throughout all phases of chronic inflammation. Although, to date, most of the work has been done in animal and *in vitro* systems there seems little doubt that with the development of monoclonal antibodies and improved cytochemical staining methods for the identification of membrane receptors and intracellular organ-elles, the next decade will see a rapid expansion of studies in patients with rheumatic diseases.

Already there is fragmentary data available which suggests that macro-phages play a number of important roles in the pathogenesis of these dis-orders. It is interesting to speculate how intrinsic or acquired defects of macrophage receptor function or biochemical processing might lead to suscep-tibility to infection, antigen persistence or impaired clearance of immune complexes. Macrophage–lymphocyte interactions may well be critical for the development of autoantibodies and mononuclear phagocytes may be the major site for expression of immune response genes. Further studies of synovial cells, which are specialized types of mononuclear phagocytes, will certainly show them to be a major source of proteolytic enzymes involved in cartilage destruction, interferon, free radicals, complement components and other amplification factors as well as the source of a wide range of monokines involved in regulation of immune processes and interaction with articular cartilage chondrocytes. Immunomodulating drugs such as levamisole may be shown to work primarily by exerting these effects on mononuclear phago-cytes. Benoxaprofen may be the prototype of a new generation of non-steroidal analgesic and anti-inflammatory drugs which exert their effects by inhibiting migration of mononuclear phagocytes. This may be a property of agents which inhibit the lipoxygenase pathway and leucotriene production rather than blocking the production of prostaglandins and other endo-peroxides.

References

1. Metchnikoff, E. (1893). *Lectures on the Comparative Pathology of Inflammation.* (London: Kegan, Paul, Trench, Truber & Co.)
2. Dannenberg, A. M. (1975). Macrophages in inflammation and infection. *N. Engl. J. Med.,* **293**, 489
3. Unanue, E. R. and Calderon, J. (1975). Evaluation of the role of macrophages in immune induction. *Fed. Proc.,* **34**, 1737
4. Pierce, C. W. and Kapp, J. A. (1978). Functions of macrophages in antibody responses *in vitro. Fed. Proc.,* **37**, 86
5. Rosenthal, A. S., Barcinski, M. A. and Blake, J. T. (1977). Determinant selection is a macrophage dependent immune response gene function. *Nature (London),* **267**, 156
6. van Furth, R. (1976). An approach to the characterization of mononuclear phagocytes involved in pathological processes. *Agents and Actions,* **6**, 91
7. Wellek, B., Hahn, H. and Opferkuch, W. (1976). Opsonizing activities of IgG, IgM and the C3b inactivator cleaved third component of complement in macrophage phagocytosis. *Agents and Actions,* **6**, 260
8. van Furth, R., Langevoort, H. L. and Schaberg, A. (1975). Mononuclear phagocytes in human pathology—proposal for an approach to improved classification. In van Furth, R. (ed.) *Mononuclear Phagocytes in Immunity, Infection and Pathology,* pp. 1–15. (Oxford: Blackwell Scientific Publications)
9. Whitelaw, D. M. and Batho, H. F. (1975). Kinetics of monocytes. In van Furth, R. (ed.) *Mononuclear Phagocytes in Immunity, Infection and Pathology,* pp. 175–188 (Oxford: Blackwell Scientific Publications)
10. van Furth, R. (1975). Modulation of monocyte production. In van Furth, R. (ed.) *Mononuclear Phagocytes in Immunity, Infection and Pathology,* pp. 161–174. (Oxford: Blackwell Scientific Publications)
11. Dannenberg, A. M., Ando, M., Shima, K. and Tsuda, T. (1975). Macrophage turnover and activation in tubercular granulomata. In van Furth, R. (ed.) *Mononuclear Phagocytes in Immunity, Infection and Pathology,* pp. 959–980. (Oxford: Blackwell Scientific Publications)
12. Blusse, van Oud, Alblas, A. and van Furth, R. (1979). Origins, kinetics and characteristics of pulmonary macrophages in the normal steady state. *J. Exp. Med.,* **149**, 1504
13. van Waarde, D., Hulsing-Hesselink, E. and van Furth, R. (1975). Humoral regulation of monocytosis during an acute inflammatory reaction. In van Furth, R. (ed.) *Mononuclear Phagocytes in Immunity, Infection and Pathology,* pp. 205–222. (Oxford: Blackwell Scientific Publications)
14. Meuret, G. and Hoffman, G. (1973). Monocyte kinetic studies in normal and disease states. *Br. J. Haematol.,* **24**, 275
15. Whitelaw, D. M. (1972). Observations on human monocyte kinetics after pulse labelling. *Cell Tissue Kinet.,* **5**, 311
16. Whitelaw, D. M. and Batho, H. F. (1972). The distribution of monocytes in the rat. *Cell Tissue Kinet.,* **5**, 215
17. van Waarde, D., Hulsing-Hesselink, E. and van Furth, R. (1978). Humoral control of monocytopoiesis by an activator and an inhibitor. *Agents and Actions,* **8**, 432
18. Barland, P., Novikoff, A. B. and Hamerman, D. (1962). Electron microscopy of the human synovial membrane. *J. Cell Biol.,* **14**, 207
19. Fell, H. B., Glauvert, A. M., Barratt, M. E. J. and Green, R. (1976). The pig synovium (1) the intact synovium *in vivo* and in organ culture. *J. Anat.,* **122**, 663
20. Barratt, M. E. J., Fell, H. B., Coombs, R. R. A. and Glauvert, A. M. (1977). The pig synovium (2) some properties of isolated intimal cells. *J. Anat.,* **123**, 47
21. Allison, A. C., Davies, P. and De Petris, S. (1971). Role of contractile microfilaments in macrophage movement and endocytosis. *Nature, New Biol.,* **232**, 153

22. Stossel, T. P. (1978). The mechanism of leucocyte locomotion. In Gallin, J. I. and Quie, P. G. (eds.) *Leucocyte Chemotaxis*, pp. 143–160. (New York: Raven Press)

23. Robinson, B. V. (1978). The pharmacology of phagocytosis. 'Trends in the drug treatment of rheumatic diseases'. *Rheum. Rehab.* (Suppl.), pp. 37–46

24. Sundquist, K. G. and Ehrnst, A. (1976). Cytoskeletal control of surface membrane mobility. *Nature (London)*, **264**, 226

25. Kvarstein, B. and Stormorken, H. (1971). Influence of acetyl salicylic acid, butazolidine. colchicine, hydrocortisone, chlorpromazine and imipramine on the phagocytosis of polystyrene latex particles by human leucocytes. *Biochem. Pharmacol.*, **20**, 119

26. Ignarro, L. J., Lint, T. F. and George, W. J. (1974). Hormonal control of lysosomal enzyme release from human neutrophils. (Effects of antonomic agents on enzyme release, phagocytosis and cyclic nucleotide levels). *J. Exp. Med.*, **139**, 1395

27. Malawista, S. E. and Bodel, P. T. (1967). The dissociation by colchicine of phagocytosis from increased O_2 consumption in human leucocytes. *J. Clin. Invest.*, **46**, 786

28. Abdou, N. I., Napombejara, C., Sagawa, A., Ragland, C., Stechschulte, D. J., Nilsson, U., Gourley, W., Watanabe, I., Lindsey, N. J. and Allen, M. S. (1977). Malakoplakia: evidence for monocyte lysosomal abnormality correctable by cholinergic agonist *in vitro* and *in vivo*. *N. Engl. J. Med.*, **297**, 1413

29. Hill, H. R. (1978). Cyclic nucleotides as modulators of leucocyte chemotaxis. In Gallin, J. J. and Quie, P. G. (eds.) *Leucocyte Chemotaxis*, pp. 179–194. (New York: Raven Press)

30. Stossel, T. P. (1973). Quantitative studies of phagocytosis. Kinetic effect of cations and heat labile opsonin. *J. Cell Biol.*, **58**, 346

31. Huber, H. and Holm, G. (1975). Surface receptors of mononuclear phagocytes: effect of immune complexes on *in vitro* function in human monocytes. In van Furth, R. (ed.) *Mononuclear Phagocytes in Immunity, Infection and Pathology*, pp. 290–301. (Oxford: Blackwell Scientific Publications)

32. Griffin, F. M. Jr., Griffin, J. A., Leider, J. E. and Silverstein, S. C. (1975). Studies on the mechanism of phagocytosis. 1. Requirements for circumferential attachment of particle bound ligands to specific receptors on the macrophage plasma membrane. *J. Exp. Med.*, **142**, 1263

33. Griffin, F. M. Jr. and Silverstein, S. C. (1975). Discrimination by the macrophage during the ingestion phase of phagocytosis. In van Furth, R. (ed.) *Mononuclear Phagocytes in Immunity, Infection and Pathology*, pp. 283–286. (Oxford: Blackwell Scientific Publications)

34. Goetzl, E. J. (1978). Regulation of the polymorphonuclear leucocyte chemotactic response by immunological reactions. In Gallin, J. I. and Quie, P. G. (eds.) *Leucocyte Chemotaxis*, pp. 161–177. (New York: Raven Press)

35. Schiffmann, E., Corcoran, B. A. and Aswanikumar, S. (1978). Molecular events in the response of neutrophils to synthetic N-f MET chemotactic peptides: demonstration of a specific receptor. In Gallin, J. I. and Quie, P. G. (eds.) *Leucocyte Chemotaxis*, pp. 97–111. (New York: Raven Press)

36. Ho, P. P. K., Young, A. L. and Southard, G. L. (1978). Methyl ester of N formylmethionyl-leucyl-phenylalanine. Chemotactic responses of human blood monocytes and inhibition of gold compounds. *Arth. Rheum.*, **21**, 133

37. Jessop, J. D., Vernon-Roberts, B. and Harris, J. (1973). Effect of gold salts and prednisolone on inflammatory cells. 1. Phagocytic activity of macrophages and polymorphs in inflammatory exudate studied by a skin window technique in rheumatoid and control patients. *Ann. Rheum. Dis.*, **32**, 294

38. Vernon-Roberts, B., Jessop, J. D. and Dore, J. (1973). Effect of gold salts and prednisolone on inflammatory cells. 2. Suppression of inflammation and phagocytosis in the rat. *Ann. Rheum. Dis.*, **32**, 301

39. Jessop, J. D. and Wilkins, M. (1979). The effect of gold salts on the phagocytic activity of synovial macrophages in organ culture. *J. Rheum.* (Suppl.), No. 5

40. Kávai, M., Lukács, K., Sonkoly, I., Páloczi, K. and Szegedi, G. Y. (1979). Circulating immune complexes and monocyte Fc function in autoimmune diseases. *Ann. Rheum. Dis.*, **38**, 79

41. Wilton, J. M. A., Gibson, T. and Chuck, C. M. (1978). Defective phagocytosis by synovial fluid and blood polymorphonuclear leucocytes in patients with rheumatoid arthritis. 1. The nature of the defect. *Rheum. Rehab.* (Suppl.), 25'

42. Landry, M. (1972). Phagocyte function and cell mediated immunity in SLE. *Arch. Dermatol.*, **113**, 147

43. Williams, B. D., Pussell, B. A., Lockwood, C. M. and Cotton, C. (1979). Defective reticuloendothelial system function in rheumatoid arthritis. *Lancet*, **1**, 1311

44. Frank, M. M., Hamburger, M. I., Lawley, I. J., Kimberley, R. P. and Plotz, P. H. (1979). Defective reticuloendothelial system Fc-receptor function in systemic lupus erythematosus. *N. Engl. J. Med.*, **300**, 518

45. Lockwood, C. M., Worlledge, S., Nicholas, A., Cotton, C. and Peters, D. K. (1979). Reversal of impaired splenic function in patients with nephritis or vasculitis (or both) by plasma exchange. *N. Engl. J. Med.*, **300**, 524

46. Svensson, B., Sturfelt, G., Nived, O., Odeberg, H., Norberg, R. and Torstensson, R. (1980). Studies on serum dependent *in vitro* monocyte function in rheumatic diseases. *Scand. J. Rheumatol.* (Suppl.), 31

47. Rosenthal, A. S., Barcinski, M. A. and Rosenwasser, L. J. (1978). Function of macrophages in genetic control of immune responsiveness. *Fed. Proc.*, **37**, 79

48. Benacerraf, B. (1978). Hypothesis to relate the specificity of T-lymphocytes and the activity of I region-specific Ir genes in macrophages and B-lymphocytes. *J. Immunol.*, **120**, 1809

49. Rosenthal, A. S., Barcinski, M. A. and Blake, J. T. (1977). Determinant selection is a macrophage dependent immune response gene function. *Nature (London)*, **267**, 156

50. Yamashita, U. and Shevach, E. M. (1978). The histocompatibility restrictions on macrophage T-helper cell interaction determine the histocompatibility restrictions on T-helper cell B-cell interaction. *J. Exp. Med.*, **148**, 1171

51. Sφnderstrop, G., Rubin, B., Sφrensen, S. F. and Svejgaard, A. (1978). Importance of HLA-D antigens for the co-operation between human monocytes and T-lymphocytes. *Eur. J. Immunol.*, **8**, 520

52. Seldin, M. F., Rich, P. R. and Rich, S. S. (1978). Self preference of secondary proliferative responses to hapten conjugated human peripheral blood mononuclear cells. *Fed. Proc.*, **37**, 1369 (Abst. 548)

53. Stastny, P. (1976). Mixed lymphocyte cultures in rheumatoid arthritis. *J. Clin. Invest.*, **57**, 1148

54. Stastny, P. (1978). Association of the B-cell alloantigen DRw4 with rheumatoid arthritis. *N. Engl. J. Med.*, **298**, 869

55. Cardella, C. J., Davies, P. and Allison, A. C. (1974). Immune complexes induce selective release of lysosomal enzymes by macrophages. *Nature (London)*, **247**, 46

56. Schorlemmer, H. V., Bitter-Suermann, D. and Allison, A. C. (1977). Complement activation by the alternative pathway and macrophage enzyme secretion in the pathogenesis of chronic inflammation. *Immunology*, **32**, 929

57. Schorlemmer, H. V. and Allison, A. C. (1976). Effects of activated complement components on enzyme secretion by macrophages. *Immunology*, **31**, 781

58. Schorlemmer, H. V., Davies, P. and Allison, A. C. (1976). Ability of activated complement components to induce lysosomal enzyme release from macrophages. *Nature (London)*, **261**, 48

59. Unanue, E. R. (1976). Secretory function of mononuclear phagocytes. *Am. J. Pathol.*, **83**, 396

60. Synderman, R. and McCarthy, G. A. (1978). The role of macrophages in the rheumatic diseases. *Clin. Rheum. Dis.*, **4**, no. 3

61. Bentley, C., Bitter-Suermann, D., Hadding, U. and Brade, V. (1976). *In vitro* synthesis of Factor B of the alternative pathway of complement activation by mouse peritoneal macrophages. *Eur. J. Immunol.*, **6**, 393
62. Gordon, S., Unkeless, J. C. and Cohn, Z. A. (1974). Induction of macrophageplasminogen activator by endotoxin stimulation and phagocytosis: evidence for a two-stage process. *J. Exp. Med.*, **140**, 995
63. Unkeless, J. C., Gordon, S. and Reiche, E. J. (1974). Secretion of plasminogen activator by stimulated macrophage. *Exp. Med.*, **139**, 834
64. Gordon, S., Newman, W. and Bloom, B. (1978). Macrophage proteases and rheumatic diseases: regulation of plasminogen activator by thymus-derived lymphocytes. *Agents and Actions*, **8**
65. Kay, A. B., Petter, D. S. and Ewart, M. R. (1973). Generation of chemotactic activity for leucocytes by the action of thrombin on human fibrinogen. *Nature (London)*, **24**, 56
66. Koboyashi, I. and Ziff, M. (1975). Electron microscopic studies of the cartilage–pannus junction in rheumatoid arthritis. *Arth. Rheum.*, **18**, 475
67. Harvey, W. *et al.* (1976). Macrophage and cartilage destruction. *Lancet*, **2** (letter), 202
68. Wahl, L. M., Wahl, S. M., Mergenhagen, S. E. and Martin, G. R. (1974). Collagenase production by endotoxin activated macrophage. *Proc. Natl. Acad. Sci. USA*, **72**, 3598
69. Werb, Z. and Gordon, S. (1975). Secretion of a specific collagenase by stimulated macrophage. *J. Exp. Med.*, **142**, 356
70. Werb, Z. and Gordon, S. (1975). Elastase secretion by stimulated macrophages. *J. Exp. Med.*, **142**, 361
71. Berger, H. Jr. (1977). Secretion of plasminogen activator by rheumatoid and non-rheumatoid synovial cells in culture. *Arth. Rheum.*, **20**, 1198
72. Harris, E. D., Mainardi, C. L. and Werb, Z. (1977). Collagenolysis in RA. In Gordon, J. L. and Hazelman, B. L. (eds.), *Rheumatoid Arthritis—Cellular Pathology and Pharmacology*, pp. 199–210. Elsevier/North Holland. (Amsterdam: Biomedical Press)
73. Evanson, J. M., Jeffrey, J. J. and Krane, S. M. (1967). Human collagenase: identification and characterization of an enzyme from rheumatoid synovium in culture. *Science*, **158**, 499
74. Brackertz, D., Hagmann, J. and Kueppers, F. (1975). Proteinase inhibitors in rheumatoid arthritis. *Ann. Rheum. Dis.*, **34**, 225
75. Abe, S. and Nagai, Y. (1973). Evidence for the presence of a complex of collagenase with alpha₂ macroglobulin in human rheumatoid synovial fluid: a possible regulatory mechanism of collagenase activity *in vivo*. *J. Biochem. (Tokyo)*, **73**, 897
76. Woolley, D. E., Crossley, M. J. and Evanson, J. M. (1977). Collagenase at sites of cartilage erosion in the rheumatoid joint. *Arth. Rheum.*, **20**, 1231
77. Deporter, D. A. (1979). The role of the macrophage in collagen resorption during chronic inflammation. A new look at an old hypothesis. *Agents and Action*, **9**, 168
78. Hamerman, D., Janis, R. and Smith, C. (1967). Cartilage matrix depletion by rheumatoid synovial cells in tissue culture. *J. Exp. Med.*, **126**, 1005
79. Fell, H. B. (1978). Synoviocytes. *J. Clin. Pathol.*, **31** (Suppl. Royal College of Pathology), **12**, 14
80. Fell, H. B. and Jubb, R. W. (1977). The destructive action of synovial tissue on articular cartilage in organ culture. In Gordon, J. L. and Hazelman, B. L. (eds.), *Rheumatoid Arthritis—Cellular Pathology and Pharmacology*, pp. 193–197. Elsevier/North Holland. (Amsterdam: Biomedical Press)
81. Fell, H. B. and Jubb, R. J. (1977). The effect of synovial tissue on the breakdown of articular cartilage in organ culture. *Arth. Rheum.*, **20**, 1359
82. Fell, H. B. and Barratt, M. E. J. (1973). The role of soft connective tissue in the breakdown of pig articular cartilage cultivated in the presence of complement-sufficient antiserum to pig erythrocytes (1). Histological changes. *Int. Arch. Allergy Appl. Immunol.*, **44**, 441

83. Dingle, J. T., Horsfield, P., Fell, H. B. and Barratt, M. E. J. (1975). Breakdown of proteoglycan and collagen induced in pig articular cartilage in organ culture. *Ann. Rheum. Dis.*, **34**, 303

84. Yamaski, K. and Ziff, M. (1977). Enhancement of *in vitro* gammaglobulin synthesis of human lymphocytes by lysosomal enzymes from PMN. *Clin. Exp. Immunol.*, **27**, 254

85. Gisler, R. H., Vischer, T. L. and Dukor, P. (1976). Trypsin increases *in vitro* antibody synthesis and substitutes for helper T-cells. *J. Immunol.*, **116**, 1354

86. Vischer, T. L. (1978). Macrophages, lymphocytes and proteases. In Panayi, G. S. and Johnson, P. M. (eds.) *Immunopathogenesis of Rheumatoid Arthritis*, pp. 131–136. (Chertsey, Surrey: Reed Books)

87. Fehr, K., Artmann, G., Velvart, M. and Boni, A. (1977). Cathepsin D. agglutinators + neutral protease agglutinators in rheumatoid arthritis. *Arth. Rheum.*, **20**, 1240

88. Mesteck, Y. J., Miller, E. J., Gay, S. and Andriopoulos, N. A. (1978). Immune response to collagen. In Panayi, G. S. and Johnson, P. M. (eds.) *Immunopathogenesis of Rheumatoid Arthritis*, pp. 63–67. (Chertsey, Surrey: Reed Books Ltd)

89. Morley, J., Bray, M. A. and Meade, H. (1978). Macrophage and prostaglandins. In Panayi, G. S. and Johnson, P. M. (eds.) *Immunopathogenesis of Rheumatoid Arthritis*, pp. 119–122. (Chertsey, Surrey: Reed Books Ltd)

90. Kurland, J. I. and Bockman, R. (1978). Prostaglandin E production by human blood monocytes and mouse peritoneal macrophages. *J. Exp. Med.*, **147**, 952

91. Goodwin, J. S., Bankhurst, A. D. and Messner, R. P. (1977). Suppression of human T cell mitogenesis by prostaglandin. Existence of a prostaglandin producing suppressor cell. *J. Exp. Med.*, **146**, 1719

92. Wahl, L. M., Olsen, C. W., Wahl, S. M., Sandberg, A. L. and Mergenhagen, S. E. (1978). Prostaglandin regulated macrophage collagenase. In Horton, J. G., Tarpley, T. M. and Davis, W. F. (eds.) *Mechanisms of Localized Bone Loss*, pp. 181–190. Special supplement to *Calcified Tissue Abstracts*, pp. 181–190

93. Webb, D. R. and Osheroff, P. L. (1976). Antigen stimulation of prostaglandin synthesis and control of immune responses. *Proc. Natl. Acad. Sci. USA*, **73**, 1300

94. Gordon, D., Bray, M. A. and Morley, J. (1976). Control of lymphokine secretion by prostaglandins. *Nature (London)*. **262**, 402

95. Klein, D. C. and Raisz, L. G. (1970). Prostaglandins: stimulation of bone resorption in tissue culture. *Endocrinology*, **86**, 1436

96. Yoneda, T. and Mundy, G. R. (1979). Monocytes regulate osteoclast activity factor production by releasing prostaglandins. *J. Exp. Med.*, **150**, 338

97. Allison, A. C., Clark, J. A. and Davies, P. (1977). Cellular interactions in fibronogenesis. *Ann. Rheum. Dis.*, **36** (Suppl.), 8

98. Babior, B. M. (1978). Oxygen dependent killing by phagocytes (Part 1). *N. Engl. J. Med.*, **298**, 659

99. Babior, B. M. (1978). Oxygen dependent killing by phagocytes (Part 2). *N. Engl. J. Med.*, **298**, 721

100. Sbarra, A. J. and Karnovsky, M. L. (1959). The biochemical basis of phagocytosis. 1. Metabolic changes during the ingestion of particles by PMN leucocytes. *J. Biol. Chem.*, **234**, 1355

101. Goldstein, I. M., Roos, D., Kaplan, H. B. and Weissmann, G. (1975). Complement and immunoglobulin stimulate superoxide production by human leucocytes independently of phagocytosis. *J. Clin. Invest.*, **56**, 1155

102. Weening, R. S., Wever, R. and Roos, D. (1975). Quantitative aspects of the production of superoxide radicals by phagocytosing human granulocytes. *J. Lab. Clin. Med.*. **85**. 245

103. Johnston, R. B. Jr., Lehmeyer, J. E. and Guthrie, L. D. (1976). Generation of superoxide anion and chemiluminescence by human monocytes during phagocytosis and on contact with surface bound immunoglobulin G. *J. Exp. Med.*, **143**, 1551

104. Curnutte, J. T., Babior, B. M. and Karnovsky, M. L. (1979). Fluoride mediated activation of the respiratory burst in human neutrophils. *J. Clin. Invest.*, **63**, 637
105. Diaz, P., Jones, D. G. and Kay, A. B. (1979). Histamine-coated particles generate superoxide O_2^- and chemiluminescence in alveolar macrophages. *Nature (London)*, **278**, 454
106. Sacks, T., Moldow, C. F., Craddock, P. R., Bowers, T. K. and Jacob, H. S. (1978). Oxygen radicals mediate endothelial cell damage by complement stimulated granulocytes. An *in vitro* model of immune vascular damage. *J. Clin. Invest.*, **61**, 1161
107. Simonchowitz, L., Mehta, J. and Spilberg, I. (1979). Chemotactic factor-induced generation of superoxide radicals by human neutrophils—effect of metabolic inhibitors and anti-inflammatory drugs. *Arth. Rheum.*, **22**, 755
108. Kinsky, R. G., Christie, G. H., Elson, J. and Howard, J. G. (1969). Extra hepatic deprivation of Kupffer cells during oestrogenic stimulation of parabiosed mice. *Br. J. Exp. Pathol.*, **50**, 438
109. Göthlin, G. and Ericsson, J. L. E. (1976). The osteoclast: review of ultrastructure, origin and structure–function relationship. *Clin. Ortho. Rel. Res.*, **120**, 201
110. Grimley, P. M. and Sokoloff, L. (1966). Synovial giant cells in rheumatoid arthritis. *Am. J. Pathol.*, **49**, 931
111. Han, A. K. and Roy, S. (1971). Synovial giant cells in rheumatoid arthritis and other joint diseases. *Ann. Rheum. Dis.*, **30**, 294
112. Mackay, J. M. K., Panayi, G., Neill, W. A., Robinson, A., Smith, W., Marmion, B. P. and Duthie, J. J. R. (1974). Cytology of rheumatoid synovial cells in culture. 1. Composition and sequence of cell populations in cultures of rheumatoid synovial fluid. *Ann. Rheum. Dis.*, **33**, 225
113. Panayi, G. S., Mackay, J. M. K., Neill, W. A., McCormick, J. N., Marmion, B. P. and Duthie, J. J. R. (1974). Cytology of rheumatoid synovial cells in culture. 2. Association of polykaryocytes with rheumatoid and other forms of arthritis. *Ann. Rheum. Dis.*, **33**, 234
114. Spector, W. G. and Mariano, M. (1975). Macrophage behaviour in experimental granulomas. In van Furth, R. (ed.) *Mononuclear Phagocytes in Immunity, Infection and Pathology*, pp. 927–942. (Oxford: Blackwell Scientific Publications)
115. Dreher, R., Keller, N. V., Hess, M. W. and Cottier, H. (1975). Enhancement of talcum-induced macrophage fusion and giant cell proliferation by delta-hydrocortisone acetate. In van Furth, R. (ed.) *Mononuclear Phagocytes in Immunity, Infection and Pathology*, pp. 943–950. (Oxford: Blackwell Scientific Publications)

10
The Relationship between Epstein–Barr Virus and the Inflammatory Arthropathies

A. G. BIRD

It is clear from the abundant evidence already presented in previous chapters of this volume that immunological disturbances are consistently found in patients with inflammatory arthropathy. The crucial question remains whether the observed phenomena represent primary pathogenic mechanisms in these diseases or not. Many of the local and systemic immunological manifestations could be the result of secondary or even immunoregulatory events super-imposed upon a primary initiation inflicted by an environmental agent in a genetically predisposed individual. Understanding of the underlying disease processes will be greatly facilitated if the diseases can be studied earlier in their evolution and if trigger factors can be identified.

The search for aetiological agents is not new. Over the years, a number of bacteria, including mycoplasma and L forms[1] have been isolated from rheumatoid synovial tissue and viruses have also been considered likely candidates as triggers. The interest in this field has been reawakened by the discovery of the association between HLA-B27 and ankylosing spondylitis and the description of antigenic cross-reactivity between B27 and *Klebsiella* species[2,3]. The concept of an environmental agent interacting with a genetically suscep-tible individual now dominates current thinking.

Viruses have generally not been isolated from affected synovial tissue and serum viral titres from affected individuals have not indicated susceptibility to any particular species[4]. However, viruses have been recently implicated in experimental adjuvant arthritis[5] and have frequently found favour as possible aetiological agents in rheumatoid arthritis[6]. The original description by

Alspaugh and Tan[7] of an antibody present in the serum of many patients with rheumatoid arthritis, which was later shown to have specificity for a nuclear antigen induced by Epstein–Barr virus (EBV), has renewed interest in the role of viruses, and EBV in particular, in rheumatoid arthritis.

THE NATURE OF RHEUMATOID ARTHRITIS-ASSOCIATED NUCLEAR ANTIGEN (RANA)

In their original description, Alspaugh and Tan[7] demonstrated a precipitating antibody in sera of patients with rheumatoid arthritis reactive with extracts of human B lymphoblastoid cell lines. This antibody was present in the sera of over 60% of patients with seropositive rheumatoid arthritis (RA) but only at a much lower incidence in normal subjects, patients with seronegative RA or with other inflammatory arthropathies. The use of indirect immunofluorescence allowed the identification of the antigen within the B lymphocyte nucleus and it became clear that RANA was only present in B cell lines which harbour the EBV[8]. The use of differential sera indicated that RANA was a separate entity from the EBV-determined nuclear antigen (EBNA) first described by Reedman and Klein[9], whose induction is a prerequisite for B lymphocyte transformation by EBV. It is now clear that RANA differs from EBNA biochemically[10] and both probably represent different nuclear antigens induced during EBV transformation of the human B lymphocyte.

These initial observations have now been confirmed by other laboratories[11,12] and using immunofluorescence it is now clear that RANA antibodies are present in the sera of the majority of cases of seropositive rheumatoid arthritis but in only 16% of normal controls and 19% of patients with other assorted arthritides. Not only does the presence of anti-RANA further support the possibility that seropositive RA is a distinct entity, but it also strongly suggests a link between EBV and RA. Prior to discussing whether such a relationship is justified and the possible implications, I would first like to describe the EBV itself, since it possesses some intrinsic properties which are of major interest.

THE RELATIONSHIP BETWEEN EPSTEIN–BARR VIRUS AND THE HUMAN B LYMPHOCYTE

Epstein–Barr virus is a member of the herpes group of viruses. Infection is restricted to cells of higher primates and in the human lymphoid system only the B cell can be infected via its surface complement receptor[13]. After B lymphocyte infection, sequential events occur with the synthesis of EBNA and later DNA cell division and secretion of immunoglobulin[14]. The cellular activation initiated by EBV results in the polyclonal activation of infected B lymphocytes with secretion of immunoglobulin of all classes and specificities[15]. Infection of human B lymphocytes *in vitro* results in the appearance of permanent lymphoblastoid cell lines which have unlimited growth potential, harbour the EBV genome and frequently secrete immunoglobulin[16]. Indeed, infection of antigen-specific B lymphocytes has enabled the establishment of permanent human B cell lines secreting immunoglobulin of desired specificity (e.g. Rhesus anti-D)[17].

The virus is ubiquitous in human society and is transmitted horizontally, infecting all human populations. Infection leads to seroconversion, usually unaccompanied by symptoms[18], or less commonly to infectious mononucleosis. During acute infectious mononucleosis EBNA-positive transformed B lymphocytes and polyclonal-secreting B lymphocytes are present in the peripheral blood[19,20] and this is reflected in a polyclonal rise in serum IgM of many specificities, including autoantibodies[21]. The haematological picture is dominated by the atypical mononuclear cells which are in fact activated T lymphocytes. These are thought to play a major role in the removal of infected B lymphocytes[22,23]. Following recovery, small numbers of B lymphocytes containing latent EBV remain in circulation and lymphoblastoid cell lines containing EBV can be isolated from seropositive individuals if immune T cells are removed[24].

There are an increasing number of case reports of chronic EBV infection which can develop into chronic lymphoproliferation and overt malignancy[25]. A family has been described with extreme susceptibility to chronic EBV infection with progression to hypogammaglobulinaemia and lymphoproliferation, and the trait is inherited as an X-linked defect[26].

In East Africa EBV is clearly associated with Burkitt's lymphoma and is present in the cells of more than 95% of the tumours in the endemic region[27]. A low incidence of Burkitt's lymphoma is also found amongst Caucasians but the majority of these cases have no evident association with EBV. The lymphocytes of the tumours are monoclonal, can be grown as lines *in vitro* and all show B cell surface marker characteristics. As well as containing EBNA the majority of Burkitt cell lines show a characteristic chromosomal translocation (t8;14). This translocation is specific for Burkitt's lymphoma[28] and does not occur after *in vitro* B cell infection with EBV. It appears that EBV infection is insufficient alone to induce lymphoma but that the interaction of EBV and the immunosuppressive effects of holoendemic malaria provide the milieu for the development of the translocation characterizing the lymphoma[29].

EBV has therefore established a close relationship with the human immune system. The outcome of disease can vary from symptomless infection in early life with lifelong latency to fatal lymphoma. Genetic or acquired immune deficiencies must generate the possibility of abnormal overreactions against, or the inadequate removal of, EBV-infected B cells and the discovery of RANA inevitably leads to speculation about a possible role for EBV in rheumatoid arthritis.

THE POSSIBLE RELEVANCE OF ANTI-RANA IN RHEUMATOID ARTHRITIS

The two most recent reports suggest that anti-RANA is present in the sera of 93% of cases of seropositive rheumatoid arthritis compared with an incidence of 16–25% in normal individuals or patients with other arthropathies[11, 12]. The antibody has specificity not only for rheumatoid arthritis (RA) but also for the presence of EBV in B lymphoblastoid cell lines. Whilst it is not conclusive, the evidence suggests that it is EBV itself that determines the specificity of RANA. Alspaugh et al.[7] failed to find RANA in EBV-negative B cell lines. EBV can transform simian and primate B cells, and these lines were also positive for RANA whereas B cells from these species transformed with other herpes viruses did not reveal the antigen. This strong relationship between RANA and EBV, and the very high prevalence of anti-RANA in RA, has inevitably promoted EBV as a strong candidate for an aetiological role in RA.

Early studies had provided little support for a link. Comparable levels of anti-viral capsid antibody (VCA) were found in normal individuals and RA patients[30, 31] and no evidence for increased anti-VCA was found in rheumatoid effusions compared with paired RA sera[32]. Following the discovery of RANA, Elson et al.[33] attempted to further evaluate EBV serology in RA. These workers postulated that if there were a direct aetiological relationship between EBV and RA, then all patients should have antibodies to EBV-determined antigens. They analysed the incidence of anti-VCA in RA patients compared with normal adults and found a similar incidence of 80%. They argued against the possibility that RA patients could become seronegative as a result of immunosuppression by demonstrating a normal immunization response to bacteriophage ϕX174. However, Purtilo[34] has observed a failure of specific anti-VCA response in patients with the X-linked predisposition to EBV and a similar specific defect could also conceivably occur in some cases of RA. It may also be unnecessary to invoke EBV as the only trigger agent to what is probably a heterogeneous disease. Ng et al.[12] have noted that sera from three patients with RA studied contained anti-RANA antibodies in the absence of anti-VCA. If RANA is specific for EBV, then the presence of anti-RANA without VCA suggests that some of these patients do indeed have an inability to mount an immune response against VCA[34]. Perhaps the dogma that anti-VCA occurs after all cases of EBV infection and persists lifelong should be questioned.

Another possible explanation for the presence of anti-RANA is that they occur as a result of polyclonal activation of B cell activation. Polyclonal activation by B cell mitogens or EBV results in the secretion of antibodies in a random non-specific fashion. Antibodies of all specificities, including auto-antibodies, are generated even in acute infectious mononucleosis[35]. Polyclonal elevation of both IgM and IgG occurs in RA, and anti-RANA could merely represent a tiny proportion of a general hyperreactivity or non-specific B cell stimulation. This explanation could certainly explain the appearance of anti-RANA in patients seronegative for VCA and, therefore, by current definition, non-immune to EBV. A strong argument against the polyclonal explanation is the relative absence of anti-RANA in other inflammatory arthritides, particularly systemic lupus erythematosus (SLE), a disease which displays even clearer evidence of *in vivo* polyclonal hyperimmunoglobulinaemia than RA. It will be of crucial importance to observe whether anti-RANA occurs in acute infectious mononucleosis where the polyclonal B cell activation is the result of EBV itself. Catalano *et al.*[11] provided further evidence against the polyclonal argument when they demonstrated that although patients with RA and anti-RANA have elevated anti-EBNA titres, titres against other viruses—notably measles, rubella, cytomegalovirus and VCA itself—are present at normal levels. This finding again argues strongly for a specific anti-EBV response in RA. Interestingly, normal individuals who possess anti-RANA have significantly elevated titres of anti-VCA compared with anti-RANA-negative normals. This finding suggests a hyperreactivity to EBV transformation antigens in these apparently normal individuals[11] and these patients should be closely followed up to see if they are at special risk of developing RA in the future.

Another possible explanation for the appearance and incidence of anti-RANA in RA is that the antibody represents a chance cross-reaction between a pathological antibody in RA and an antigen induced by EBV in B lymphocytes. The cross-reaction would imply that immunization with RANA was not the reason for the appearance of anti-RANA. Evidence for cross-reactions in RA has been provided by Hannestad[36]. He has shown that a proportion of classical rheumatoid factors not only have specificity for IgG but also with antinuclear determinants. These findings raise the possibility that some rheumatoid factors may not be the result of immunization with IgG but rather with nuclear antigens. Williams *et al.*[37] has recently speculated further on this possibility. If anti-RANA was indeed a cross-reacting antibody it could still point the way to a causal agent in rheumatoid arthritis, but this need not necessarily be EBV. It remains an intriguing possibility that RANA has no relationship with EBV even in lymphoblastoid cell lines containing both RANA and EBV. Whilst it is clear that acute B lymphocyte infection with EBV leads to activation of a large proportion of B lymphocytes[15] the percentage finally transformed and immortalized as cell lines is very small and evidence for very restricted transformation has been presented[38]. If EBV only immortalized human (and simian) B lymphocytes of one particular differentiation phase then RANA, or even EBNA, could represent a B cell nuclear differentiation antigen rather than an EBV-determined antigen. If this were the case, then anti-RANA could be induced as a result of B lymphocyte transformation by an agent like EBV that activates or transforms B cells of that same maturation phase. This agent could be a viral or even bacterial activator and such an explanation could account for the compelling disparity between anti-RANA and anti-VCA seen in some patients with RA. The high titres of anti-EBNA coexisting with anti-RANA noted by Catalano *et al.*[11] make this differentiation antigen hypothesis less likely than the more obvious one that RANA is determined by EBV infection.

If we accept the most likely and most interesting possibility that RANA is associated with EBV infection, then what pathological role could EBV play in RA? The latent and polyclonal-activating properties of EBV could account for many of the immunological features of RA. The polyclonal B cell-activating properties of EBV would account for the hyperimmunoglobulin-aemia found both in the serum and synovial fluid of affected joints in RA patients. No thorough study searching for the presence of EBV-activated or transformed cells in rheumatoid synovium has yet been performed, but some indirect evidence is already available. Pathological numbers of activated and immunoglobulin-secreting B lymphocytes are present in the peripheral blood of RA patients[39]. Slaughter *et al.*[40] report that *in vitro* infection of RA blood B lymphocytes with EBV results in synthesis of significant amounts of rheuma-toid factor. More importantly, B lymphocytes from RA patients frequently transform *in vitro* in the absence of superinfection with EBV. This phenom-enon is unusual in normal individuals unless immune T lymphocytes are previously removed[23] and suggests either that increased numbers of EBV-infected cells are present in RA blood or that T cell surveillance is impaired.

Peripheral blood lymphocytes, whilst freely available, are probably less representative than synovial lymphocytes and a search for EBV-transformed cells and EBV antigens, including RANA, in diseased synovium should be a matter of priority. However, the majority of lymphocytes in diseased synovium or synovial fluid are not activated B cells but T lymphocytes[41]. This T lymphocyte response could be the result of alteration of the major histo-compatibility complex on B cells by drugs or a virus[42] such as EBV. T cells will then react against the altered antigens on the B lymphocytes in a similar way to that seen in experimental graft-versus-host reaction (GVHR) or allogeneic effect. GVHR induces, in animals, lymphoid enlargement, secondary poly-clonal B cell activation, formation of immune complexes and infiltration of tissues with cytotoxic T lymphocytes and eventually lymphoma. The histo-logical picture in rheumatoid synovium is reminiscent of GVHR and could be the result of a reaction against small numbers of EBV-transformed lympho-cytes expressing viral antigens. This possibility again emphasizes the necessity of a thorough examination of RA synovium for the presence of EBV-transformed cells.

Epstein–Barr virus therefore demonstrates many properties that make it an agent worthy of consideration as an environmental trigger for RA. The description of anti-RANA and its selectivity for RA encourages further speculation of an association of EBV with RA, but certain inconsistencies remain and lack of experimental data still causes doubts which may be soon resolved. Even if RANA does not lead directly to the discovery of the elusive trigger it should certainly stimulate further directions of research, and at the very least has provided a marker of surprising specificity for seropositive rheumatoid arthritis.

References

1. Pearse, P. E. (1969). Bacterial forms in the blood and joint fluids of arthritic subjects. *Ann. Rheum. Dis.*, **28**, 270
2. Ebringer, A., Cawdell, D. and Ebringer, A. (1979). *Klebsiella pneumoniae* and acute anterior uveitis in ankylosing spondylitis. *Br. Med. J.*, **1**, 383
3. Seager, K., Bashir, H. V., Geczy, A. F., Edmonds, J. and De Vere-Tindall, A. (1979). Evidence for a specific B27-associated cell surface marker on lymphocytes of patients with ankylosing spondylitis. *Nature (London)*, **277**, 68
4. Phillips, P. E. (1979). Virologic studies in rheumatoid arthritis. *Rheumatology*, **6**, 353
5. Chang, Y. H. and Hoffman, W. (1977). Adjuvant polyarthritis. III. Evidence in support of viral etiology. *Arth. Rheum.*, **16**, 1507
6. Denman, A. M. (1977). Viruses, poisons and arthritis, *Rheumatol. Rehab.*, **16**, 205
7. Alspaugh, M. A. and Tan, E. M. (1976). Serum antibody in rheumatoid arthritis reactive with a cell-associated antigen. *Arth. Rheum.*, **16**, 711
8. Alspaugh, M. A., Jenson, F. C., Rabin, H. and Tan, E. M. (1978). Lymphocytes transformed by Epstein–Barr virus. Induction of nuclear antigen reactive with antibody in rheumatoid arthritis. *J. Exp. Med.*, **147**, 1018
9. Reedman, B. M. and Klein, G. (1973). Cellular localization of an Epstein–Barr virus (EBV associated complement fixing antigen) in producer and non-producer lymphoblastoid cell lines. *Int. J. Cancer*, **17**, 21
10. Baron, D. and Strominger, J. L. (1978). Partial purification and properties of the Epstein–Barr virus-associated nuclear antigen. *J. Biol. Chem.*, **253**, 2875
11. Catalano, M. A., Carson, D. A., Slovin, S. F., Richmann, D. D. and Vaughan, J. H. (1979). Antibodies to Epstein–Barr virus-determined antigens in normal subjects and in patients with seropositive rheumatoid arthritis. *Proc. Natl. Acad. Sci. USA*, **76**, 5825
12. Ng, K. C., Brown, K. A., Perry, J. D. and Holborow, E. J. (1980). Anti-RANA antibody: a marker for seronegative and seropositive rheumatoid arthritis. *Lancet*, **1**, 447
13. Jondal, M., Klein, G., Oldstone, M. B. A., Bokish, V. and Yefenof, E. (1976). Surface markers on human B and T lymphocytes. VIII. Association between complement and Epstein–Barr virus receptors on human lymphoid cells. *Scand. J. Immunol.*, **5**, 401
14. Einhorn, L. and Ernberg, I. (1978). Induction of EBNA precedes the first cellular S phase after EBV infection of human lymphocytes. *Int. J. Cancer*, **21**, 157
15. Bird, A. G. and Britton, S. (1979). A live human B cell activator operating in isolation of other cellular influences. *Scand. J. Immunol.*, **5**, 507
16. Adams, A. and Klein, G. (1973). Superinfection with Epstein–Barr virus of human lymphoid cell lines of different origins. *Nature, New Biol.*, **242**, 234
17. Koskimies, D. S. (1980). Human lymphoblastoid cell line producing specific antibody against Rh-Antigen D. *Scand. J. Immunol.*, **11**, 73
18. Biggar, R. J., Henle, G., Böcker, J., Lenette, E. T., Fleisher, G. and Henle, W. (1978). Primary Epstein–Barr virus infections in African infants. II. Clinical and serological observations during seroconversion. *Int. J. Cancer*, **17**, 244
19. Klein, G., Svedmyr, E., Jondal, M. and Persson, P. E. (1976). EBV-determined nuclear antigen (EBNA) positive cells in the peripheral blood of infectious mononucleosis patients. *Int. J. Cancer*, **17**, 21
20. Bird, A. G. and Britton, S. (1979). A new approach to the study of human B lymphocyte function using an indirect plaque assay and a direct B cell activator. *Immunol. Rev.*, **45**, 41

21. Wollheim, F. A. and Williams, R. C. (1966). Studies on the macroglobulins of human serum. I. Polyclonal immunoglobulin class M (IgM). Increases in infectious mononucleosis. *N. Engl. J. Med.*, **274**, 61

22. Svedmyr, E. and Jondal, M. (1975). Cytotoxic effector cells specific for B cell lines transformed by Epstein–Barr virus infection are present in patients with infectious mononucleosis. *Proc. Natl. Acad. Sci. USA*, **72**, 1622

23. Moss, D. J., Rickinson, A. B. and Pope, (1978). Long term T cell mediated immunity to Epstein–Barr virus infection in man. *Int. J. Cancer*, **22**, 662

24. Nilsson, K., Klein, G., Henle, W. and Henle G. (1971). The establishment of lymphoblastoid cell lines from adult and foetal human lymphoid tissue and its dependance on EBV. *Int. J. Cancer*, **8**, 443

25. Virelizier, J. L., Lenoir, G. and Griscelli, C. (1978). Persistent Epstein–Barr virus infection in a child with hypergammaglobulinaemia and immunoblastic proliferation associated with a selective defect in immune interferon secretion. *Lancet*, **2**

26. Purtilo, D. T., De Florio, D., Hutt, L. M., Bhawan, J., Yang, J. P. S., Otto, R. and Edwards, W. (1977). Variable phenotypic expression of an X-linked recessive lymphoproliferative syndrome. *N. Engl. J. Med.*, **297**, 1077

27. Lindahl, T., Klein, G., Reedman, B. M., Johansson, B. and Singh, S. (1974). Relationship between Epstein–Barr virus (EBV–DNA and the EBV-determined nuclear antigen (EBNA) in Burkitt lymphoma biopsies and other lymphoproliferative diseases. *Int. J. Cancer*, **13**, 764

28. Manolov, G. and Manolova, Y. (1972). Marker band in one chromosome 14 from Burkitt's lymphoma. *Nature (London)*, **237**, 33

29. Klein, G. (1979). Lymphoma development in mice and humans: diversity of initiation is followed by a convergent cytogenetic evolution. *Proc. Natl. Acad. Sci. USA*, **76**, 2442

30. Stevens, D. A., Stevens, M. B., Newell, G. R., Levine, P. H. and Waggoner, D. E. (1972). Epstein–Barr virus (herpes-type virus) antibodies in connective tissue diseases. *Arch. Intern. Med.*, **130**, 23

31. Phillips, P. E., Waxman, J., Hirshant, Y. and Kaplan, M. H. (1976). Virus antibody levels and delayed hypersensitivity in rheumatoid arthritis. *Ann. Rheum. Dis.*, **35**, 153

32. Cremer, N. F., Hurwitz, Quismorio, F. P., Lenette, E. H. and Friou, G. J. (1974). Antiviral antibodies in rheumatoid synovial fluid and cryoprecipitate. *Clin. Exp. Immunol.*, **18**, 27

33. Elson, C. J., Crawford, D. H., Bucknall, R. C., Allen, C., Thompson, J. L., Epstein, M. A., Hall, N. D. and Bacon, P. A. (1980). Infection with EB virus and rheumatoid arthritis. *Lancet*, **1**, 105

34. Purtilo, D. T. (1980). Epstein–Barr virus-induced oncogenesis in immune-deficient individuals. *Lancet*, **1**, 300

35. Sutton, R. N. P., Emond, R. T. D., Thomas, D. B. and Doniach, D. (1974). The occurrence of autoantibodies in infectious mononucleosis. *Clin. Exp. Immunol.*, **17**, 427

36. Hannestad, K. (1978). Certain rheumatoid factors react with both IgG and an antigen associated with cell nuclei. *Scand. J. Immunol.*, **7**, 127

37. Williams, R. C. (1979). A second look at rheumatoid factor and other autoantibodies. *Am. J. Med.*, **67**, 179

38. Steel, C. M., Philipson, J., Arthur, E., Gardiner, S. E., Newton, M. S. and McIntosh, M. S. (1977). Possibility of E.B. virus preferentially transforming a subpopulation of human B lymphocytes. *Nature (London)*, **270**, 729

39. Strelkauskas, A. J., Callery, R. T., McDowell, J., Borel, Y. and Schlossmann, S. F. (1978). Direct evidence for loss of human suppressor cells during active autoimmune disease. *Proc. Natl. Acad. Sci. USA*, **75**, 5150

40. Slaughter, L., Carson, D. A., Jensen, F. C., Holbrook, T. L. and Vaughan, J. H. (1978). *In vitro* effects of Epstein–Barr virus on peripheral blood mononuclear cells from patients with rheumatoid arthritis and normal subjects. *J. Exp. Med.*, **148**, 1429

41. Tannenbaum, H. and Schur, P. H. (1974). The role of lymphocytes in rheumatic diseases. *J. Rheumatol.*, **1**, 392
42. Gleichmann, E., Gleichmann, H. and Wilke, W. (1976). Autoimmunisation and lymphomagenesis in parent Fi combinations differing at the major histocompatibility complex: model for spontaneous disease caused by altered self antigens? *Transplant, Rev.*, **31**, 157

11
Virus–Host Interactions and the Connective Tissue Diseases

A. M. DENMAN

INTRODUCTION

The immunopathological features of rheumatoid arthritis and other inflammatory disorders characterized by chronic inflammation and autoimmune reactions and termed 'connective tissue diseases' for convenience have been elucidated in considerable detail. Unfortunately this knowledge has not enabled us to identify the causes of the vast majority of these diseases. Indeed it is now apparent that a wide variety of insults provoke a spectrum of inflammatory and immunological responses which are remarkably similar irrespective of the provoking cause; this depressing truth applies both to animal models and human disease. For example experimental infection with African trypanosomiasis[1] provokes the same polyclonal hypergammaglobulinaemia accompanied by autoantibodies to nucleic acids, red cells, and lymphocyte antigens as is commonly regarded as characteristic of autoimmune diseases. Similarly, experimental infection or immunization with a variety of cocci including streptococci, pneumococci, meningococci, and micrococci induces an antibody response which is not only restricted in heterogeneity and range of specificities against the immunizing bacterial antigens but also against other antigens with which the animals are simultaneously immunized[2]. Furthermore mice immunized in this way produce autoantibodies against immunoglobulins and against a complex carbohydrate antigen expressed on the surface of non-dividing lymphocytes. These lymphocytotoxins are presumably provoked by cross-reacting bacterial antigens. Obviously, microbial infections disturb the immune system in a fundamental manner thereby

221

provoking both autoantibody production and a degree of immunodeficiency and are the consequence of persistent infection by bacteria or the inability to degrade bacterial products. Investigators pursuing the aetiology of the connective tissue diseases must accept that microbial infections produce an array of immunological abnormalities which is equally confusing for the infected host and for the medical scientist. In contrast primary infection with Epstein–Barr virus directly induces the proliferation of B lymphocytes and thereby provokes an array of autoantibodies which in patients with infectious mononucleosis may rival that seen in patients with autoimmune disease of unknown causes[3]. This is an example of an infectious agent which infects lymphocytes and may thereby stimulate a primary if ephemeral lymphoproliferative process in susceptible individuals.

Despite the failure to detect an infectious agent to account for rheumatoid arthritis and most forms of connective tissue diseases such observations provide an important incentive for continuing to pursue an infectious aetiology. By analogy with the effects of known infections, microbial agents could provoke a continued inflammatory and immune response by one of two mechanisms. On the one hand, persistent infection could provoke a variety of inflammatory and autoimmune responses resulting from continued infection by the responsible agent. The agent might be a novel hitherto undetected micro-organism or one endemic in the community which provokes a continued response because of some defect in the patient's ability to eliminate or control such infections. Alternatively the inciting agent may have the ability to grow in cells of the immune system and thereby provoke a variety of lymphoproliferative disorders including the production of autoantibodies. At present it is reasonable to contemplate the possibility that a variety of bacterial and viral infections could operate through either of these mechanisms. The search for an infectious aetiology of the connective tissue diseases would be greatly helped if their fundamental nature could be determined by distinguishing between a reactive response to microbial persistence and a primary immunoproliferative process induced by infection[4]. The evidence favouring a microbial aetiology in general and a viral aetiology in particular[5,6] has been recently reviewed. The purpose of this review is to consider the evidence that viruses could cause rheumatoid arthritis and other connective tissue diseases through persistent infection of target cells or by inducing a primary lymphoproliferative disorder.

VIRAL INFECTIONS AS AN ESTABLISHED CAUSE OF ARTHRITIS

Transient arthritis accompanies a variety of viral infections[7]. For example an illness resembling serum sickness with polyarthralgia, polyarthritis, rash and fever has been particularly noted in patients with hepatitis B infection. The association between this infection and polyarteritis nodosa is also well recognized and, more recently, cryoprecipitates containing hepatitis B antigen and antibody have been detected in patients with essential mixed cryoglobulinaemia[8]. Acute transient arthritis may accompany common infectious viral diseases of childhood such as rubella, mumps, and varicella[7]. Transient arthralgias or overt arthritis are also encountered in patients with infectious mononucleosis, and infections by echovirus, adenovirus and influenza virus. It is usually assumed that the arthritis results from the deposition of circulating immune complexes but it is equally possible that the reticuloendothelial cells, including macrophages in the synovial membrane, are a site of predilection for viral growth[9, 10]. In these instances the association with a viral illness is apparent from the clinical features of the disorder and the diagnosis can be confirmed serologically. An important form of chronic arthritis which is possibly of viral aetiology has been detected in residents of Lyme, Connecticut. This arthritis is characterized by recurrent attacks of asymmetrical polyarticular pain and swelling affecting primarily large but also small joints. Geographical clustering provided the clue not only that this is a hitherto undiscovered variety of arthritis, but also for unearthing the epidemiological evidence that the disease may result from an infectious agent transmitted by a tick vector, namely *Ixodes scapularis*[11]. The polyarthritis is preceded by an annular skin lesion, erythema chronicum migrans, and is often accompanied by neurological abnormalities and disturbances of cardiac conduction. The absence of subcutaneous nodules and rheumatoid factor, and the asymmetrical pattern of joint involvement, clearly distinguish this disorder from classical rheumatoid arthritis[12]. Nevertheless the chronic arthritis sometimes necessitates synovectomy as a result of pannus formation and erosion of cartilage. Patients developing arthritis are also more prone to develop cryoglobulins containing IgM and a reduction of serum complement levels. Circulating immune complexes can also be detected early in the disease, particularly in the most severely affected patients. Furthermore immune complexes tend to persist in patients whose central nervous system and heart are affected but disappear in patients whose disease is characterized by chronic arthritis[13–15]. It is also noteworthy that chronic arthritis develops more frequently in individuals with the B lymphocyte alloantigen DR2[12]. This epidemic is intriguing for those concerned with the possible viral aetiology of rheumatoid arthritis. Firstly the joint involvement has some features in common with inflammatory arthritis of unknown aetiology. Secondly the evidence for an infectious aetiology is primarily epidemiological and no infectious agent has been successfully isolated from the tissues or blood of patients with this disorder. Finally there are hints that genetic factors determine the pattern of host response to an infectious agent widely disseminated in family groups living in susceptible communities. The relationship between infection rate, incubation period, and clinically detectable disease is now recognized as highly variable with different agents[16].

GENETIC FACTORS

The self-limited nature of the arthritis accompanying acute viral infections has been taken as evidence against a viral aetiology for most forms of chronic arthritis on the grounds that with very few exceptions[17] the acute arthritis does not give rise to chronic, persistent arthritis. Furthermore there is little evidence that rheumatoid arthritis clusters within families or communities in a manner consistent with an infectious aetiology. Nevertheless such arguments are not insurmountable. A prolonged incubation period may obscure any obvious association of this kind and there are many experimental models of viral immunopathology in which a prolonged latent period precedes the onset of overt disease. This is particularly true of viruses which induce demyelinating diseases of the central nervous system. In man it is reasonable to speculate that diseases may be provoked by virus which are universally encountered in early childhood but which provoke inflammatory responses only in a small number of individuals with the appropriate genetic background. A particularly important group of viruses which persist lifelong after primary infection are the DNA herpes viruses, including Epstein–Barr virus, cytomegalovirus and herpes simplex virus.

The analysis of genetically determined susceptibility to inflammatory arthritis has now passed from speculation to detecting markers for this susceptibility. There have been two principal approaches to this problem. The first concerns the detection of autoantibodies in family members of patients with connective tissue diseases. Lymphocytotoxins, that is autoantibodies reactive with circulating lymphocytes[18], are found in a variety of disorders and thus their presence does not provide any guide to the likely aetiology of those disorders with which these antibodies are associated. Nor is there convincing evidence that these autoantibodies are responsible for the alleged disturbances of lymphocyte regulation which have been sought for in patients with connective tissue diseases. However lymphocytotoxins have been detected in patients with systemic lupus erythematosus and their relatives which react with lymphocyte antigens clustering in normal families and which are presumably related to D-locus antigens[19]. These findings suggest immunization to a genetically determined but as yet uncharacterized antigen associated with B lymphocytes. The second approach utilizes inherited HLA antigens as genetic markers of disease susceptibility. The well-known associations[20, 21] between HLA antigens of the D series and diseases such as rheumatoid arthritis and juvenile chronic arthritis provide evidence of this kind. However the nature of many inherited lymphocyte antigens has not been clarified even when possessing these antigens clearly points to disease susceptibility. For example in one study chronic polyarthritis but not rheumatoid factor was detected in four families in which the proband presented with juvenile chronic arthritis[22]. The striking clinical feature was the different pattern of arthritis observed even in members of the same family. This pattern was also affected by the age of onset. Histocompatibility testing suggested to the authors that susceptibility was controlled by a dominant allele with variable penetrance and expression, an inexact interpretation which leaves every possibility open. There are several ways in which the genetic markers could be related to the host response to virus infections[23]. One possibility already alluded to in the context of bacterial infections is that virus-coded antigens on the surface of infected cells induce antibodies which cross-react with some D-locus or other lymphocyte antigens. A second possibility is that the vigour with which T lymphocytes react with viral antigens expressed on the surface of infected cells is genetically controlled by immune response genes for which HLA antigens are convenient markers.

HOST DEFENCES AGAINST VIRUS INFECTION

If commonly encountered viruses produce chronic immunopathological disorders only in susceptible individuals this susceptibility must be based either on a defect in the normal host defences against such infections or on the ability of some viruses or virus strains to evade these responses. Traditionally these defences to virus infections have been divided into two categories[24]. The first consists of humoral immunity and involves antibody in the blood and extracellular compartments, antibody secreted across mucous membranes, and antibody synthesized at sites of viral persistence. The neutralization of virus and the lysis of infected cells by antibody is usually dependent on complement. This form of defence is particularly important in limiting the spread of infection from the portal of entry. Conversely, cell-mediated immunity is particularly relevant to controlling the growth of virus infection established in the tissues. This form of immunity also limits the dissemination of viruses whose genome is permanently incorporated in host cells and which are liable therefore to periodic reactivation; thus immunity against DNA herpes viruses is primarily cell-mediated. However these distinctions were based initially on observations in patients with gross forms of immunodeficiency; patients with congenital absence of the thymus are, for example, highly susceptible to vaccinia virus and patients with hypogammaglobulinaemia to enterovirus infections. However such distinctions over-simplify the situation. Whilst some forms of host defence are of particular importance in controlling particular virus infections, most such infections provoke a variety of responses which act synergistically. In reviewing the elaborate range of these defences, two principal kinds of abnormalities can be envisaged which could predispose to chronic inflammatory disorders in man. The first is a defect which prevents the elimination of what is usually an evanescent infection. An extreme example is chronic myositis from persistent echovirus infections in patients with hypogammaglobulinaemia[25]. It is interesting to speculate that more subtle forms of immunodeficiency predispose to inflammatory myositis in general. The second kind of abnormality is one based upon an excessive response to a viral infection producing a true hypersensitivity disorder. The established precedent for such a situation in clinical medicine is confined to those rare patients who develop encephalitis or demyelinating syndromes after viral infections or immunization.

The importance of specific immunity mediated by cytotoxic T lymphocytes has been fully established in experimental animals. Indeed the need for T lymphocytes to recognize and destroy virus-infected host cells is central to the organization of immune responses. Pre-T lymphocytes arise from bone marrow precursor cells which are programmed to respond to specific viral antigens. Thus antigen is presumed to select this category of lymphocyte in the same way that antigen selects antibody-producing cells programmed to respond to the antigen in question. After migrating to the thymus pre-T lymphocytes learn to recognize the entire repertoire of histocompatibility antigens expressed on the surface of that individual[26]. After education in the thymus the mature T lymphocytes migrate to other lymphoid organs. T lymphocytes recognize and react with virus-infected cells which express viral antigens in association with self-antigens. There has been considerable debate about the nature of this association and in particular as to whether cytotoxic T lymphocytes recognize altered self-antigens or viral antigens and self-antigens as contiguous but separate antigens on the cell membrane. This issue is being resolved by defining the antigens recognized by cytotoxic T lymphocytes in molecular terms. For example it is essential for influenza viral antigens to be incorporated into the target cell membrane if these cells are to be lysed by specifically sensitized lymphocytes[27, 28]. Similarly, artificial membranes have been used to define the essential features of virus-infected cells necessary to stimulate this kind of immune response[29, 30]. Synthetic phospholipid vesicles (liposomes) only stimulate a cytotoxic T lymphocyte response to target cells infected by vesicular stomatitis virus if viral glycoproteins are incorporated into the membrane and not simply absorbed to its surface. An important extension of these observations is the observation that genetic factors determine the intensity of the T lymphocyte response generated by sensitization to viral-altered host cells. The ability of different strains of inbred mice to respond to target cells infected with viruses such as vaccinia, sendai, and lymphocytic choriomeningitis virus is controlled by genes which map to the major murine histocompatibility regions[31]. Moreover unresponsiveness is dominant over responsiveness. Such observations have obvious implications for the pathogenesis of virus infections in individuals with different genetic backgrounds. Those virus infections which result in tissue damage not through the direct cytopathic effect of the invading virus but from the immune response mounted by the host to infected cells will be predictably more severe if the T response is unusually vigorous. Conversely viruses which damage tissues directly, and whose extent is normally limited by an efficient host response, will be more damaging in individuals with an impoverished T lymphocyte response.

There is less evidence in man than in other species that cytotoxic T lymphocytes contribute to host defence against virus infections. It is possible to elicit responses of this kind *in vitro* but usually with systems which involve *in vitro* sensitization. In most experimental protocols the cells are first exposed to virus-infected target cells in order to induce sensitization and the cytotoxic potential of the sensitized cells is then demonstrated using fresh target cells. Whilst cytotoxicity against virus-infected cells can be generated relatively easily in this manner there is little evidence that cytotoxic T lymphocytes are the most important component of this response. Nevertheless there is some experimental evidence relating to Epstein–Barr, influenza and measles virus infections that human T lymphocytes also react with virus-altered HLA antigens and not with viral antigens in isolation[32]. There are also some indications that the briskness of such HLA-restricted responses is genetically controlled in man. Thus cytotoxic T lymphocyte responses against autologous lymphocytes infected with influenza virus are impoverished if the donor lymphocytes are obtained from HLA A2 positive individuals[33]. However the interpretation of such experiments is still open to doubt as apparent genetic differences in immune responses of this nature may reflect the efficiency with which viral antigens are expressed on the target cell membrane or the efficiency which other mediators of target cell destruction are generated. The relationship between T lymphocyte responses and viral infections in man needs further study.

The importance of antibody in host defence against virus infections is unchallengeable. However there is increasing speculation that defects in co-operative defence mechanisms involving antibody may lead to persistent or atypical infections. Circulating immune complexes formed between many infectious viruses and antibody are neutralized only if these complexes are solubilized by complement and thereby rendered susceptible to phagocytosis and degradation by circulating monocytes or fixed macrophages of the reticuloendothelial system. The importance of both early and late components of the classical complement pathway in this context is now established. The dependence of antibody-mediated lysis of virus-infected cells on the alternative complement pathway has also recently been shown[34]. HeLa cells acutely infected with measles virus are lysed by antibody and isolated components of the alternative pathway with an efficiency comparable with that produced by whole serum. Moreover these components are able to lyse measles-infected cells sensitized with specific antibody without the need for other serum proteins. In addition host defence against many virus infections depends upon the non-specific killing of antibody-sensitized target cells by K cells. The importance of this co-operative mechanism has been shown in a variety of animal experiments of which the most convincing depend upon the abrogation of antiviral immunity by drugs such as cyclophosphamide or by other immunosuppressive manoeuvres and its restoration by infusing specific antibody and K cells[35]. The K cells are equally efficient whether these are obtained from specifically sensitized or normal donors. Appropriate experimental designs have also shown that K cells are important in protecting humans from viral infection. Some such experiments have relied upon assays of K cell activity in, for example, recurrent herpes simplex virus infections and demonstrating that recovery from such infections is associated with normal K cell activity whereas susceptibility can be correlated with impaired K cell function. An alternative method is to generate antiviral activity *in vitro* by exposing blood lymphocytes to infected target cells. Surprisingly, many of these experiments, which were designed to show the importance of cytotoxic T lymphocytes, have shown instead that the antiviral effect is mediated by antibody and K cells. This has been demonstrated with respect to vaccinia[36, 37] and measles viruses[37–40].

Another form of antiviral immunity which has assumed increasing importance is mediated by 'natural killer' (NK) cells. Human blood lymphocytes display spontaneous cytotoxicity towards several established cell lines *in vitro* and, as this cytotoxicity can be demonstrated without any initial experimental sensitization of the effector cells, this kind of cell killing has been regarded as a form of surveillance against virus-transformed cells. Several attempts have been made to characterize these cells and it appears that NK cells are morphologically distinctive, being large lymphocytes with pale and characteristically granular cytoplasm. These cells are derived from several lymphocyte populations but possess the common property of displaying Fc receptors[41]. There are several lines of evidence indicating that these cells are functionally important. Patients with the Chediak–Higashi syndrome have normal humoral immunity and delayed-type hypersensitivity reactions but are susceptible to bacterial infections because of defective granules in their polymorphonuclear lymphocytes. Patients who survive this complication usually succumb to lymphoproliferative disorders. This susceptibility has been attributed to an associated deficiency of NK cells[42]. There has also been a report indicating that NK cells may be essential for host defence against virus infections as well as against virus-transformed cells which are potentially malignant. Patients with severe recurrent herpes simplex virus infections have been shown to possess defective NK cell activity measured by the ability of their blood mononuclear cells to kill a target cell line *in vitro*[43]. The relationship between this type of cytotoxic cell and other mediators of immune reactions is still debated. There is evidence that interferon regulates the production of NK cell activity[44] but it is unlikely that interferon is the sole mechanism by which cytotoxic ability is conferred on this cell population. There is also evidence that some cytotoxic activity in human peripheral lymphocyte cultures usually attributed to NK cells may be mediated not by these cells but by antibody secreted *in vitro* as the result of recent infection; this antibody may coat the virus-infected target cells in such experimental systems, thereby rendering these susceptible to lysis by K cells[45].

Clearly there are considerable difficulties in deciding the relative importance of different antiviral mechanisms in host defence against specified viruses. Furthermore the range and complexity of these mechanisms suggests several ways in which genetically determined immunodeficiency could account for viral persistence. The techniques for measuring each form of host defence still need amplifying and standardization before a realistic search for possible defects can be made in patients with connective tissue diseases. Most studies of this kind have been solely concerned with tests for sensitization to viral antigens measured by lymphocyte transformation *in vitro*; moreover the results are hard to interpret. For example hyporesponsiveness to viral antigens has been reported in patients with rheumatoid arthritis[46] but it is not clear whether this reflects primary immunodeficiency or the non-specific effects of disease activity. Similarly patients with systemic lupus erythematosus have been reported to show an increased reactivity to viral antigens reported in terms of both serum antibody concentrations and lymphocyte transformation. However such patients react strongly to a variety of tissue antigens in general and there is little guarantee that the alleged antiviral activity does not simply reflect contamination of viral antigens with tissue antigens at the time of preparation[47]. A more promising approach to detecting defects in viral immunity is to seek such evidence before the onset of disease, or in other words in appropriate family studies. An interesting possibility of this kind is suggested by the well-known association between complement defects and various kinds of inflammatory connective tissue disease. A depression in both serum C4 concentration and total haemolytic activity has been reported in asymptomatic relatives of children with systemic lupus erythematosus although only in those relatives with circulating antinuclear antibodies[48]. It is important that this and other forms of antiviral immunity be systematically examined in extended surveys of this kind.

STRATEGY OF VIRAL PERSISTENCE

There are a variety of ways in which viruses may evade the host immune response and replicate in unusual sites or to abnormally high titres. Many of these mechanisms depend upon subtle forms of immunodeficiency which are either induced by virus infection or amplified as a result of infection. Some of these mechanisms involve T lymphocytes. For example the amount of interferon induced by virus infections varies in different hosts and is genetically determined. Furthermore the efficiency with which interferon protects susceptible cells is also genetically controlled. Thus cultured macrophages from those inbred mouse strains which are resistant to infection by orthomyxoviruses can be protected by smaller amounts of interferon than are necessary to protect similar cultures from susceptible mouse strains[49]. However this is not the complete explanation since other genetic factors also influence the resistance of mononuclear phagocytes to virus infection[50]. There are strong indications that similar defects determine human susceptibility to some human virus infections. Interferon production in patients with frequently recurring herpes simplex infections appears to be deficient when tested during the interval between successive exacerbations of infection[51]. This abnormality is therefore detected at a time when it is not attributable to non-specific disease activity. Similarly, cellular immunity judged by lymphocyte responses to challenge with viral antigen *in vitro* is impaired in children congenitally infected with cytomegalovirus and in their mothers[52]. There is as yet no evidence that similar defects predispose to connective tissue diseases but in multiple sclerosis, a noteworthy example of a chronic immunopathological disorder, there is some indication that interferon production may be deficient[53]. This finding indicates that defects of this nature may be unsuspected unless systematically sought.

Antibody is also commonly of limited efficacy and especially in established infections. It is well documented, for example, that congenital cytomegalovirus infection may be transmitted to the fetus even when substantial antibody titres to the virus can be detected in the mothers[54]. Moreover antibody may facilitate viral growth in a variety of ways. Antibody may lead to the disappearance of viral antigens from the surface of infected cells in a process known as modulation, thereby rendering the cells resistant to cell-mediated immune mechanisms. This has been nicely demonstrated in tissue culture cells infected with measles antibody[55]. In addition an altered pattern of measles virus synthesis has been revealed in cells exposed to specific antibody by the latter's indirect effect on viral polypeptide synthesis[56]. Antibody also enhances viral growth in macrophages which are a favoured site of viral persistence in many infections[57]. Viruses may also abet their own escape from antibody neutralization by rendering the infected cells inaccessible to antibody. For example antibody binding to infected cells is depressed in cultured cells infected with influenza virus.

Another point of importance is the possibility that certain strains of virus are particularly adept at invading the host response. One of the most convincing examples of persistent inflammatory diseases in man of proven viral aetiology is subacute sclerosing panencephalitis resulting from measles infection of the central nervous system. Although high antibody titres are encountered in the blood and cerebrospinal fluid of patients with this disorder, no antibody is synthesized against the major virus polypeptide known as M polypeptide[58]. Theoretically this defect could arise either from a failure of the infecting measles virus strain to synthesize this protein or from the failure of the immune system to recognize this antigen. Although this point has not been finally resolved, it appears more likely that there is deficient synthesis of the M polypeptide by measles virus in the brain cells of patients with this disorder[59]. Temperature-sensitive (t.s.) mutants of a large number of viruses have been isolated which grow at lower temperatures than those optimal for the growth of the wild strains from which these mutants are derived. The original purpose in isolating t.s. mutants was for their value in analysing the interactions between host cells and viruses but there has been great interest in the possibility that the growth of t.s. mutants generated *in vivo* may have unusual immunopathological consequences. This possibility has been investigated experimentally in the context of chronic demyelinating diseases of the central nervous system. BALB/c mice inoculated with t.s. mutants of vesicular stomatitis virus develop a subacute neurological disease characterized by focal demyelination and perivascular infiltration with mononuclear cells and plasma cells[60]; t.s. mutants can be regularly isolated from the lesions and these do not revert to the wild type of virus from which the t.s. mutant was derived[61]. The ability of t.s. mutants to produce persistent atypical disease may in part depend upon the ability of such mutants to evade host immune responses. However it is difficult to make generalizations in this context. Cells experimentally infected with t.s. mutants of vaccinia virus, for example, are more susceptible to lysis by sensitized lymphocytes than similar cells infected with wild type virus[62]. Other virus mutants can be generated *in vitro* or *in vivo* which do not undergo a complete cycle of replication but lead to the production of a defective interfering particle. Only small amounts of infective virus are produced in such persistent infected cells and few viral antigens are expressed on the cell surface. As a result these infected cells are less likely to attract the attention of cytotoxic T lymphocytes or to activate other cytolytic mechanisms, thereby rendering the persistently infected cells relatively resistant to the normal mechanisms which destroy cells infected by conventional viruses. Moreover simultaneous infection by defective and complete virus particles of the same strain may also help to protect the latter from immune elimination[63]. The immune response also provokes the production of mutant viruses with a heightened capacity to evade host defences. A notable example is Visna virus. This retrovirus causes a chronic inflammatory disease of the central nervous system of sheep after a prolonged incubation period. Despite the emergence of both humoral and cell-mediated immune responses to the virus the animals remain persistently infected for many years. Not only does antibody enhance the production of mutant viruses but these mutants may grow preferentially in host cell exposed to antibody[64]. Furthermore, Visna virus is also resistant to interferon, thereby helping to explain the ineffectual nature of the cell-mediated immune response[65]. It is intriguing that a retrovirus closely related to Visna induces chronic arthritis in goats[66]. Ironically, whilst interferon is an important form of host defence in limiting both primary virus infection and reactivation, it may also help to perpetuate infection by t.s. mutants and other forms of defective virus[67, 68]. Many persistent infections by such mutants which do not damage the host cells are turned into lethal, cytopathic infections when the defectively infected cultures are exposed to an antiserum which neutralizes interferon. Furthermore, prior treatment with interferon helps to establish defective infections[69]. These observations encourage the speculation that, just as antibody may modulate viral antigens from chronically infected cells *in vivo* and so protect these cells from destruction by various lymphocyte populations, so interferon may allow the reservoir of continued virus growth to persist at too low a level to attract an efficient immune response against the persistently infected cells. There are no direct experimental observations to show that these mechanisms are relevant to the pathogenesis of connective tissue diseases. However, it is important to reflect that, whilst conventional techniques for isolating viruses have been almost uniformly disappointing, the methods employed would not be expected to detect defective agents able to persist in only a small percentage of cells in the affected tissues.

LYMPHORETICULAR CELLS AS A SITE OF VIRAL PERSISTENCE

There are two principal reasons for speculating that lymphocytes and cells of the monocyte–macrophages series could harbour the putative agent in many connective tissue diseases. Firstly these cells are infected during the pathogenesis of many known virus infections[24] and intermittent infection of blood lymphocytes commonly accompanies persistent viral infections. Secondly the immunological aberrations which abound in patients with rheumatoid arthritis and diffuse connective tissue diseases could theoretically be attributed to viral infection of lymphocyte subpopulations which are of critical importance in the initiation and control of immune responses. There is good evidence that an impressive number of commonly encountered viruses can either be induced to grow in lymphocytes cultured *in vitro* or can be isolated from blood lymphocytes during the course of natural infections (Table 11.1). There are several points to be made about these observations. Most studies have concentrated on showing that lymphocytes infected *in vitro* support a complete cycle of virus replication leading to the release of fresh infectious particles. Less consideration has been given to the possibility that incomplete or defective virus growth may lead to the synthesis of virus-specific proteins but not of fully infectious progeny. Incomplete growth of this kind has indeed been detected in lymphocytes infected with influenza A virus[75]. However there have been few attempts to determine whether or not other viruses will abortively infect human lymphocytes. In addition not all the different strains of common viruses have been studied. Thus, whilst influenza and para-influenza viruses generally do not grow in human lymphocytes, one strain of parainfluenza type I virus recovered from the brain of a patient with multiple sclerosis did replicate in the cultured monocytes and lymphocytes of normal human donors[76]. *In vivo* mutation of viruses responsible for persistent infection may produce adaptive changes which allow the mutant virus to grow atypically in lymphoreticular cells. The susceptibility of human lymphocytes may also vary with the age of the donor. Normal herpes simplex virus only grows in adult human lymphocytes which have been appropriately stimulated

Table 11.1   Virus infection of human lymphocytes

Source	Virus	Susceptible population	Immune response Cell-mediated*	Humoral†	References‡
Natural infection of blood lymphocytes	measles	not characterized	depressed	nil	70
	rubella	not characterized	depressed	depressed	72
	Epstein–Barr	B lymphocytes	depressed	derepressed	3
	cytomegalovirus	lymphocytes and monocytes	depressed	nil	74
Experimental in vitro infection of blood lymphocytes	measles	T and B lymphocytes	depressed	'helper' T cells	71
	rubella	T lymphocytes; monocytes	depressed	unknown	73
	influenza	incomplete in lymphocytes	nil	variable	75
	parainfluenza	some strains in monocytes	unknown	unknown	76
	alphaviruses	some strains in monocytes	unknown	unknown	77
	herpes simplex	T and B lymphocytes	depressed	'helper' T cells	78–82
	Epstein–Barr	B lymphocytes	nil	derepressed	3
	cytomegalovirus	possibly in monocytes	nil	nil	78
Experimental in vitro infection of lymphoblastoid cell lines	measles	T and B lymphocytes			83
	herpes simplex	T and B lymphocytes			84
	cytomegalovirus	T and B lymphocytes			85–87

* Cell-mediated immune responses: in vivo skin test reactions and in vitro lymphocyte responses to mitogens
† Humoral response: specific antibody responses
‡ Selected references from the recent literature

with mitogens such as phytohaemagglutinin. However, cord blood lymphocytes support the growth of this virus without any need for such stimulation[81].
This observation emphasizes that circulating lymphocytes may disseminate
infection acquired at a particularly susceptible age[88]. In addition opportunistic infection of circulating lymphocytes may occur when these cells are
simultaneously infected by a second virus. Thus herpes simplex virus does not
normally grow in human B lymphocytes but can be induced to do so if the cells
are simultaneously exposed to certain strains of EB virus[80]. It is also noteworthy that viruses may produce latent infection of human lymphocytes
which is not readily detected by conventional techniques. Measles virus, for
example, infects resting human lymphocytes without inducing detectable viral
antigens on the cell surface or the appearance of new infectious particles.
However the latent infection can readily be activated if the infected cells are
exposed to phytohaemagglutinin which activates both the host lymphocytes
and the resident virus[89]. Most *in vitro* experiments have only demonstrated
short-term infection of lymphocytes and, correspondingly, there is scant
evidence that virus can be recovered from circulating lymphocytes for prolonged periods after the initial infection. In contrast persistent infection can be
demonstrated *in vitro* using permanent lymphoblastoid cell lines transformed
by EB virus. These experiments are interesting because the cultures usually
produce only a low yield of infectious virus; moreover the infection of
lymphoblastoid cell lines by measles virus favours the emergence of a heterogeneous population of t.s. mutants[83]. The relevance of these *in vitro* experiments to immunopathological events is purely speculative but concerns the
proposition that the *in vivo* infection of lymphocyte precursor cells in central
lymphoid organs may favour not only persistent infection but also the emergence of mutant strains. There have been few attempts to isolate viruses from,
or to rescue defective virus particles from, lymphocytes in the blood and
tissues of patients with rheumatoid arthritis and inflammatory connective
tissue diseases. Most such attempts have concentrated on fresh or cultured
material from affected synovial membranes. However experiments have been
attempted in which it was postulated that latent virus infection of lymphocytes
may be detected by viral interference. This is a phenomenon in which cells
infected with a particular virus fail to permit superinfection with the same or a
closely related virus[90]. Herpes simplex virus invariably grows in appropriately
stimulated lymphocyte cultures from normal donors. In contrast lymphocytes
isolated from rheumatoid synovial effusions or from the blood of many
patients with various inflammatory connective tissue diseases fail to support
the growth of this virus[91, 92]. Whilst various trivial explanations for this
observation can be excluded there is as yet scant evidence that this resistance
to the growth of herpes simplex virus is attributable to viral interference.
Nevertheless in one such disorder, namely Behçet's syndrome, the failure of
blood lymphocytes to support the growth of this virus can be correlated with
chromosome abnormalities which are consistent with a viral aetiology[93].

VIRAL IMMUNOSUPPRESSION

There is ample evidence that viruses interfere with immune responses in experimental animals by a variety of mechanisms. Whilst the majority of such infections depress cell-mediated or humoral immune responses, some viruses interfere with tolerance induction or may even increase the intensity of immune reactions. Murine leukaemia viruses are particularly liable to suppress immune responses and the extent of the immunosuppression is genetically determined[94]. Thus genetic restrictions have been noted in the ability of Friend leukaemia virus to suppress lymphocyte responsiveness *in vitro* caused by viral activation of a suppressor cell[95]. However other viruses may also show an unexpected ability to interfere with the generation of biologically important immune responses. Thus vesicular stomatitis virus blocks the induction of acute graft-versus-host disease in mice[96]. A variety of mechanisms have been invoked to explain viral immunosuppression. These include the generation of suppressor cells[97], the immunosuppressive effects of interferon generated in viral infections[98], and the suppressive effects of other factors generated as a result of interferon production[99]. However viral immunosuppression in man appears to be more closely related to the ability of the viruses responsible to grow in lymphocytes sub-populations which are indispensable for the generation of immune responses. Herpes simplex virus, for example, ablates antibody synthesis by human cells *in vitro* because the virus selectively infects a small percentage of helper T lymphocytes[82]. Similar observations involving both natural infections and *in vitro* experiments suggest that measles virus affects immune responses through its direct action on selected lymphocyte populations. Although measles virus infects only a very small percentage of circulating lymphocytes *in vitro*, these cells are critically important in the generation of cell-mediated immune responses[70]. Similarly, *in vitro* suppression of lymphocyte reactivity by this virus does not appear to depend upon suppressor cells, monocytes, or interferon but on infection of human lymphocytes proliferating at an early stage in the immune response[100–102]. In general the direct inactivation of lymphocytes rather than indirect effects account for those examples of viral immunosuppression of human lymphocytes that have been most fully analysed. There are several factors which determine the susceptibility of a minority of lymphocytes at risk of infection. To some extent the availability of binding sites for viruses such as measles[71] or of Fc receptors for viruses such as herpes simplex govern this susceptibility[103]. However, since only a small percentage of cells with these characteristics are either susceptible to infection or to immunosuppression following infection, other unknown factors must also be responsible.

There are also a number of interesting animal models of viral immunosuppression which may have their counterpart in man. A virus related to murine cytomegalovirus causes extensive destruction of murine T lymphocytes *in vivo*[104]. A virus has also been described in chickens which causes extensive destruction of lymphoid cells by its ability to infect and destroy those cells which bear IgM receptors[105, 106]. The factors which limit the extent to which DNA herpes viruses grow in human lymphocytes have not yet been clarified.

These observations indicate a variety of ways in which atypical infections or *in vivo* mutation could produce unusual immunopathological reactions in man.

CONNECTIVE TISSUE DISEASES AND LYMPHOPROLIFERATIVE DISORDERS

The clonal theory of immunity postulates that antigens select the progeny of a single antibody-producing precursor cell or clone programmed to produce antibody of the appropriate specificity. In its original form it was proposed that autoreactive cells are eliminated in the thymus. This theory has needed modification for two principal reasons. Firstly T lymphocytes recognize chemical and microbial antigens in association with self-antigens so that self-recognition is indispensable for generating normal immune responses[25]. Secondly in man as in other species B lymphocytes can be detected with auto-reactivity for self-antigens such as immunoglobulins, red cells, and nucleic acids. Thus autoimmune disease arises not from the *de novo* generation of autoreactive B lymphocytes but from the uncontrolled proliferation of pre-existing autoreactive B lymphocytes following the breakdown of normal suppressor mechanisms. The single cell or clonal origin of many malignant myeloproliferative and lymphoproliferative diseases has been established beyond doubt[107]. Much of the evidence for this view depends upon studying the isoenzymes of glucose-6-phosphate dehydrogenase (G6PD) in neoplastic and apparently normal cells. G6PD production is controlled by the X chromosome and in females one of the two *X* genes is active in each somatic cell. Some black females heterozygous at this locus for the usual *B* gene and a common variant. the *A* gene, have a mosaic of two cell populations, one producing type B G6PD and the other type A G6PD. The progeny of a single neoplastic stem cell or clone produce type A or type B enzyme but not both, whereas the progeny of normal multiple-stem cells express a mixture of both isoenzymes. It is not altogether surprising that cells which are clearly malignant such as the granulocytes in chronic myeloid leukaemia or the B lympho-cytes in Burkitt's lymphoma should be clonal by this and other criteria. What is more surprising was the discovery that the apparently normal bone marrow progeny in a disease like chronic myeloid leukaemia, namely the circulating red cells, platelets, and monocytes are also derived from the malignant clone. Furthermore the disease polycythaemia vera, which has been variously re-garded as a disorder of stem cell regulation or the consequence of excessive erythropoietin production, has also been shown to be a clonal, myeloproliferative disease. It is also apparent that many B lymphocytes in patients with chronic myeloid leukaemia are derived from the malignant clone even though these cells synthesize immunoglobulin containing all the major heavy-chain classes and both kappa and lambda light chains[108]. These observations reinforce those made in normal individuals in whom all the major heavy-chain classes have also been detected in a monoclonal antibody response[109]. Thus the detection of heterogeneity in antibody response by immunochemical criteria does not necessarily constitute evidence against a single stem cell or clonal origin. It is also evident that a clonal disease such as multiple myeloma may originate as a mutation of a precursor cell before its differentiation into a conventional B lymphocyte[110]. The evolution of angioimmunoblastic lymphadenoneuropathy, commonly regarded as a reactive lymphoproliferative disorder provoked by hyperimmunization, into an unequivocal lymphoma emphasizes the difficulty of drawing a firm distinction between malignant and non-malignant lymphoproliferative disorders[111]. There are no studies indicating that diseases of alleged autoimmune nature such as rheumatoid arthritis and systemic lupus erythematosus are lymphoproliferative disorders involving a single or a limited number of clones. Nevertheless the view has been cogently expressed that the diseases resembling systemic lupus erythematosus in inbred mouse strains such as NZB mice result primarily from disorders of stem cell regulation and that abnormalities such as defects in T lymphocyte function and suppressor cell function, and the presence of circulating lymphocytotoxins, are all reflections of this same basic disorder[112]. There is good evidence also that B lymphocyte hyperreactivity is a major consequence of this disordered regulation and that its culmination in autoimmune disease can be prevented in F_1 hybrids between NZB mice and CBA/N strain mice which have an X-chromosome-linked defect in their ability to mount an immune response to T-independent antigens[113]. Since B cell development is arrested in such hybrids, autoimmune phenomena do not emerge. Other stem cell defects in autoimmune strains of mice have been detected by *in vitro* techniques used to study the maturation of B cells and their progeny[114]. Two obvious questions arise in the context of the human autoimmune diseases and chronic inflammatory diseases. Firstly, is there any evidence that rheumatoid arthritis and systemic lupus erythematosus for example result from the abnormal or unregulated proliferation of bone marrow stem cells? It has to be admitted that there is no direct evidence for this view. Indeed it has not yet been shown that the alleged disorders of immune responsiveness and its regulation in such patients is of fundamental pathogenetic importance and not merely the consequence of continued inflammatory disease. Nor is it likely that the simple application of the techniques which allowed the clonal nature of malignant myeloproliferative disorders to be established will provide such direct evidence in chronic inflammatory diseases. Possibly a minority population of B lymphocytes and other cells derived from abnormal stem cells could be identified by such techniques but this task has not yet been methodically attempted. The second question concerns the possibility that viral infections of stem cells or the differentiated progeny of these cells could allow the autonomous proliferation of B lymphocytes producing autoantibodies to, for example, immunoglobulins and nucleic acids. There are several ways in which such infection could operate. Virus might selectively inactivate suppressor lymphocytes thereby allowing the proliferation of autoreactive B lymphocytes. Viruses might selectively infect autoreactive B lymphocytes thereby stimulating their continued proliferation. Finally opportunistic infection by endogenous or exogenously acquired viruses might transform B lymphocytes already reacting with totally unrelated antigens. The susceptibility to infection of stem cells at different stages of maturation has been mapped in considerable detail in experimental animals. The increasing availability of techniques for cloning and characterizing the progeny of the human bone marrow stem cells makes it feasible to contemplate similar studies with human material. Two kinds of virus infection which could theoretically derepress human B lymphocytes are considered next.

RETROVIRUSES AND CONNECTIVE TISSUE DISEASES

Retroviruses (RNA tumour viruses, oncogenic C type viruses) have been cited more commonly than any other virus group as a possible cause of the connective tissue diseases. This enthusiasm owes more to the premature extrapolation of results in laboratory animals than to any firm observations in human disease. In particular the ready detection of retroviruses or their products in NZB mice prompted speculation about a possible retroviral aetiology for human systemic lupus erythematosus. Furthermore burgeoning interest in the possible retroviral aetiology of human leukaemias encouraged the view that the abnormal proliferation of autoantibody-producing cells might result from similar infection. However a clear distinction must be made between endogenous viruses whose genome is incorporated in the DNA of the mammalian cell and other retroviruses. Endogenous viruses are inherited by vertical transmission in the germ line. In contrast retroviral infections may be acquired by horizontal infection and detecting evidence of exogenous, acquired retroviral infection has different connotations than the detection of activated endogenous infection. For example there is molecular evidence that a lymphoproliferative disease of turkeys is associated with infection by a retrovirus which does not originate in the affected turkey and is distinct from the usual endogenous group of viruses which causes avian leukosis and sarcoma[115]. Similarly the leukaemias and lymphomas of cats are caused by a horizontally transmitted retrovirus, feline leukaemia virus[116]. Infection by this virus has many interesting features for those concerned with a viral aetiology for the connective tissue diseases. Usually, primary infection by this virus causes a relatively mild or subclinical acute infection even in laboratory animals in whom acquisition of the infection is regularly monitored. Most cats recover uneventfully and only a small percentage of infected animals develop leukaemias or lymphomas and then only after an interval of months or years. It is obvious that analogous infection in man would not produce a pattern which could be readily recognized by conventional epidemiological studies. However there is only scant evidence that retroviruses are involved in human connective tissue diseases. There have been claims that immune complexes containing retroviral antigens and antibody can be detected by immuno-fluorescence in the kidneys of patients with systemic lupus erythematosus[117]. There is also evidence that antigens related to retroviruses are widely expressed in the tissues and placentas of patients with this disease[118]. Unfortunately it is also clear that the mere detection of retroviruses or retroviral products in murine or human autoimmune disease does not necessarily imply that these viruses are the cause of the disease. The cells of most mammalian species contain the genome of retroviruses and indeed 0.1% of mammalian cell DNA may code for retroviral information[119]. There has been speculation that vertically transmitted retroviral information may play a physiological role in the generation of normal immune responses but there is no experimental evidence to support such contentions. Conversely the highly conserved sequences in the retroviral RNA from different mammalian species suggests that replication in mammalian cells may depend upon integration with a mammalian DNA sequence which is common to all species and is indispensable for viral replication[120]. In addition it has been shown that virus-specific sequences of the retrovirus, murine sarcoma virus, are represented within the normal mouse genome in a manner analogous with a cellular gene[121]. Such observations emphasize that retroviral genes are intimately and regularly associated with mammalian gene and the events which control the expression of mammalian genes or gene segments also allow the activation of retroviral genes and their products. Although it has proved more difficult to detect evidence of endogenous retroviral infection in man than in other species, there are many indications that it is present[122]. Quite apart from the many failures to confirm the observation that retroviral antigens can be detected on cell surfaces or in immune complexes in patients with systemic lupus erythematosus[123–126], it seems more likely that the problem will not be the failure to detect such antigens in due course but to determine the pathological significance of such findings. In the meantime it is essential to design strategies which will allow the discovery of retroviral infection in patients with such diseases to be put in proper perspective. In particular criteria will have to be devised for ascribing pathogenic significance to such infections.

It is possible that a primary abnormality in the regulation of retroviral information allows the abnormally high expression of viral antigens. This possibility has been accepted in inbred mouse strains with spontaneous autoimmune disease. Thus it seems likely that a single autosomal gene regulates the high expression of retroviruses in NZB mice[127]. In addition inbred mouse strains can be classified as G IX-positive or G IX-negative depending upon whether or not thymocytes from these strains express this major envelope glycoprotein of murine leukaemia virus. The development of immune complex glomerulonephritis and lymphoproliferative disorders in inbred mouse strains depends upon the expression of this antigen although this is not the only genetic factor involved[128]. The importance of other genes is emphasized by the observation that the gene controlling the production of endogenous retrovirus in NZB mice segregates independently from the genes predisposing to the autoimmune diseases characteristic of these animals[129, 130]. These observations reinforce the conclusion that the expression of endogenous retroviral information is only one of a complex of genetic factors involved in the pathogenesis of autoimmune disease in inbred mouse strains and that these diseases are not simply the result of viral activation in isolation. Such observations reinforce the conclusions in human studies of systemic lupus erythematosus that genetic and environmental factors cannot as yet be disentangled. Another possibility is that a defect in immune function in some individuals could also allow the abnormal expression of retroviral information thereby increasing the risk of uncontrolled B lymphocyte proliferation. Certainly there is normally natural immunity to retroviruses. Cats exposed to feline leukaemia virus develop antibodies to the retroviral enzyme reverse transcriptase[131]. Similarly antibody directed against the major glycoproteins of murine leukaemia viruses can be detected in the serum of mice with dormant infection by these agents[132]. Lymphocyte-mediated immunity to retroviruses can be detected in naturally infected mice[133] and can also be induced by the *in vitro* sensitization of T-lymphocytes[134]. There has been much speculation that deficient cell-mediated immunity may allow retroviruses to induce malignant disease. This may be genetically determined as, for example, in AKR mice which develop spontaneous lymphomas and fail to produce interferon on challenge with murine leukaemia viruses[135]. These speculations are relevant to the problems of autoimmune disease only if experimental evidence can be derived to support the possiblity that retroviruses infect and thereby induce the proliferation of immunologically competent lymphocytes. There are interesting indications that murine leukaemia virus binds preferentially to T lymphocytes, thereby providing both a portal of infection for the agent and also a mitogenic signal for the infected cells[136]. Virally transformed clones of T lymphocytes may give rise to autonomous populations of alloreactive and autoreactive lymphocytes which are not responsive to normal homeostatic control[137]. Possibly B lymphocytes contain retroviral genes which are capable of transforming the cell if these genes are expressed at abnormally high levels. Endogenous retrovirus in B cell genes could theoretically be activated by complementation with exogenously acquired viral infections[138] or by exposure to chemicals or drugs[139]. It is also interesting to speculate that antibodies in human disease against DNA polymerases are attempts by the host to suppress enzymes concerned in the expression of activated retroviruses[140].

At present there is no firm evidence linking retroviral infection with connective tissue diseases. Nevertheless it is possible to envisage a series of investigations which will eventually test this contention. Firstly the detection and characterization of retroviruses associated with human cells will allow the distinction to be made between vertically acquired endogenous and horizontally acquired exogenous infection. Secondly the contribution of such retroviral antigens to immune complex disease will be clarified as more specific monoclonal antibodies become available to characterize the antigens in these complexes. Finally the ability to quantitate the host responses to these antigens of both an immunological and a non-immunological nature will allow the postulated genetic susceptibility to retroviral infections to be properly evaluated.

EPSTEIN–BARR VIRUS

Epstein–Barr (EB) virus transforms B lymphocytes *in vitro* and *in vivo*, thereby immortalizing the infected cells[3]. Moreover the transformed B lymphocytes can be induced to produce specific antibody including rheumatoid factor. Thus EB virus could theoretically cause lymphoproliferative diseases of B lymphocytes accompanied by autoimmune phenomena. In addition the clinical outcome of EB virus infections is highly variable and is influenced by a variety of host factors. Primary infection in infancy is clinically silent and induces a limited range of antibodies compared with those encountered in adolescent patients and young adults with infectious mononucleosis[141, 142]. EB virus infects and transforms a minority population of circulating B lymphocytes. Once acquired the virus persists indefinitely, most probably in those cells which were initially infected[143, 144]. This process is restricted by host immune responses to which T lymphocytes make the most critical contribution. T lymphocytes, particularly from patients with infectious mononucleosis but also from all individuals who have at some time acquired EB virus infection, are sensitized against the virus; this is shown by the ability of the immune T lymphocytes to restrict the transformation of B lymphocytes *in vitro*[145, 146] and to limit the subsequent proliferation of the transformed cells[147]. These attributes of immune T lymphocytes appear to persist indefinitely after primary infection whether or not this was manifested clinically as infectious mononucleosis[148]. The mechanisms by which immune T lymphocytes control EB virus infection in part involve interferon[149]. However, such lymphocytes limit viral transformation of lymphocytes which are already infected[150]. Suppressor T lymphocytes may also help to limit the proliferation of B lymphocytes[151]. Whilst a rise in antibody titres to EB virus accompanies many lymphoproliferative disorders which may develop later in life, it is likely that this increase reflects the coincidental reactivation of passenger virus.

Primary EB virus infections may be unusually severe in susceptible individuals and is attributable to various forms of specific immunodeficiency to this virus. Fatal immunoblastic proliferation has been reported in a child with a selective defect in interferon production[152] and severe autoimmune haemolytic anaemia developed in another patient who was unable to generate a cytotoxic T lymphocyte response to EB virus-infected cells[153]. However, fatal infectious mononucleosis has also developed in patients without any obvious defects in measurable immune responses to EB virus itself or to EB virus-transformed B cells[154, 155]. Primary EB virus infection has also caused unexplained fatal polyclonal B cell lymphoma in contradistinction to the clonal disease Burkitt's lymphoma, which is also strongly suspected to result from EB virus infection[156]. Indeed the defect in the majority of patients with atypical EB viral infection has not been characterized but studies in families with a high incidence of fatal lymphoproliferative syndromes following EB virus infection strongly suggests that this susceptibility is related to an X-linked recessive trait[157, 158]. EB virus is therefore an infectious agent of man which induces a variety of disorders in susceptible individuals. Moreover there is a variable time interval between the primary infection and the onset of disease. These theoretical considerations for implicating EB virus in the pathogenesis of autoimmune diseases have been tested by serological observations in patients with rheumatoid arthritis[159]. An antibody has been detected in patients with this disease which reacts specifically with an antigen in B lymphocytes induced by EB virus. These observations have been confirmed; for example in one study this antibody was detected in 16% of normal controls but in over 90% of patients with classical rheumatoid arthritis and may therefore prove of some diagnostic value[160]. However these observations do not prove that EB virus causes rheumatoid arthritis. The sera of patients with this and other inflammatory connective tissue disorders react with a variety of tissue antigens; thus the antigen induced in B lymphocytes transformed by EB virus may simply be a host cell antigen expressed at a certain stage only in the growth cycle of these cells and with which sera from rheumatoid patients fortuitously react. In addition there are no data indicating that the development of these antibodies to B cell antigens follows sequentially after the first appearance of antibodies to EB virus. Moreover patients with rheumatoid arthritis and positive tests for rheumatoid factor do not invariably show serological evidence of previous EB virus infection and there is no precedent for the idea that EB virus infection could be acquired without seroconversion.

On balance, therefore, there is no firm evidence linking EB virus infection with the pathogenesis of rheumatoid arthritis. Nevertheless the complicated relationship between persistent infection by this agent and the host response encourages speculation that known or unknown DNA herpes viruses could cause lymphoproliferative autoimmune diseases in man. In particular there is an experimental basis for the hypothesis that virus infection of B lymphocytes could induce autoimmune lymphoproliferative disorders.

CONCLUSIONS

There are ample precedents from animal models and from human disease that virus infection can cause the immunopathological abnormalities which characterize patients with rheumatoid arthritis and other connective tissue diseases. Moreover the complexities of the immune response to viruses and the variety of ways in which these can be circumvented could explain why commonly encountered but usually ephemeral infections might cause persistent inflammatory disease in susceptible individuals. This could occur in two principal ways. Firstly, persistent virus infection in target organs could induce a variety of aberrant immune responses including autoimmune reactions. Persistent infection of lymphoreticular cells could contribute to these aberrations. Secondly, viruses may induce the autonomous proliferation of a limited number of clones programmed to produce autoantibodies. Whilst some forms of immune response to common viruses have been studied in patients with connective tissue diseases, the complete spectrum of such responses has not been systematically analysed. For example it is not known whether or not the pattern of virus growth in synovial macrophages resembles that in cells of the monocyte–macrophage series isolated from other sites. The genetic control of these responses also needs to be analysed. This is particularly important since otherwise it is difficult to decide whether abnormal immune responses in general are primary or the secondary non-specific result of disease activity. The reported defects of suppressor cell function, for example in patients with systemic lupus erythematosus, will be more meaningful if the claim that these are genetically determined can be substantiated[161]. Such defects could predispose to allergic disease after viral infections; thus there are hints that genetic factors may explain susceptibility to arthritis after rubella immunization[162]. Similarly the continued circulation of immune interferon in patients with connective tissue diseases[163] may simply reflect a continued inflammatory response after infection and could be a good marker for a genetically controlled predisposition to make an exaggerated response to common viral infections. At present interest in specific viruses which may be implicated in these disorders centres on retroviruses and EB viruses. So far the grounds for these suspicions are tenuous. Moreover the mere detection of ubiquitous viruses does not prove that these play a pathological role; this problem is compounded by the recent recognition that defective infection by such agents as adenovirus[164] and herpes simplex virus[165] is a universal occurrence. In order to prove the pathogenicity of any isolate it will be necessary to show the type of agent, the site of replication, and the pattern of immune response compatible with this interpretation.

The failure to detect viruses or other microbial infections in rheumatoid synovial membranes and other inflammatory lesions in the connective tissue diseases may reflect the inappropriate selection of starting material, the difficulty of rescuing viruses in the presence of an excess of defective interfering factors[166, 167] and many other factors. The history of microbiology started with the realization that free-living organisms could cause disease. It took many years from the first discovery of bacteriophages for the concept of infection by obligate intracellular parasites, namely viruses, to obtain universal acceptance[168]. The third phase of microbial advance depends upon elucidating the precise relationship between structural genes, integrated viral genes, whether horizontally or vertically acquired, and the factors which suppress and control the expression of both kinds of genes. Indeed the distinction between genetic and viral factors in the aetiology of diseases such as systemic lupus erythematosus has now become increasingly semantic; delineating these control mechanisms is a task of greater and more pressing importance.

References

1. Kobayakawa, T., Louis, J., Izui, S. and Lambert, P. H. (1979). Autoimmune response to DNA, red blood cells, and thymocyte antigens in association with polyclonal antibody synthesis during experimental African trypanosomiasis. *J. Immunol.*, **122**, 296
2. Grooten, J., Baetselier, P., de Vercauteren, E. and Hamers, R. (1980). Anti-micrococcus antibodies recognize an antigenic marker of confluent mouse lymphoid cell lines. *Nature (London)*, **285**, 401
3. Epstein, M. A. and Achong, B. G. (eds.) (1979). *The Epstein–Barr Virus.* (Berlin, Heidelberg and New York: Springer)
4. Bennett, J. C. (1978). The infectious etiology of rheumatoid arthritis. *Arth. Rheum.*, **21**, 531
5. Marmion, B. P. (1978). Infection, autoimmunity and rheumatoid arthritis. *Clin. Rheum. Dis.*, **4**, 565
6. Denman, A. M. (1980). The viral aetiology of rheumatoid arthritis. In Hill, A. G. S. (ed.) *Topical Reviews in Rheumatic Disorders*, pp. 133–243. (Bristol: Wright)
7. Hyer, F. H. and Gottlieb, N. L. (1978). Rheumatic disorders associated with viral infection. *Sem. Arth. Rheum.*, **8**, 17
8. Levo, Y., Gorevic, P. D., Kassab, H. J. Zucker-Franklin, D. and Franklin, E. C. (1977). Association between hepatitis B virus and essential mixed cryoglobulinemia. *N. Engl. J. Med.*, **296**, 1501
9. Murphy, F. A., Buchmeier, M. J. and Rawls, W. E. (1977). The reticuloendothelium as the target in a virus infection. *Lab. Invest.*, **37**, 502
10. Schleupner, C. J., Olsen, G. A. and Glasgow, L. A. (1979). Activation of reticuloendothelial cells following infection with murine cytomegalovirus. *J. Infect. Dis.*, **139**, 641
11. Steere, A. C., Malawista, S. E., Snydman, D. R., Shope, R. E., Andiman, W. A., Ross, M. R. and Steele, F. M. (1977). Lyme arthritis. An epidemic of oligoarticular arthritis in children and adults in three Connecticut communities. *Arth. Rheum.*, **20**, 7
12. Steere, A. C., Gibofsky, A., Patarroyo, M. E., Winchester, R. J., Hardin, J. A. and Malawista, S. E. (1979). Chronic Lyme arthritis. *Ann. Intern. Med.*, **90**, 896
13. Hardin, J. A., Steere, A. C. and Malawista, S. E. (1979). Immune complexes and the evolution of Lyme arthritis. *N. Engl. J. Med.*, **301**, 1358
14. Steere, C., Hardin, J. A., Ruddy, S., Mummaw, J. G. and Malawista, S. E. (1979). Lyme arthritis. *Arth. Rheum.*, **22**, 471
15. Hardin, J. A., Walker, L. C., Steere, A. C., Trumble, T. C., Tung, K. S. K., Williams, R. C., Ruddy, S. and Malawista, S. E. (1979). Circulating immune complexes in Lyme arthritis. *J. Clin. Invest.*, **63**, 468

16. Anderson, R. M. and May, R. M. (1979). Population biology of infectious diseases. *Nature (London)*, **280**, 361
17. McCormick, J. N., Duthie, J. J. R., Gerber, H., Hart, H., Baker, S. and Marmion, B. P. (1978). Rheumatoid polyarthritis after rubella. *Ann. Rheum. Dis.*, **37**, 266
18. DeHoratius, R. J. (1980). Lymphocytotoxic antibodies. In Schwartz, R. S. (ed.) *Progress in Clinical Immunology*. Vol. 4, pp. 151–174. (New York, London, Toronto, Sydney and San Francisco: Grune & Stratton)
19. Persselin, J. E., Messner, R. P., De Horatius, R. J. and Troup, G. M. (1977). Antilymphocyte antibodies in systemic lupus erythematosus: familial clustering of lymphocyte antigens. *J. Rheumatol.*, **4**, 11
20. Stastny, P. and Fink, C. W. (1979). Different HLA-D associations in adult and juvenile rheumatoid arthritis. *J. Clin. Invest.*, **63**, 124
21. Thomsen, M., Morling, N., Snorrason, E., Svejgaard, A. and Sorensen, S. F. (1979). HLA-DW4 and rheumatoid arthritis. *Tissue Antigens*, **13**, 56
22. Rossen, R. D., Brewer, E. J., Sharp, R. M., Ott, J. and Templeton, J. W. (1980). Familial rheumatoid arthritis. *J. Clin. Invest.*, **65**, 629
23. Zinkernagel, R. M. (1979). Associations between major histocompatibility antigens and susceptibility to disease. *Ann. Rev. Microbiol.*, **33**, 201
24. Mims, C. A. (1976). *The Pathogenesis of Infectious Disease*. (New York, San Francisco and London: Academic Press)
25. Webster, A. D. B. (1979). Infections in immunodeficient patients. In Tyrrell, D. A. J. (ed.) *Aspects of Slow and Persistent Virus Infections*, pp. 255–265. (The Hague: Martinus Nijhoff)
26. Williamson, A. R. (1980). Three-receptor clonal expansion model for selection of self-recognition in the thymus. *Nature (London)*, **283**, 527
27. Kurrie, R., Wagner, H., Röllinghoff, H. and Rott, R. (1979). Influenza virus-specific T cell-mediated cytotoxicity. *Eur. J. Immunol.*, **9**, 107
28. Liberti, P. A., Hackett, C. J. and Askonas, B. A. (1979). Influenza virus infection of mouse lymphoblasts alters the binding affinity of anti-H-Z antibody requirement for viral neuraminidase. *Eur. J. Immunol.*, **9**, 751
29. Chamberlain, B. K., Nozaki, Y., Tanford, C. and Webster, R. E. (1978). Association of the major coat protein of fd bacteriophage with phospholipid vesicles. *Biochem. Biophys. Acta*, **510**, 18
30. Loh, D., Ross. A. H., Hale, A. H., Baltimore, D. and Eisen, H. N. (1979). Synthetic phospholipid vesicles containing a purified viral antigen and cell membrane proteins stimulate the development of cytotoxic T lymphocytes. *J. Exp. Med.*, **150**, 1067
31. Zinkernagel, R. M., Althage, A., Cooper, S., Kreeb, G., Klein, P. A., Sefton, B., Flaherty, L., Stimpfling, J., Shreffler, D. and Klein, J. (1978). Ir-genes in H-2 regulate generation of anti-viral cytotoxic T cells: mapping to *K* or *D* and dominance of unresponsiveness. *J. Exp. Med.*, **148**, 592
32. Kreth, H. W., ter Meulen, V. and Eckert, G. (1979). Demonstration of HLA restricted killer cells in patients with acute measles. *Med. Microbiol. Immunol.*, **165**, 203
33. McMichael, A. (1978). HLA restriction on human cytotoxic T lymphocytes specific for influenza virus. Poor recognition of virus associated with HLA A2. *J. Exp. Med.*, **148**, 1458
34. Sissons, J. G. P., Schreiber, R. D., Perrin, L. H., Cooper, N. R., Müller-Eberhard, H. J. and Oldstone, M. B. A. (1979). Lysis of measles virus-infected cells by the purified cytolytic alternative pathway and antibody. *J. Exp. Med.*, **150**, 445
35. Hirsch, R. L., Griffin, D. E. and Johnson, R. T. (1979). Interactions between immune cells and antibody in protection from fatal Sindbis virus encephalitis. *Infect. Immun.*, **23**, 320
36. Perrin, L. H., Zinkernagel, R. M., and Oldstone, M. B. A. (1977). Immune response in humans after vaccination with vaccinia virus: generation of a virus-specific cytotoxic activity by human peripheral lymphocytes. *J. Exp. Med.*, **146**, 949

37. Perrin, L. H., Reynolds, D., Zinkernagel, R. and Oldstone, M. B. A. (1978). Generation of virus-specific cytolytic activity in human peripheral lymphocytes after vaccination with vaccinia virus and measles virus. *Med. Microbiol. Immunol.*, **166**, 71

38. Galama, J. M. D., Lucas, C. J. and Vos, A. (1978). Lymphocyte-mediated cytotoxicity to cells infected with measles virus. *Cell. Immunol.*, **38**, 365

39. Galama, J. M. D., Lucas, C. J. and Vos, A. (1978). Lymphocyte-mediated cytotoxicity to cells infected with measles virus. *Cell. Immunol.*, **38**, 365

40. Galama, J. M. D., Vos, A. and Lucas, C. J. (1979). Lymphocyte-mediated cytotoxicity to autologous cells infected with measles virus. II: Specificity of the cytotoxic reaction and characterization of the effector cells involved. *Cell. Immunol.*, **48**, 296

41. Timonen, T., Saksela, E., Ranki, A. and Häyry, P. (1979). Fractionation and morphological and functional characterization of effector cells responsible for human natural killer activity against cell-line targets. *Cell. Immunol.*, **48**, 133

42. Roder, J. C., Haliotis, T., Klein, M., Korec, S., Kett, J. R., Ortaldo, J., Herberman, R. B., Katz, P. and Fauci, A. S. (1980). A new immunodeficiency disorder in humans involving NK cells. *Nature (London)*, **284**, 533

43. Ching, C. and Lopez, C. (1979). Natural killing of herpes simplex virus type I—infected target cells: normal human responses and influence of antiviral antibody. *Infect. Immun.*, **26**, 49

44. Huddlestone, J. R., Merigan, T. C. and Oldstone, M. B. A. (1979). Induction and kinetics of natural killer cells in humans following interferon therapy. *Nature (London)*, **282**, 417

45. Greenberg, S. B., Six, H. R., Drake, S. and Crouch, R. B. (1979). Cell cytotoxicity due to specific influenza antibody production *in vitro* after recent influenza antigen stimulation. *Proc. Natl. Acad. Sci. USA*, **76**, 4622

46. Wolf, R. E. (1978). Hyporesponsiveness of lymphocytes to virus antigens in rheumatoid arthritis. *Arth. Rheum.*, **21**, 238

47. Pincus, T., Steinberg, A. D., Blacklow, N. R. and Decker, J. L. (1978). Reactivities of systematic lupus erythematosus sera with cellular and virus antigen preparations. *Arth. Rheum.*, **21**, 873

48. Lehman, T. J. A., Hanson, V., Singsen, B. H., Kornreich, H. K., Bernstein, B. and King, K. K. (1979). Serum complement abnormalities in the antinuclear antibody-positive relatives of children with systematic lupus erythematosus. *Arth. Rheum.*, **22**, 954

49. Haller, O., Arnheiter, H., Lindenmann, J. and Gresser, I. (1980). Host genes influence sensitivity to interferon action selectively for influenza virus. *Nature (London)*, **283**, 660

50. Haller, O., Arnheiter, H. and Lindenmann, J. (1979). Natural, genetically determined resistance towards influenza virus in hemopoietic mouse chimeras. *J. Exp. Med.*, **150**, 117

51. Kirchner, H., Schwenteck, M., Northoff, H. and Schöpe, E. (1978). Defective *in vitro* lymphoproliferative responses to herpes simplex virus in patients with frequently recurring herpes infections during the disease-free interval. *Clin. Immunol. Immunopathol.*, **11**, 267

52. Starr, S. E., Tolpin, M. D., Friedman, H. M., Paucker, K. and Plotkin, S. A. (1979). Impaired cellular immunity to cytomegalovirus in congenitally infected children and their mothers. *J. Infect. Dis.*, **140**, 500

53. Neighbour, P. A. and Bloom, B. R. (1979). Absence of virus-induced lymphocyte suppression and interferon production in multiple sclerosis. *Proc. Natl. Acad. Sci. USA*, **76**, 476

54. Stagno, S., Reynolds, D. W., Huang, E.-S., Thames, S. D., Smith, R. J. and Alford, C. A. (1977). Congenital cytomegalovirus infection. Occurrence in an immune population. *N. Engl. J. Med.*, **296**, 1254

55. Oldstone, M. B. A. and Tishon, A. (1978). Immunologic injury in measles virus infection. *Clin. Immunol. Immunopathol.*, **9**, 55

56. Fujinami, R. S. and Oldstone, M. B. A. (1979). Antiviral antibody reacting on the plasma membrane alters measles virus expression inside the cell. *Nature (London)*, **279**, 529

57. Peiris, J. S. M. and Porterfield, J. S. (1979). Antibody-mediated enhancement of flavivirus replication in macrophage-like cell lines. *Nature (London)*, **282**, 509

58. Hall, W. W., Lamb, R. A. and Choppin, P. W. (1979). Measles and subacute sclerosing panencephalitis virus proteins: lack of antibodies to the M protein in patients with subacute sclerosing panencephalitis. *Proc. Natl. Acad. Sci USA*, **76**, 2047

59. Hall, W. W. and Choppin, P. W. (1979). Evidence for lack of synthesis of the M polypeptide of measles virus in brain cells in subacute sclerosing panencephalitis. *Virology*, **99**, 443

60. Rabinowitz, S. C., Johnson, T. C. and Dal Canto, M. C. (1979). Subacute infection with temperature-sensitive vesicular stomatitis virus mutant G41 in the central nervous system of mice. I. Clinical and virologic studies. *J. Infect. Dis.*, **139**, 26

61. Dal Canto, M. C., Rabinowitz, S. G. and Johnson, T. C. (1979). Subacute infection with temperature-sensitive vesicular stomatitis virus mutant G41 in the central nervous system of mice. II, Immunofluorescent morphologic and immunologic studies. *J. Infect. Dis.*, **139**, 36

62. Keller, F., Drillien, R. and Kirn, A. (1979). Effect of cell-mediated immune factors on the replication of an attenuated temperature-sensitive mutant of vaccinia virus. *Infect. Immun.*, **26**, 841

63. Welsh, R. M. and Buchmeier, M. J. (1979). Protein analysis of defective interfering lymphocytic choriomeningitis virus and persistently infected cells. *Virology*, **96**, 503

64. Dubois-Dalcq, M., Narayan, O. and Griffin, D. E. (1979). Cell surface changes associated with mutation of Visna virus in antibody-treated cell cultures. *Virology*, **92**, 353

65. Carroll, D., Ventura, P., Haase, A., Rinaldo, C. R. C., Overall, J. C. and Glasgow, L. A. (1978). Resistance of Visna virus to interferon. *J. Infect. Dis.*, **138**, 614

66. Crawford, T. B., Adams, D. S., Cheevers, W. P. and Cork, L. C. (1980). Chronic arthritis in goats caused by a retrovirus. *Science*, **207**, 997

67. Youngner, J. S., Preble, O. T. and Jones, E. V. (1978). Persistent infection of L cells with vesicular stomatitis virus: evolution of virus populations. *J. Virol.*, **28**, 6

68. Sekellick, M. and Marcus, P. I. (1979). Persistent infection. II: Interferon-inducing temperature-sensitive mutants as mediators of cell sparing: possible role in persistent infection by vesicular stomatitis virus. *Virology*, **95**, 36

69. Ramseur, J. M. and Friedman, R. M. (1978). Prolonged infection of L cells with vesicular stomatitis virus. *Virology*, **85**, 253

70. Whittle, H. C., Dossetor, J., Oduloju, A., Bryceson, A. D. M. and Greenwood, B. M. (1978). Cell-mediated immunity during natural measles infection. *J. Clin. Invest.*, **62**, 678

71. Bankhurst, A. D., Maki, D. and McLaren, L. C. (1980). Binding sites for measles virus antigens on human B and T lymphocytes. *Cell. Immunol.*, **50**, 243

72. Buimovici-Klein, E. and Cooper, L. Z. (1979). Immunosuppression and isolation of rubella virus from human lymphocytes after vaccination with two rubella vaccines. *Infect. Immun.*, **25**, 352

73. Logt, J. T. M. van cler, Loon, A. M. van and Veen, J. van der (1980). Replication of rubella virus in human mononuclear blood cells. *Infect. Immun.*, **27**, 309

74. Rinaldo, C. R., Black, P. H. and Hirsch, M. S. (1977). Interaction of cytomegalovirus with leukocytes from patients with mononucleosis due to cytomegalovirus. *J. Infect. Dis.*, **136**, 667

75. Brownson, J. M., Mahy, B. W. J. and Hazleman, B. L. (1979). Interaction of influenza A virus with human peripheral blood lymphocytes. *Infect. Immun.*, **25**, 749

76. Verini, M. A. and Lief, F. S. (1979). Interaction between 6/94 virus, a parainfluenza type I strain, and human leukocytes. *Infect. Immun.*, **24**, 734

77. Levitt, N. H., Miller, H. V. and Edelman, R. (1979). Interaction of alphaviruses with human peripheral leukocytes: *in vitro* replication of Venezuelan equine encephalomyelitis virus in monocyte cultures. *Infect. Immun.*, **24**, 642

78. Rinaldo, C. R., Richter, B. S., Black, P. H., Callery, R., Chess, L. and Hirsch, M. S. (1978). Replication of herpes simplex virus and cytomegalovirus in human lymphocytes. *J. Immunol.*, **120**, 130

79. Plaeger-Marshall, S. and Smith, J. W. (1978). Inhibition of mitogen and antigen-induced lymphocyte blastogenesis by herpes simplex virus. *J. Infect. Dis.*, **138**, 506

80. Kirchner, H. and Schröder, C. H. (1979). Replication of herpes simplex virus in human B lymphocytes stimulated by Epstein-Barr virus. *Intervirology*, **11**, 61

81. Trofatter, K. F., Daniels, C. A., Williams, R. J. and Gall, S. A. (1979). Growth of Type 2 herpes simplex virus in newborn and adult mononuclear leukocytes. *Intervirology*, **11**, 117

82. Pelton, B. K., Duncan, I. B. and Denman, A. M. (1980). Herpes simplex virus depresses antibody production by affecting T-cell function. *Nature (London)*, **284**, 176

83. Ju, G., Udem, S., Rager-Zisman, B. and Bloom, B. R. (1978). Isolation of a heterogeneous population of temperature-sensitive mutants of measles virus from persistently infected human lymphoblastoid cell lines. *J. Exp. Med.*, **147**, 1637

84. Rinaldo, C. R., Richter, B. S., Black, P. H. and Hirsch, M. S. (1979). Persistent infection of human lymphoid and myeloid cell lines with herpes simplex virus. *Infect. Immun.*, **25**, 521

85. Furukawa, T. (1978). Persistent infection with human cytomegalovirus in a lymphoblastoid cell line. *Virology*, **94**, 214

86. Tocci, M. J. and St. Jeor, A. C. (1979). Persistence and replication of the human cytomegalovirus genome in lymphoblastoid cells of B and T origin. *Virology*, **96**, 664

87. Furukawa, T., Yoshimura, N., Jean, J.–H. and Plotkin, S. A. (1979). Chronically persistent infection with human cytomegalovirus in human lymphoblasts. *J. Infect. Dis.*, **139**, 211

88. Summers, B. A., Greisen, H. A. and Appel, M. J. G. (1978). Possible initiation of viral encephalomyelitis in dogs by migrating lymphocytes infected with distemper virus. *Lancet*, **2**, 187

89. Lucas, C. J., Ubels-Postma, J. C., Rezee, A. and Galama, J. M. D. (1978). Activation of measles virus from silently infected human lymphocytes. *J. Exp. Med.*, **138**, 940

90. Diet, N. H. and Libikova, H. (1979). Selective resistance to togaviral superinfection in mice with tolerant lymphocytic choriomeningitis virus infection. *Acta Virol.*, **23**, 385

91. Denman, A. M., Pelton, B. K., Appleford, D. and Kingsley, M. (1976). Virus infections of lympho-reticular cells and auto-immune diseases. *Transplant. Rev.*, **31**, 79

92. Appleford, D. J. A. and Denman, A. M. (1979). Fate of herpes simplex virus in lymphocytes from inflammatory joint effusions. I: Failure of the virus to grow in cultured lymphocytes. *Ann. Rheum. Dis.*, **38**, 443

93. Denman, A. M., Fialkow, P. J., Pelton, B. K., Salo, A. C., Appleford, D. J. and Gilchrist, C. (1981). Lymphocyte abnormalities in Behçet's syndrome. *Clin. Exp. Immunol.* (In press)

94. Friedman, H. and Secter, S. (1979). Interaction of leukemia viruses with cells of the immune response system. *Transplant. Proc.*, **11**, 1060

95. Humar, V. and Bennett, M. (1979). Immunosuppression by Friend leukemia virus is H-2 restricted by alloreactive T lymphocytes. *Proc. Natl. Acad. Sci. USA*, **76**, 2415

96. Umetsu, D. T., Romano, T. J., Bloom, B. R. and Thorbecke, G. J. (1979). Diminution by vesicular stomatitis virus of acute graft vs host mortality in mice. *Cell. Immunol.*, **46**, 416

97. Bendinelli, M., Matteucci, D., Toniolo, A. and Friedman, H. (1979). Suppression of *in vitro* antibody response by spleen cells of mice infected with Friend-associated lymphatic leukemia virus. *Infect. Immun.*, **24**, 1

98. Kadish, A. S., Tansey, F. A., Yu, G. S. M., Doyle, A. T. and Bloom, B. R. (1980). Interferon as a mediator of human lymphocyte suppression. *J. Exp. Med.*, **151**, 637

99. Johnson, H. M. and Ohtsuki, K. (1979). Suppression of *in vitro* antibody response by ribosome-associated factor(s) from interferon-treated cells. *Cell. Immunol.*, **44**, 125

100. Lucas, C. J., Galama, J. M. D. and Ubels-Postma, J. (1977). Measles virus-induced suppression of lymphocyte reactivity *in vitro*. *Cell. Immunol.* **32**, 70

101. Lucas, C. J., Ubels-Postma, J., Galama, J. M. D. and Rezee, A. (1978). Studies on the mechanism of measles virus-induced suppression of lymphocyte functions *in vitro*. *Cell. Immunol.*, **37**, 448

102. Zweiman, B., Lisak, R. P., Waters, D. and Koprowski, H. (1979). Effects of purified measles virus components on proliferating human lymphocytes. *Cell. Immunol.*, **47**, 241

103. Menezes, J. and Bourkas, A. E. (1980). Herpesvirus–lymphoid cell interactions: comparative studies on the biology of herpes simplex virus-induced Fc receptors in B, T, and 'null' lymphoid cell lines. *J. Virol.*, **33**, 115

104. Cross, S. S., Parker, J. C., Rowe, W. P. and Robbins, M. L. (1979). Biology of mouse thymic virus, a herpesvirus of mice and the antigenic relationship to mouse cytomegalovirus. *Infect. Immun.*, **26**, 1186

105. Hirai, K., Kato, N., Fujiura, A. and Himakura, S. (1979). Further morphological characterization and structural proteins of infectious bursal disease virus. *J. Virol.*, **32**, 323

106. Hirai, K. and Calnek, B. W. (1979). *In vitro* replication of infectious bursal disease virus in established lymphoid cell lines and chicken B lymphocytes. *Infect. Immun.*, **25**, 964

107. Fialkow, P. J., Denman, A. M., Singer, J., Jacobson, R. J. and Lowenthal, M. N. (1978). Human myeloproliferative disorders: clonal origin in pluripotent stem cells. In *Differentiation of Normal and Neoplastic Hematopoietic Cells*, pp. 131–144. (Cold Spring Harbor)

108. Fialkow, P. J., Denman, A. M., Jacobson, R. J. and Lowenthal, M. N. (1978). Chronic myelocytic leukaemia. *J. Clin. Invest.*, **62**, 815

109. Krueger, R. G., Fair, D. S. and Kyle, R. A. (1979). Monoclonal IgM, IgA, and IgC in the serum of a single individual: immunofluorescence identification of cells producing the immunoglobulins. *Eur. J. Immunol.*, **9**, 606

110. Kubagawa, H., Vogler, L. B., Capra, J. D., Conrad, M. E., Lawton, A. R. and Cooper, M. D. (1979). Studies on the clonal origin of multiple myeloma. *J. Exp. Med.*, **150**, 792

111. Mazur, E. M., Lovett, D. H., Enriquez, R. E., Breg, W. R. and Papac, R. J. (1979). Angioimmunoblastic lymphadenopathy evolution to a Burkitt-like lymphoma. *Am. J. Med.*, **67**, 317

112. Dixon, F. J. (1979). The pathogenesis of murine systematic lupus erythematosus. *Am. J. Pathol.*, **97**, 10

113. Taurog, J. L., Moutsopoulos, H. M., Rosenberg, Y. J., Chused, T. M. and Steinberg, A. D. (1979). CBA/N X-linked B-cell defect prevents NZB B-cell hyperactivity in F_1 mice. *J. Exp. Med.*, **150**, 31

114. Kincade, P. W., Lee, G., Fernandes, G., Moore, M. A. S., Williams, N. and Good, R. A. (1979). Abnormalities in clonable B lymphocytes and myeloid progenitors in autoimmune NZB mice. *Proc. Natl. Acad. Sci. USA*, **76**, 3464

115. Gazit, A., Yaniv, A., Ianconescu, M., Perk, K., Aizenberg, B. and Zimber, A. (1979). Molecular evidence for a type C retrovirus etiology of the lymphoproliferative disease of turkeys. *J. Virol.*, **31**, 639

116. Francis, D. P. and Essex, M. (1978). Leukemia and lymphoma: infrequent manifestations of common viral infections–a review. *J. Infect. Dis.*, **138**, 916

117. Panem, S., Ordonez, N. G., Katz, A. I., Spargo, B. H. and Kirsten, W. H. (1978). Viral immune complexes in systemic lupus erythematosus. *Lab. Invest.*, **39**, 413

118. Panem, S. and Reynolds, J. T. (1979). Retrovirus expression in normal and pathogenic processes of man. *Fed. Proc.*, **38**, 2674

119. Lerner, R. A. (1978). Recombinant origins of leukemogenic murine viruses. *Am. J. Pathol.*, **93**, 10

120. Kominami, R. and Hatanaka, M. (1979). Conserved region of mammalian retrovirus RNA. *J. Virol.*, **32**, 925

121. Tronick, S. R., Robbins, K. C., Canaani, E., Devare, S. C., Andersen, P. R. and Aaronson, S. A. (1979). Molecular cloning of Moloney murine sarcoma virus: arrangement of virus-related sequences within the normal mouse genome. *Proc. Natl. Acad. Sci. USA*, **76**, 6314

122. Thiry, L. (1979). Evidence for the presence of retrovirus markers in man. In Tyrrell, D. A. J. (ed.) *Aspects of Slow and Persistent Virus Infections*. Vol. 2: *New Perspectives in Clinical Microbiology*, pp. 153–163. (The Hague: Martinus Nijhoff)

123. Phillips, P. E. and Hargrave-Granda, R. (1978). Type C oncornavirus isolation studies in systemic lupus erythematosus. II: Attempted detection by viral RNA-dependent DNA polymerase assay. *Ann. Rheum. Dis.*, **37**, 225

124. Phillips, P. E., Sellers, S. A. and Cotronei, S. L. (1978). Type C oncornavirus isolation studies in systemic lupus erythematosus. III: Isolation of a putative retrovirus by triple cell fusion. *Ann. Rheum. Dis.*, **37**, 234

125. Aulakh, G. S., Hicks, J. T., Martin, W. J. and Phillips, P. E. (1978). Search for type-C oncornavirus-related genetic information in tissues from patients with systemic lupus erythematosus. *Arth. Rheum.*, **21**, 880

126. Hicks, J. T., Aulakh, G. S., McGrath, P. P., Washington, G. C., Kim, E. and Alepa, F. P. (1979). Search for Epstein-Barr and type C oncornaviruses in systemic lupus erythematosus. *Arth. Rheum.*, **22**, 845

127. Levy, J. A., Joyner, J., Nayar, K. T. and Kouri, R. E. (1979). Genetics of xenotropic virus expression in mice. *J. Virol.*, **30**, 754

128. Obata, Y., Tanaka, T., Stockert, E. and Good, R. A. (1979). Autoimmune and lympho-proliferative disease in $(B6–G_{IX}^+ \times 129) F_1$ mice: relation to naturally occurring antibodies against murine leukemia virus-related cell surface antigens. *Proc. Natl. Acad. Sci. USA*, **76**, 5289

129. Datta, S. M., Manny, N., Andrzejewski, C., André-Schwartz, J. and Schwartz, R. S. (1978). Genetic studies of autoimmunity and retrovirus expression in crosses of New Zealand Black Mice. I: xenotropic virus. *J. Exp. Med.*, **147**, 854

130. Datta, S. K., McConahey, P. J., Manny, N., Theofilopoulos, A. N., Dixon, F. J. and Schwartz, R. S. (1978). Genetic studies of autoimmunity and retrovirus expression in crosses of New Zealand Black Mice. II: The viral envelope glycoprotein gp70. *J. Exp. Med.*, **147**, 872

131. Jacquemin, P. C., Saxinger, C., Gallo, R. C., Hardy, W. D. and Essex, M. (1978). Antibody response in cats to feline leukemia virus reverse transcriptase under natural conditions of exposure to the virus. *Virology*, **91**, 472

132. Callahan, R. M., Marx, P. A. and Wheelock, E. F. (1979). Group-specific cytolytic antibody directed against the major glycoprotein (gp70) of murine leukemia viruses in serum of mice with dormant FLV infections. *Virology*, **97**, 55

133. Kende, M., Hill, R., Dinowitz, M., Stephenson, J. R. and Kelloff, G. J. (1979). Naturally occurring lymphocyte-mediated immunity to endogenous type-C virus in the mouse. *J. Exp. Med.*, **149**, 358

134. Taniyama, T. and Holden, H. T. (1979). *In vitro* induction of T-lymphocyte mediated cytotoxicity by infectious murine type C oncornaviruses. *J. Exp. Med.*, **150**, 1367

135. Blank, K. J. and Murasko, D. M. (1980). Induction of interferon in AKR mice by murine leukaemia viruses. *Nature (London)*, **283**, 494

136. Fathman, C. G. and Weissman, I. L. (1980). Production of alloreactive T-cell lymphomas. *Nature (London)*, **283**, 404

137. Proffitt, M. R., Hirsch, M. S. and Black, P. H. (1977) Viruses, autoimmunity, and murine leukaemia. In Tald, N. (ed.) *Autoimmunity*, pp. 385–401. (New York: Academic Press)

138. Markham, P. D., Ruscetti, F., Salahuddin, S. Z., Gallagher, R. E. and Gallo, R. C. (1979). Enhanced induction of growth of B lymphoblasts from fresh human blood by primate type-C retroviruses. *Int. J. Cancer*, **23**, 148

139. Cooper, G. M., Okenquist, S. and Silverman, L. (1980). Transforming activity of DNA of chemically transformed and normal cells. *Nature (London)*, **284**, 418

140. Altaner, C. and Cebecauer, L. (1977). DNA polymerase activity and antibody against it in sera of patients with systemic lupus erythematosus. *Biomedicine*, **26**, 42

141. Biggar, R. J., Henle, G., Böcker, J., Lennette, E. L., Fleisher, G. and Henle, W. (1978). Primary Epstein-Barr virus infections in African infants. *Int. J. Cancer*, **22**, 244

142. Fleisher, G., Henle, W., Henle, G., Lennette, E. T. and Biggar, R. J. (1979). Primary infection with Epstein-Barr virus in infants in the United States. *J. Infect. Dis.*, **139**, 553

143. Katsuki, T., Hinuma, Y., Saito, T., Yamamoto, J., Hirashima, Y., Sudoh, H., Deguchi, M. and Motokawa, M. (1979). Simultaneous presence of EBNA-positive and colony-forming cells in peripheral blood of patients with infectious mononucleosis. *Int. J. Cancer*, **23**, 746

144. Robinson, J., Frank, A., Henderson, E., Schweitzer, J. and Miller G. (1979). Surface markers and size of lymphocytes in human umbilical cord blood stimulated into deoxyribonucleic acid synthesis by Epstein-Barr virus. *Infect. Immun.*, **26**, 225

145. Rickinson, A. B., Crawford, D. and Epstein, M. A. (1979). Inhibition of the *in vitro* outgrowth of Epstein-Barr virus-transformed lymphocytes by thumus-dependent lymphocytes from infectious mononucleosis patients. *Clin. Exp. Immunol.*, **28**, 72

146. Thorley-Lawsson, D. A., Chess, L. and Strominger, J. L. (1977). Suppression of *in vitro* Epstein-Barr virus infection. A new role for adult human T lymphocytes. *J. Exp. Med.*, **146**, 495

147. Moss, D. J., Rickinson, A. B. and Pope, J. H. (1978). Long term T-cell mediated immunity to Epstein-Barr virus in man. I: Complete regression of virus-induced transformation in cultures of seropositive donor leukocytes. *Int. J. Cancer*, **22**, 662

148. Rickinson, A. B., Moss, D. J., Pope, J. H. and Ahlberg, N. (1980). Long-term T-cell-mediated immunity to Epstein-Barr virus in man. IV: Development of T-cell memory in convalescent infectious mononucleosis patients. *Int. J. Cancer*, **25**, 59

149. Lai, P. K., Alpers, M. P. and MacKay-Scollay, E. M. (1977). Epstein–Barr herpesvirus infection: inhibition by immunologically induced mediators with interferon-like properties. *Int. J. Cancer*, **20**, 21

150. Thorley-Lawson, D. A. (1980). The suppression of Epstein–Barr virus infection *in vitro* occurs after infection but before transformation of the cell. *J. Immunol.*, **124**, 745

151. Tosato, G., Magrath, I., Koski, I., Dooley, N. and Blaese, M. (1979). Activation of suppressor T cells during Epstein–Barr-virus-induced infectious mononucleosis. *N. Engl. J. Med.*, **301**, 1133

152. Virelizier, J. L., Lenoir, G. and Griscelli, C. (1978). Persistent Epstein–Barr virus infection in a child with hypergammaglobulinaemia and immunoblastic proliferation associated with a selective defect in immune interferon secretion. *Lancet*, **2**, 231

153. Smith, H. and Denman, A. M. (1978). A new manifestation of infection with Epstein–Barr virus. *Br. Med. J.*, **2**, 248

154. Britton, S., Andersson-Anvret, M., Gergely, P., Henle, W., Jondal, M., Klein, G., Sandstedt, B. and Svedmyr, E. (1978). Epstein–Barr virus immunity and tissue distribution in a fatal case of infectious mononucleosis. *N. Engl. J. Med.*, **298**, 89

155. Crawford, D. H., Epstein, M. A., Achong, B. G., Finerty, S., Newman, J., Liversedge, S., Tedder, R. S. and Stewart, J. W. (1979). Virological and immunological studies on a fatal case of infectious mononucleosis. *J. Infect.*, **1**, 37

156. Robinson, J. E., Brown, N., Andiman, W., Halliday, K., Francke, U., Robert, M. F., Andersson-Anvret, M., Horstmann, D. and Miller, G. (1980). Diffuse polyclonal B-cell lymphoma during primary infection with Epstein–Barr virus. *N. Engl. J. Med.*, **302**, 1293

157. Purtilo, D. T., De Florio, D., Hutt, L. M., Bhawan, J., Yang, J. P. S., Otto, R. and Edwards, W. (1977). Variable phenotypic expression of an X-linked recessive lymphoproliferative syndrome. *N. Engl. J. Med.*, **297**, 1077

158. Purtilo, D. T., Hutt, L., Bhawan, J., Yang, J. P. S., Cassel, C., Allegra, S. and Rosen, F. S. (1978). Immunodeficiency to the Epstein–Barr virus in the X-linked recessive lymphoproliferative syndrome. *Clin. Immunol. Immunopathol.*, **9**, 147

159. Tan, E. M. (1979). The possible role of Epstein–Barr virus in rheumatoid arthritis. *Rev. Infect. Dis.*, **1**, 997

160. Ng, K. C., Brown, K. A., Perry, J. D. and Holborow, E. J. (1980). Anti-RANA antibody: a marker for seronegative and seropositive rheumatoid arthritis. *Lancet*, **1**, 447

161. Miller, K. B. and Schwartz, R. S. (1979). Familial abnormalities of suppressor-cell function in systemic lupus erythematosus. *N. Engl. J. Med.*, **301**, 803

162. Tingle, A. J., Ford, D. K., Price, G. E. and Kettyls, D. W. G. (1979). Prolonged arthritis in identical twins after rubella immunization. *Ann. Intern. Med.*, **90**, 203

163. Hooks, J. J., Moutsopoulos, H. M., Geis, S. A., Stahl, N. I., Decker, J. L. and Notkins, A. L. (1979). Immune interferon in the circulation of patients with autoimmune disease. *N. Engl. J. Med.*, **301**, 5

164. Jones, K. W., Kinross, J., Maitland, N. and Norval, M. (1979). Normal human tissues contain RNA and antigens related to infectious adenovirus type 2. *Nature (London)*, **277**, 274

165. Brown, S. M., Subak-Sharpe, J. H., Warren, K. G., Wroblewska, Z. and Koprowski, H. (1979). Detection of complementation of defective or uninducible (herpes simplex type 1) virus genomes in human ganglia. *Proc. Natl. Acad. Sci. USA*, **76**, 2364

166. Wilson, G. and Miller, G. (1979). Recovery of Epstein–Barr virus from non-producer neonatal human lymphoid cell transformants. *Virology*, **95**, 351

167. Rustigian, R., Winston, S. H. and Darlington, R. W. (1979). Variable infection of vero cells and homologous interference after co-cultivation with He La cells with persistent defective infection by Edmonston measles virus. *Inf. Immun.*, **23**, 775

168. Hughes, S. M. (1977). *The Virus: a History of the Concept.* (London: Heinemann; New York: Science History Publications)

Index